Evelyn,

I hope you find this a
fascinating read. Let's
spread the word and support
our veterans.

All the best,

Adam Montgomery

THE INVISIBLE INJURED

McGill-Queen's/Associated Medical Services Studies in the History of Medicine, Health, and Society

SERIES EDITORS: J.T.H. Connor and Erika Dyck

Volumes in this series have financial support from Associated Medical Services, Inc. (AMS). Associated Medical Services Inc. was established in 1936 by Dr Jason Hannah as a pioneer prepaid not-for-profit health care organization in Ontario. With the advent of medicare, AMS became a charitable organization supporting innovations in academic medicine and health services, specifically the history of medicine and health care, as well as innovations in health professional educa-tion and bioethics.

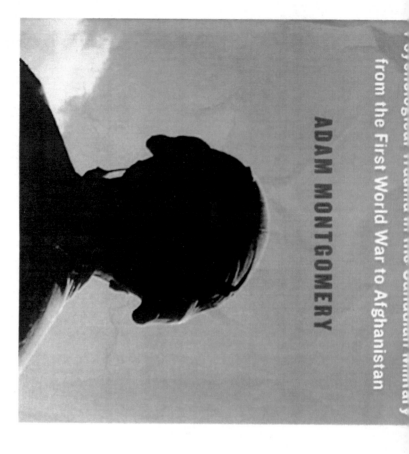

from the First World War to Afghanistan

ADAM MONTGOMERY

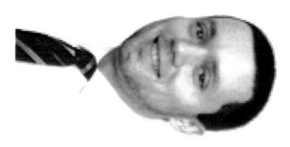

Museum

An evening with author
and military historian
Adam Montgomery

THE
INVISIBLE
INJURED

Tuesday,
May 16
7 pm
Centennial

THE INVISIBLE INJURED

Psychological Trauma
in the Canadian Military
from the First World War to Afghanistan

ADAM MONTGOMERY

McGill-Queen's University Press
Montreal & Kingston · London · Chicago

© McGill-Queen's University Press 2017

ISBN 978-0-7735-4995-1 (cloth)
ISBN 978-0-7735-4996-8 (ePDF)
ISBN 978-0-7735-4997-5 (ePUB)

Legal deposit second quarter 2017
Bibliothèque nationale du Québec

Printed in Canada on acid-free paper that is 100% ancient forest free
(100% post-consumer recycled), processed chlorine free.

This book has been published with the help of a grant from the
Canadian Federation for the Humanities and Social Sciences, through
the Awards to Scholarly Publications Program, using funds provided
by the Social Sciences and Humanities Research Council of Canada.

McGill-Queen's University Press acknowledges the support of the
Canada Council for the Arts for our publishing program. We also
acknowledge the financial support of the Government of Canada
through the Canada Book Fund for our publishing activities.

Library and Archives Canada Cataloguing in Publication

Montgomery, Adam, 1982–, author
    The invisible injured : psychological trauma in the Canadian military
from the First World War to Afghanistan / Adam Montgomery.

(McGill-Queen's/Associated Medical Services studies in the history of
medicine, health, and society ; 46)
Includes bibliographical references and index.
Issued in print and electronic formats.
ISBN 978-0-7735-4995-1 (cloth). – ISBN 978-0-7735-4996-8 (ePDF). –
ISBN 978-0-7735-4997-5 (ePUB)

    1. Veterans – Mental health – Canada – History. 2. Soldiers – Mental
health – Canada – History. 3. Psychic trauma – Canada – History.
4. Psychic trauma – Treatment – Canada – History. 5. Canada. Canadian
Armed Forces – History. I. Title. II. Series: McGill-Queen's/Associated
Medical Services studies in the history of medicine, health, and
society ; 46

RC552.P67M65 2017   616.85'212   C2016-908169-9
                                               C2016-908170-2

This book was typeset by True to Type in 10.5/13 Sabon

For the past and present members of the Canadian military,
and for Sapper Albert Thurlow Shadd,
whose war demons troubled, but never conquered him.

Contents

Acknowledgments

I am indebted to numerous people for their help during the research and writing of this book. First and foremost, I wish to thank Dr Erika Dyck, for her unwavering support and guidance, and for helping me to "see the forest for the trees" on numerous occasions. I would also like to thank Drs Valerie Korinek, Bill Waiser, and Camelia Adams, for their constructive input throughout this process, as well as Dr Mark Humphries. Thanks also to the Social Sciences and Humanities Research Council for helping fund the research from which this book is derived.

I'd also like to express my thanks and gratitude to Kyla Madden, who has been kind and patient while leading me through the publication process. Her insightful comments and suggestions have certainly helped make this book more organized, cogent, and complete. Scott Howard's dedication, savvy editing skills, and well-timed humour made him a joy to work with, and for that I will always be grateful. Ryan Van Huijstee was a thorough and instructive organizer who likewise deserves credit for helping bring everything together. Thank you to everyone else at McGill-Queen's University Press for helping mould my manuscript into a finished product, and for making the adventure of publishing my first book a rewarding and memorable experience.

Many veterans and Canadian Armed Forces members aided me as I shaped and wrote this book, and I would like to acknowledge several who were crucial to its completion. Thanks to Dr Allan English and Brigadier-General (ret.) Joe Sharpe for providing me with their recollections, input, and certain material unavailable elsewhere. Dr English and General Sharpe were also kind in connecting me with numerous people that were a part of the story this book tells. English and Sharpe's assistance allowed me to gather more stories, piece together key events, and penetrate more deeply into Canadian military culture, and for that I am in their debt. Thank you also to Lieutenant-Colonel (ret.) Stéphane Grenier, for his reminiscences, insightful thoughts about trauma, and correspondence throughout the past many months. Most kind thanks as well are owed to Master Warrant Officer (ret.) Barry Westholm, for sharing his story, discussing the ins and outs of military bureaucracies, and pointing me in the right direction several times.

To all Forces members, serving and retired, who freely and courageously shared their personal battles with trauma and subsequent journey, I wish to say: this work could not have been done without you. Thank you.

David Pugliese and Chris Cobb at the *Ottawa Citizen* were instrumental in helping me grasp the important relationship between the Canadian media and the Department of National Defence. Thank you to both men for taking the time to share some interesting anecdotes from their reporting on the military over the past two decades. I am also indebted to Affinity Production Group for providing me with a copy of their heart-wrenching film, *Witness the Evil*, and to Brian McKeown at Howe Sound Films for sending and discussing with me his insightful production, *War Wounds and Memory*. Gareth Jones was also kind enough to answer several questions I had about his role as an Ombudsman's investigator during the early 2000s.

I'd also like to express my gratitude to Dr John Weaver, a mentor and friend throughout my academic journey at McMaster University and beyond. His kind and encouraging words bolstered my morale when I needed it most, and he has been a true role model as I have worked my way through the transition from student to scholar. Dr Lucas Richert has been a loyal comrade. Our numerous, fruitful discussions over the past several years have provided me with much inspiration, and I am honoured to call him a friend. Thanks also to Dr Dustin McNichol for the many conversations about philosophy, literature, and the writing of history; they provided me with food for thought at crucial times.

Lastly, I would like to thank my family for their ongoing support, and for always believing in me. Thank you especially to Stephanie Bellissimo for being my rock and friend throughout the past five years, and for always reminding me that there was a light at the end of the tunnel. I am blessed to have her as my partner. To anyone I may have overlooked: my sincerest thanks for your help.

Abbreviations

APA	American Psychiatric Association
ARTAL	Adjustment Reaction to Adult Life
BOI	Croatia Board of Inquiry
CAF	Canadian Armed Forces
CAR	Canadian Airborne Regiment
CBC	Canadian Broadcasting Corporation
CDS	Chief of the Defence Staff
CEF	Canadian Expeditionary Force
CF	Canadian Forces (used interchangeably with CAF and "Forces")
CFB	Canadian Forces Base
CISD	Critical Incident Stress Debriefing
CMHA	Canadian Mental Health Association
CNCMH	Canadian National Committee for Mental Hygiene
CPA	Canadian Psychiatric Association
CPC	Canadian Pension Commission
CSC	Correctional Service Canada
CSS	Combat Service Support
DND	Department of National Defence
DPNH	Department of Pensions and National Health
DSCR	Department of Soldiers' Civil Reestablishment
DSM	*Diagnostic and Statistical Manual of Mental Disorders*
DVA	Department of Veterans Affairs
GAP	Group for the Advancement of Psychiatry
GSR	Gross Stress Reaction
GWS	Gulf War Syndrome
IPSC	Integrated Personnel Support Centre

JPSU	Joint Personnel Support Unit
MHC	Military Hospitals Commission
MHCHC	Military Hospitals and Convalescent Homes Commission
MND	Minister of National Defence
MOD	(British) Ministry of Defence
MPCC	Military Police Complaints Commission
NATO	North Atlantic Treaty Organization
NDHQ	National Defence Headquarters
NIMH	(United States) National Institute for Mental Health
NVC	New Veterans Charter
OSI	Operational Stress Injury
OSISS	Operational Stress Injury Social Support
OTSSC	Operational Trauma and Stress Support Centre
PPCLI	Princess Patricia's Canadian Light Infantry (battalion numbers placed before, e.g., 2PPCLI)
PSC	Peer Support Coordinator
PTSD	post-traumatic stress disorder
RCAMC	Royal Canadian Army Medical Corps
RDC	Research Diagnostic Criteria
SCONDVA	Standing Committee on National Defence and Veterans' Affairs
SISIP	Service Income Security Insurance Plan
TLD	third location decompression
UN	United Nations
UNAMIR	United Nations Assistance Mission for Rwanda
UNEF	United Nations Emergency Force
UNPROFOR	United Nations Protection Force
VA	(United States) Veterans Administration
VAC	Veterans Affairs Canada
VTC	Veterans Treatment Court
VVAW	Vietnam Veterans Against the War

THE INVISIBLE INJURED

Trauma, Culture, and History

Barry Westholm joined the Canadian Armed Forces (CAF) in 1982 in London, Ontario. Unlike numerous comrades, Westholm was not a "base brat" from a military family. Instead, he deemed himself an "accidental soldier."[1] As a youth that got into "a fair bit of trouble," the military helped him occupy his idle hands and satiate his need for adventure.[2] He trained first at Canadian Forces Base (CFB) Cornwallis in Nova Scotia, then at CFB Borden in Ontario, and ultimately finished his apprenticeship training as a vehicle technician at CFB North Bay in Ontario, in 1985.[3] After completing his training, Westholm was stationed at Canadian Forces Europe in Lahr, West Germany, in 1987, where he remained for three years, giving him the opportunity to witness first-hand the fall of the Berlin Wall in November 1989.

Although the Cold War was over by 1991, the 1990s brought no rest for the CAF, which saw its personnel committed to numerous peacekeeping missions around the world. In 1992, Westholm went on his first United Nations (UN) mission as part of the United Nations Transitional Authority in Cambodia. While in Cambodia, he experienced the "sickly sweet smell of decaying bodies, garbage, excrement, [and] filth," toured the killing fields of Pol Pot, and, on one occasion, had a rocket-propelled grenade pointed at the window of his truck. Yet, in spite of these harrowing moments, it was during his second UN mission in 1995–96, as part of the United Nations Mission in Haiti, that he began "a new life" as a result of mental trauma.

Westholm's trade is a unique one in the CAF, something known as Combat Service Support (CSS). A CSS soldier must be able to conduct highly delicate technical tasks directly in the line of, or under, enemy fire, and be prepared to join the fight at a moment's notice. A CSS soldier frequently has to operate independently or in a team of two, far away from committed military (infantry) support. As a vehicle technician, some of Westholm's duties in Haiti included operating a wrecker to repair, extricate, and return damaged military equipment to base. One fateful day, he received a call to drive to Île de la Gonâve, a small island off the Haitian coast, to help move two UN trucks that were mired on the island's only causeway and blocking access to a vital port.[4] The task began as a quintessential CSS mission – a crew of two people, with Westholm the crew commander, dispatched kilometres away from their base to provide support to two damaged vehicles. But while travelling along the island's unstable shore, Westholm's truck sank directly into the mixture of coral and pebbles, rendering it immobile. Thinking still of his directive, he bargained with some of the locals to call in the island's only bulldozer to extricate his truck. Unfortunately, the local man operating the bulldozer was quite drunk, and when he was "tantalizingly close," drove it underwater, leaving the bulldozer immobile too, and placing Westholm and his colleague in both a metaphorical and literal quagmire.[5]

Now, with their only bulldozer wrecked, many locals began gathering, some seething with anger, armed with rocks and machetes. With only one comrade present, Westholm worried about their chances of getting out of the situation unscathed, or even alive. Believing that they were in imminent danger, he sent his colleague to seek help from nearby American troops. He was now alone with only a nine-millimetre pistol and ten bullets to defend himself and his equipment. In his own words, Westholm felt like "prey with wolves around me." As the crowd closed in, he bantered with the group's de facto leader, attempting to keep the conversation light-hearted and downplay his anxiety. Although outwardly calm, he now believed he was "looking at a medieval type of death," and anxiously considered his remaining options. Given the crowd's size and his limited ammunition, he believed his chances of survival were small. He thus decided on his final plan: "I was going to shoot the guy I was talking to, and another upstart beside him. Those two were gone … a third [would be shot] if I could, and then I was going to kill myself."[6]

With the situation's grim reality in focus, Westholm spent – he estimates – almost fifteen minutes trying to keep the angry mob at bay. As he negotiated for his life, he surprisingly found himself thinking of childhood Christmases, seeing himself in "perfect clarity" in front of the tree in flannel pajamas. He also had visions and memories of his own son in Ontario, wondering if he would ever see him again. Back in real time, he considered what condition his body would be in when discovered by UN troops, "if they discovered it" at all. Westholm rested his hand near his pistol's grip, leaving the hammer cocked and safety off. With the tension now at its highest point, he locked eyes with the group's leader and began to pull out his sidearm to execute his final, desperate act: kill as many of the group's aggressors as possible and then commit suicide, to avoid being beaten, hacked, or possibly burned to death. It was the last decision he felt he would ever make. Then, just at the moment when he had made peace with the finality of his predicament, United States Special Forces and Canadian troops appeared in the distance, bringing with them enough equipment and personnel to scatter the angry crowd, de-escalate the situation, and save Westholm's life. Still mindful of his original mission, Westholm proceeded to pull his truck out of the sunken shore. He eventually extricated the UN vehicles and unblocked the island's causeway, which nonetheless was left heavily damaged by the work. Mission accomplished and broken vehicles in tow, he made his way towards the United States Army landing craft to return to the main island of Haiti and home base. He arrived back at the Canadian camp at about 11:00 p.m. Knowing the situation back on Île de la Gonâve was still volatile, with an angry populace, a damaged causeway, and a bulldozer underwater, Westholm briefed his platoon commander on the incident and shortly after went to sleep, feeling relieved about his last minute rescue.

Several hours later, at 2:15 a.m, Westholm was woken by his captain, who asked him if the earlier incident might have been one of the causes of a riot currently in progress. Westholm replied in the affirmative, and his captain left. Sitting up in his bunk, he began to think about the unprocessed events of the previous day. Now, unshielded by the adrenalin that had propelled him through the encounter, the flood of thoughts and emotions about his near death at the hands of the angry mob hit him like a punch to the stomach. The concurrent thoughts of bargaining for his life and family Christmases which he had experienced with such clarity on Île de la Gonâve now overwhelmed him, and he began to vomit. Westholm recounted: "I staggered out of that tent and went right to the portable toilet and puked my guts out, and sat there shaking like a leaf, like 'wow,' because I could not process the amount of stuff that had happened out there, and the officer when he came in had brought it all to the forefront."[7]

Westholm felt tired the next day, but carried on with his duties. In his dream that night he relived the entire event, waking up screaming around a quarter past two in the morning. He leapt from his cot and began to vomit again. Almost twenty years later, as I interviewed him, Westholm recalled waking up at 2:00 a.m. many nights for years, like a programmed alarm clock. But despite the harrowing nature of the causeway incident, upon arriving back in Canada, Westholm chalked up his anxiety to the general difficulties of his "high impact job." Nonetheless he began to notice a severe degradation in his mental capacity. His short-term memory was significantly reduced, as was his ability to multitask and focus. He became worried. He assumed his issues were connected to the handling of chemicals as a mechanic, and the job's physical stresses, including intense paratrooper training. Over the next several years, his symptoms, including sleeplessness, nightmares, intense anxiety, and feelings of fight-or-flight ("Why am I scared at the mall?") caused him to seek help from military physicians and psychologists on numerous occasions. He was given a MRI, CT scan, and other tests for physical injuries, but no definitive diagnosis was made. By 1999, after much "disjointed" support, feeling exhausted and frustrated at having made no headway, Westholm said "fuck it," and attempted to cope as best he could on his own, immersing himself completely in work and avoiding the problems that plagued his mind. In his own words, "The military became my crutch … All I really did was military, military, military, military … Everything else was sort of put on the sideline."[8] Ultimately, he did what many colleagues would do – and have done – in his situation: "soldier on." It was not until 2007, a full twelve years after the incident, that he was finally diagnosed: post-traumatic stress disorder.

HISTORICAL CONNECTIONS

Although Westholm's experiences are unique in many respects, they are also representative of the history – hitherto untold – of psychological trauma in the Canadian Forces after the Cold War.[9] That history was shaped by several factors: first, by individual soldiers like Westholm, and other men and women, prominent and unknown, who were affected first-hand by the way PTSD was viewed by rank-and-file soldiers, military leaders, politicians, and Canadian society during the late twentieth century. It was also a history formed by institutions, including of course the CAF, but also Canadian psychiatry and journalism. Finally, at a social level, it was a story about the socio-economic outcomes of trauma, consequences encapsulated in PTSD, a disorder with links to other, historical manifestations of overwhelming anxiety.

Westholm's journey from health to illness, and the familiar journey of numerous other CAF members during the 1990s and 2000s, illuminates some of the key issues this book relates. First, it illustrates a general lack of understanding within CAF ranks during the 1990s about what PTSD and psychological trauma were; a dearth of knowledge reflected by the attribution of PTSD's myriad symptoms to physical rather than mental injury. In some cases, troops and leaders expressed outright denial about the possibility of psychological injuries. Second, Westholm's difficulties resulted from a military culture that instilled a highly masculinized warrior ethos, emphasizing the physical prowess, stamina, and bravery of its members, thus stigmatizing both physical and mental "weakness." Third, and connected to this ethos, were the socio-economic implications that affected anyone who presented mental difficulties – implications that resulted in ostracism at best, and release from the Forces at worst.

Unlike their civilian counterparts, soldiers are subject to what is called the "Universality of Service" principle. Also known as the "Soldier First" principle, Universality of Service states that CAF members must "at all times and under any circumstances perform any functions that they may be required to perform," including a wide range of military tasks and deployment overseas.[10] As the term "Soldier First" suggests, a member is expected to, above all else, be a deployable soldier ready to serve the nation at a moment's notice. Breach of this principle, even due to physical or mental ailments, can lead to discharge from the Forces. While Universality of Service is necessary to ensure that the CAF is ready for any tasks the nation requires, it has proven to be a thorny issue for those diagnosed with mental disorders of a protracted nature. Those released from the CAF during the late twentieth and early twenty-first century sometimes found their career terminated before pension eligibility, meaning their post-service life began with ongoing illness and no pension or compensation for service-related injuries. It may surprise readers unfamiliar with Canadian military history to learn that Westholm and other veterans who served after the Korean War were, until 2001, not even categorized as "veterans" by Veterans Affairs Canada, leaving them without many of the economic benefits of their forebears.

For soldiers afflicted with psychological injuries, their diagnosis was as much a *social* and *economic* issue as a medical one, and was subject to larger factors beyond their control. Psychological trauma and its most well-known manifestation, PTSD, became prominent issues in the CAF and Canadian society during the 1990s and 2000s, but their appearance is part of a longer story, and it is one that has been shaped by military matters, medical and political interests, gender norms and expectations, and individual soldiers' experiences.

TRAUMA, MEDICINE, AND HISTORY

Standing at the crossroads of psychiatric, military, gender, and cultural histories, mental trauma provides historians and the public a window into the societies and individuals affected by it, as well as the authorities who attempt to explain its myriad manifestations. Since trauma was first systematically studied in the nineteenth century, medical knowledge, patient experiences, and societal views of trauma have been refracted through different prisms, each shaped by cataclysmic events such as the First World War. Given the sheer scale and number of collectively traumatic events throughout the twentieth century, it is, as historians Mark Micale and Paul Lerner remarked, "scarcely surprising that trauma has emerged as a highly visible and widely invoked concept."[11] To trace the history of trauma is to trace the vicissitudes of a chaotic world and humanity's moral failings. By the late twentieth and early twenty-first century, conceptualizations of trauma escaped from the pages of medical journals and entered popular culture, becoming not just a clinical entity, but also often a metaphor for life's struggles.[12] Discussions of exactly what constitutes "trauma" and its biological, psychological, and social effects have led to prolonged and widely publicized controversies across the Western world.

Although physicians first became interested in trauma during the 1870s, it was not until a century later, with the third edition of the *Diagnostic and Statistical Manual of Mental Disorders* (DSM-III) in 1980, that the American Psychiatric Association (APA) officially recognized an entity called "Post-Traumatic Stress Disorder."[13] The timing was no coin-

cidence. Coming on the heels of the Vietnam War and its divisive effect
on American society, PTSD's official recognition was due in large part to
the lobbying efforts of antiwar psychiatrists, lay activists, and alienated
veterans.[14] PTSD located the source of Vietnam veterans' baffling postwar symptoms in external events such as war and social alienation, thus
"promising to free individual veterans of the stigma of mental illness,
and guaranteeing them (in theory, at least) sympathy, medical attention,
and compensation."[15] Although initially tailored for Vietnam veterans,
over the succeeding decades the PTSD concept created a "consciousness
of trauma" in Western society, bridging the gap between civilian traumas such as rape and natural disasters, and the traumas of war.[16] Trauma's psychological effects had previously been explored, usually during
and after major wars, but most researchers lost interest as each war's
memory faded and its veterans were absorbed into postwar economies.
Official recognition of a disorder called PTSD, on the other hand,
allowed for sustained and targeted studies into trauma's causes, which
proved a "tremendous boon" to clinical research in the human sciences.[17] Popular interest in trauma followed suit. As the 1980s progressed, an enormous medical literature about PTSD developed, and
academic societies were created to share research.[18] But despite the
fact that PTSD's recognition quickly led to medical interest in trauma,
it was war trauma – and in the Canadian case, peacekeeping trauma –
that captivated the public and made PTSD an enduring subject
of discussion.

HISTORY, WAR, AND MEMORY

Clinical discussions of trauma in the 1980s and 1990s dovetailed with
historical reappraisals of, and new approaches toward, past conflicts –
most notably the First World War. Paul Fussell's 1975 book, *The Great
War and Modern Memory*, first explored the way British soldiers on the
Western Front utilized literary traditions to understand and cope with
the horrors of modern war.[19] Himself an American ex-infantry officer
wounded during the Second World War, it was fitting that Fussell was
first to investigate how the Western Front was "remembered, conven-
tionalized, and mythologized" by its participants.[20] He argued that the
Great War was such an overwhelming experience for its combatants
that it gave rise to a new, modern form of understanding – one
that was essentially ironic.[21] Soldiers' experiences of the Somme and

Passchendaele, he believed, altered ideas of modern "progress" and changed forever the way that war was conceptualized.

Fussell's study was partly stimulated by his interest in past soldier-authors' experiences, which helped him to answer the very personal question, "Was my war unique, or merely commonplace and barely worth special notice?"[22] Written while the Vietnam War still raged, his book was meant to demonstrate to American readers some of the "psychological and intellectual dimensions of 'combat.'"[23] By exploring the traumatic nature of war on its participants, he hoped "that the effect of the book ... might persuade them [Americans] that even Gooks had feelings, that even they hated to die, and like us called for help or God or Mother when their agony became unbearable."[24] Fussell's literary history of war, modernity, and memory set the stage for future examinations of the construction of social memory. Responses to Fussell's work, notably Jay Winter's *Sites of Memory, Sites of Mourning* (1995), and in the Canadian context Jonathan Vance's *Death So Noble* (1997), contributed to a fresh analysis of how collective war trauma both forms and disrupts constructions of national identity and memory.[25] All three works demonstrated that in the search for a unified collective remembrance, literal and metaphorical traumas often clashed with ideas of the "good war" and myths about a war's purpose.[26] This book expands on their analyses, highlighting how in Canada the traumatized veteran has been the living embodiment of the gritty, brutal, and harrowing nature of war and peacekeeping; a representation repeatedly at odds with collectively sanitized narratives linked with medical and political projects. Traumatized soldiers' experiences and the story of trauma's evolution provide an inroad into how national identities and social memories are shaped, and equally important, how such beliefs conflict with the everyday struggles veterans face upon their return to civilian life.

WAR, SOCIETY, AND MASCULINITY STUDIES

As scholars reappraised ideas of war and memory, a concurrent literature developed in the 1980s, 1990s, and 2000s exploring the historical shaping of masculinity. Although taken up largely by male historians, it was a woman who first investigated the subject of war, psychiatry, and masculinity in significant depth. Elaine Showalter's 1985 work *The Female Malady* uncovered historical representations of "feminine madness and masculine rationality," and devoted an entire chapter to discussing how shell-shocked soldiers presented a challenge to English psychiatry and notions of manliness during the First World War.[27] Her book was a stinging feminist critique of British psychiatry, and she extended her gender analysis to investigate how masculinity itself was pathologized using feminine constructs. Showalter argued that the war was "a crisis of masculinity and a trial of the Victorian masculine ideal."[28] In her view, numerous men were placed in overwhelmingly stressful situations and reacted with "the symptoms of hysteria," a "feminine" disorder.[29] As the war progressed, psychiatrists explored the possibility that men's problems had origins that might be more deeply rooted in their psyches than previously understood: a possibility that had a profound impact on conceptualizations of trauma throughout the rest of the century.[30]

Showalter's work was the first to critically examine how psychiatric knowledge both shaped and was coloured by masculine ideals during wartime. Her discussion went beyond strictly medical concerns, highlighting the socio-cultural aspects of war trauma and the medical theories underpinning it. By situating "shell shock" in a particular time and setting, her book provided further impetus for scholars to reappraise medical categories and use a cultural lens to deconstruct how experiences of trauma and gender intersected.[31]

Historian of gender and psychiatry Mark Micale's 2008 work *Hysterical Men*, which tracked hysteria's conceptualization across the centuries, highlighted the socio-political and medical discourses that created a willful blind spot in the minds of physicians afraid to acknowledge male nervous illness.[32] Frightened that men were not the paragons of rationality which centuries of intellectual thought had claimed, medical men "failed to constitute their own gender as a field of critical, systematized study."[33] That failure, Micale stated, was all the more surprising given the "rampant counter-evidence [about male nervous illness] in the clinic and the laboratory, on the streets and the battlefields."[34] Physicians' refusal to turn their gaze inward reflected a fear that male hysteria could uncover "feminine" elements within the male psyche.[35] To be self-aware was thus deemed an "unmasculine" quality;[36] Micale uncovered a "chronic inability to reflect nonheroically, without evasion and self-deception, on oneself individually and collectively."[37] This failure had lasting effects on interpretations of shell shock during the First World War – an affliction contemporaries frequently linked with hysteria.[38] Micale's work displayed the highly gendered manner in which psychiatric thought and practice operated throughout the nineteenth and early twentieth century. Importantly, *Hysterical Men* showed that it was only late in the twentieth century that medicine no longer played "a commanding role in producing the dominant fictions of masculinity."[39]

TRAUMA, PSYCHIATRY, AND CANADIAN MILITARY HISTORY

Discussions of war's effects on societal norms and culture were broadened by the rise of trauma as a tool of historical analysis. Since the 1980 codification of PTSD as a mental disorder, scholars from several historical subfields and other disciplines have attempted to piece together the social, medical, and cultural meanings of trauma.[40] Along with the rise of trauma debates in Canadian medical and popular culture, particularly since the 1990s, there has been a rise in the number of historical studies linking contemporary ideas of trauma with earlier medical manifestations like shell shock.[41] Prior to 1990 one looks in vain for mentions of PTSD in Canadian historical studies. For example, Tom Brown's 1984 essay "Shell Shock in the Canadian Expeditionary Force" highlighted the links between the shell shock "epidemic" during the First World War and the professional development of psychiatry and psychology, but made no mention of PTSD.[42] Terry Copp and Bill McAndrew's groundbreaking 1990 monograph *Battle Exhaustion*, which explored military psychiatrists' efforts to treat battle exhaustion in the Canadian Army during the Second World War, made only one brief mention of "Post-traumatic stress syndrome."[43] Nonetheless, that lone mention was crucial: it was the first time Canadian historians linked post-1980 conceptions of trauma with earlier battlefield manifestations like shell shock and battle exhaustion.[44]

Terry Copp's 1998 essay on post-Second World War veterans' psychological illness traced the subject's history from shell shock "to Post-Traumatic Stress Disorder," demonstrating the link historians then began making between older and newer conceptualizations of trauma.[45] Copp acknowledged the rise of trauma research and discussions in Canadian print media amidst the many peacekeeping operations of the 1990s, calling PTSD research a "growth industry."[46] Later, a 2010 collection edited by Copp and Mark Humphries about combat stress in Commonwealth soldiers across the twentieth century showed that by the new millennium, views about the universal nature of trauma had caused scholars to rethink shell shock, battle exhaustion, and PTSD. Each manifestation was now viewed as an amorphous example of a similar and timeless phenomenon. Debates and controversies ensued.[47]

One seminal study arising from the post-1980 rise of PTSD research, which still provokes responses from authors across the Western world, was Allan Young's 1995 book *The Harmony of Illusions*. Young's controversial thesis suggested that PTSD was not timeless, but instead was "glued together by the practices, technologies, and narratives with which it is diagnosed, studied, treated, and represented by the various interests, institutions, and moral arguments that mobilized these efforts and resources."[48] He particularly took aim at the belief that PTSD could be found in many times and places. Instead, he argued that the theory of a traumatic memory, emerging in the nineteenth century and enshrined later in the *DSM-III*, was a modern creation unknown and unavailable to earlier societies. Young did not deny the reality of PTSD, but rather affirmed that PTSD was a separate phenomenon from earlier medical diagnoses like hysteria, brought together by a specific set of medical practices, research, and patients' realities. Nor did he cast doubt on trauma's reality; instead, he cautioned against the expansive diagnosing of PTSD under circumstances not directly related to war. Feelings of guilt, for example, were not necessarily a part of shell shock. For historians, the most important element of Young's book was that it critically examined clinical practices, trauma theories, and historical negotiations between physicians and patients. His work displayed the importance of understanding how traumatic experiences "penetrate people's life world, acquire facticity, and shape the self-knowledge of patients, clinicians, and researchers."[49]

Young's analysis complemented another crucial work that asked scholars to rethink the dynamic relationship between patient and physician, as well as culture's effect on the shaping of illness symptoms. Edward Shorter's *From Paralysis to Fatigue* demonstrated that through numerous exchanges, whether at the cultural level in mass media, or at the micro level in the doctor's office, "historical eras shape their own symptoms of illness."[50] More than two decades after its publication, Shorter's work still provides important food for thought, especially for those studying the history of trauma, given the evident changes in trauma's presentation, and representation, throughout the past century. Like Young, Shorter pointed to the historically contingent nature of psychosomatic illnesses, arguing that as cultural shifts occur, the legitimacy of a particular disease, as well as its symptom patterns, changes along with it.[51]

Canadian historical scholarship on war trauma has been influenced by the above authors, but thus far few studies have emerged. Mark Humphries's 2010 journal article "War's Long Shadow" was the first to combine developments in these subfields, examining Canadian veterans' experiences of postwar trauma and pension concerns from medical, gender, and socio-political perspectives.[52] But in spite of Humphries's initiative, little has followed it. Copp and Humphries's edited collection brought together a vast array of historical documents and perspectives on trauma and combat stress, but their exploration of war trauma in Canada did not thoroughly address post-1980 developments. More importantly for this book, it also did not appraise Canada's challenges with peacekeeping trauma after the Cold War.[53]

Since the 1980s, Canadian military historians have led the charge to explore psychological trauma in Canadian history, but the aforementioned studies have largely focused on the First and Second World Wars, and no book-length study about Canadian military trauma across the twentieth and early twenty-first century has been attempted.[54] Moreover, aside from Humphries's article, no Canadian historian has produced a comprehensive analysis of war trauma which utilizes developments in gender and cultural history.[55] Previous works, which illuminated medical practices and theories of psychological trauma during and immediately after wartime, centred more on physicians than patients.[56] With regard to peacekeeping experiences, there have been even fewer efforts to explore trauma's effects on individual peacekeepers and Canadian conceptions of national identity. Journalist Carol Off's book *The Ghosts of Medak Pocket* (2004), about Canadian peacekeeping experiences in the Balkans during the 1990s, is one of the only book-length studies that examines peacekeeping trauma, and then only tangentially.[57] Likewise, political scientist Sandra Whitworth's *Men, Militarism and UN Peacekeeping* (2004) presented a critique of UN operations and explored the gendered elements of peacekeeping relations, but trauma was relegated to only a small section of her larger narrative.[58]

NEW OPPORTUNITIES

Taking advantage of a unique and open moment in Canadian military history, this book traces how trauma has been interpreted by the military, Canadian society, and the individuals affected by it. At the cultural level, it is an examination of how physicians and patients entered into a dialogue of ideas about how trauma was constructed and understood at the experiential level. It is also a history of the socio-politics of trauma. This story draws heavily from the concerns expressed by soldiers traumatized by war and peacekeeping operations in the post-1991 era, exploring their socio-economic motives and contributions to national identity.

PTSD and conceptions of trauma changed over time. Tracking these changes reveals medical and cultural shifts in consciousness against the larger backdrop of military operations and an evolving Canadian society. Although medical knowledge and societal attitudes toward psychological trauma shifted between the early twentieth and early twenty-first century, stigmas about the mentally ill veteran persisted, as did the socio-economic troubles that dogged veterans as they reintegrated into civilian life. While the general trend was one of increasing understanding and sympathy, veterans from the First World War through to those returning from the Afghanistan War shared many of the same socio-economic challenges. Indeed, the language of illness and the shame associated with trauma remained consistent despite changes in military operations, medicine, and technology. Although shifts in psychiatric theory and orientation after 1980 helped to formally recognize veterans' mental suffering, the clinical road to recovery often neglected the socio-economic realities of postwar and civilian life.

Soldiers' battles with traumatic events symbolize the nation's struggle to reconcile its complex history, one that has made Canadians both battle-tested warriors and harbingers of peace in troubled areas of the globe. The plight of veterans, and how Canadians rationalize it, represents society's attempts to honour and memorialize noble deeds, as well as our attempt to forget about the darker threads in our national tapestry. Historically, veterans' experiences were accepted or discarded amidst the construction of social memories based on a "combination of invention, truth, and half-truth."[59] But even when unpalatable or inconvenient to prevalent societal views, their experiences refused to be fully submerged. Ultimately, the traumatized veteran, whether afflicted with "shell shock," "battle exhaustion," or "PTSD," represented the dangerous, harrowing, and enduring legacies of military operations across many times and places.

This book contributes to discussions of trauma and military history in several key respects. First, it engages with debates about how trauma is shaped across different eras, showing that although certain manifestations of trauma, such as persistent nightmares, were common to every era, shell shock and its successors were rooted in particular times and places.[60] Like Peter Leese, and Allan Young before him, I view each trauma manifestation as a similar but distinct "idiom of sickness."[61] Here I am particularly indebted to Edward Shorter's aforementioned book, which aptly observed, among other things, that the Parkinsonian shaking displayed by First World War shell shock sufferers had all but disappeared by the Second World War just twenty years later.[62] Such observations should give historians, physicians, and the public reason to pause when assessing the tangled and multifactorial relationship between PTSD and its predecessors. Put simply, I believe PTSD is just another (re)presentation of trauma in a continuing cultural and medical project that aims to bring trauma's numerous social and health effects under a neatly encapsulated umbrella.[63] Exploring each historical phenomenon in its own right allows historians to penetrate particular socio-cultural trappings and see the complex connections between individual lived experiences, medical theories, and societal views and representations, essentially spotlighting the shadowy realms where trauma resides. Historically, each trauma manifestation was an individual illness, but considered together they reveal how Canadians, over one hundred years, have understood war and its psychological effects on soldiers. By examining trauma thus, this book brings the Canadian experience across the *longue durée* into international discussions of trauma history, something not yet undertaken by Canadian historians in a monograph-length study.

Equally important, this work also adds to an incipient trauma history field in Canada, bringing together military, medical, and social histories. Veterans' experiences speak volumes about the social experience of trauma, and, from a cultural standpoint, about the construction of masculinity and its intimate ties to military culture. The military represents one of the last bastions of "traditional" masculinity. As such, exploring its connections to trauma opens up further opportunities for understanding how military culture interacts with and shapes medical and lay perspectives on illness. Most importantly, this book provides an in-depth examination of how trauma and peace-keeping both intermingled and conflicted with medical theories and cultural discussions after the Cold War – again something no Canadian historian has attempted beyond article-length studies. By bringing the historical narrative into the late twentieth and early twenty-first century, this book opens up new avenues for future researchers and demonstrates the benefits of a comparative, multifaceted approach to the history of trauma in the military and Canadian civil society. It also opens up opportunities for comparative histories to further analyze "universal" experiences of trauma, moving beyond the idiosyncratic experiences of veterans and toward comparisons of military and civilian trauma in Canada.

This book is organized into six chapters, each revolving around particular wars or peacekeeping missions. War, and later peacekeeping, heralded the rise of popular discussions about psychological trauma in Canada. While civilian trauma captured the attention of medico-psychological researchers beginning in the 1870s, it was the strain and horror of military conflicts that haunted many men and brought their mental troubles into popular consciousness. Shell shock, battle exhaustion, and PTSD were real entities, but the symptom patterns, patient experiences, and medical terminology were shaped anew during each generation by historically contingent socio-cultural and political factors.[64]

The first chapter examines organized medicine's interest in psychological trauma from the 1870s through to 1914, and explores the Canadian Army's experience with shell shock during the First World War. Medical theories about shell shock evolved alongside popular conceptions of manliness and proper soldiering. These ideas coincided with Canadian psychiatry and psychology's early professionalization efforts. Shell shock became in many respects a metaphorical battleground on which differing medico-psychological theories competed with one another, before psychological theories explaining trauma gradually took precedence over organic, physical ones. Utilizing contemporary medical literature and newspaper sources such as the *Globe*, the opening chapter shows how popular sympathies toward shell-shocked soldiers clashed with medical and military dictates that deemed such behaviour illegitimate and feminine. After the war, physicians were the gatekeepers of pensions, and believed in the importance of a pull-up-your-bootstraps work ethic. Those unable to adapt to postwar life were viewed as weak, effeminate, and undeserving of compensation. Thus physicians successfully denied numerous shell-shocked veterans pensions, supposedly for their own good.

Chapter 2 discusses the Canadian Army's experience with "battle exhaustion" during the Second World War. Allied military psychiatrists and higher authorities attempted to prevent another shell shock epidemic by bringing battlefield trauma and psychological difficulties under the new, all-encompassing term of "battle exhaustion." Ostensibly a transient condition curable through rest and recuperation, battle exhaustion reflected a shift in medical thinking toward socio-psychological interpretations of war trauma. By the end of the Second World War, there developed a general consensus that every man had his breaking point. But that belief was a double-edged sword. If a "neurosis" continued after the war, it was, they believed, predominantly caused by earlier life events and upbringing. War was just the trigger. Freudian and other psychodynamic approaches emphasizing an individual's life history colluded to produce a conviction among Department of Veterans Affairs physicians that "neurotic" veterans should not be awarded pensions. Such men, they believed, must be prevented from shirking their duties as fathers, breadwinners, and leaders of postwar society. Once again many veterans were deemed to be weak, inadequate, and failed men by state-employed psychiatrists who were heavily influenced by contemporary beliefs about both traditional manhood and what battle exhaustion revealed about a man's inherent weakness. The second chapter concludes with a description of how Canadian psychiatry benefitted from an increased interest in psychiatric illness as a result of the Second World War and its role in raising awareness of mental disorder within civilian society. After demobilization, prominent military psychiatrists brought their wartime expertise with mental disorders into their civilian practices, in the process helping psychiatry to carve out a role for itself outside of the asylum. The post-1945 period saw, among other things, the creation of the Canadian Psychiatric Association and the expansion of the Canadian Mental Health Association, events which helped shape how psychiatric illness was approached and treated in Canadian society for the next several decades. As it had done with technology, the Second World War had the effect of stimulating new approaches to mental illness throughout Canada and the Western world.

Chapter 3 explores the creation of post-traumatic stress disorder as a legitimate medical condition in the late 1970s, following in the wake of the Vietnam War and psychiatrists' recognition of trauma's effect on American soldiers. The Vietnam War stimulated considerable public discussions about trauma, while the televised and highly visible traumatized soldiers cultivated popular sympathy and frustration about the impact of war on their mental state. The war's divisive nature, and the traumas experienced by so many Vietnam vets, dovetailed with a revolution in American psychiatry. In the 1970s a group of biologically oriented, anti-Freudian APA members campaigned to rewrite the *Diagnostic and Statistical Manual of Mental Disorders*, American psychiatrists' bible. Their success, culminating in the manual's 1980 third edition, set psychiatry on a vastly different trajectory; one which encouraged greater efforts into targeted and empirical research. Influenced by an eclectic group of radical antiwar psychiatrists, war veterans, and trauma researchers, the APA agreed to acknowledge a new conceptualization of trauma – "Post-traumatic Stress Disorder." For the first time psychiatrists officially recognized a consequence of trauma that originated from without, rather than within those afflicted. But given PTSD's socio-political origins, physicians in Canada and elsewhere at first largely dismissed it as an American, Vietnam War-specific condition.

Although not strictly a Canadian story, chapter 3 traces the medical developments and professional politics behind the creation of PTSD, as well as the Vietnam War's role in stimulating its formation. Those events are crucial for understanding how revolutionary the PTSD concept really was, and the contingent ways in which medical conditions are defined and given authority. It was only after 1980, with the vast changes in psychiatry's orientation and the creation of an organized, seemingly systematic understanding of trauma, that PTSD slowly seeped into Western culture and assumed a persistent place in medical and popular discussions.

Chapter 4 traces the history of Canada's peacekeeping operations and its contribution to national identity after the 1956 Suez Crisis, primarily through oral interviews with former peacekeepers, government documents, newspapers, and television broadcasts. By the Cold War's end, a specific vision of peacekeeping – characterized by Canadian soldiers gallantly keeping warring factions at bay in a clearly defined zone of separation – took hold. Nonetheless, after 1991 peacekeeping operations frequently entailed plunging into harrowing situations in which combatants respected neither their enemies nor the peacekeepers sent to prevent further bloodshed. The Canadian military and public were psychologically unprepared for the horrific events that occurred in places like the former Yugoslavia throughout the 1990s. Amidst numerous scandals throughout the decade – most notably the 1993 murder of a teenage boy in Somalia by Canadian peacekeepers – the CAF and Department of National Defence (DND) went into a protective posture. Politicians and military leaders deemed peacekeeping trauma another potential scandal, and thus attempted to downplay and deny it. Against the backdrop of distressing military operations and a military culture that stigmatized psychological problems, trauma became the site of battles between old and new interpretations of war trauma and masculinity, and between different popular perceptions of peacekeeping and the nation's role in international politics.

Analyzing transcribed soldiers' testimonies from the Croatia Board of Inquiry (BOI) and oral interviews with board members and former peacekeepers, the fifth chapter explores the rise of PTSD in the Canadian national consciousness as a result of peacekeeping trauma.[65] With almost 100 testimonies totalling approximately 2,000 pages, BOI documents and peacekeepers' recollections display soldiers' personal battles with trauma and the vagaries of military culture. Throughout the mid- to late 1990s, a series of prominent events – such as Lieutenant-General Roméo Dallaire's public struggle with PTSD, as well as the numerous disclosures of rank-and-file soldiers during BOI testimonies – caused a distinct shift in views of psychological trauma. Canadian military leaders, politicians, and the general public began to realize that trauma could result from peacekeeping as well as war. Moreover, a disorder once deemed a uniquely American affliction gradually became linked in Canada with peacekeeping trauma, something hitherto unheard of. Discussed throughout its proceedings on national newscasts and in newspapers in late 1999, the BOI presented a challenge to historically suppressed discussions of men's psychological problems and forced an acknowledgment of the reality of peacekeeping trauma.

The sixth and final chapter discusses the battle between military reformers and an "old guard" after the Canadian Forces' entry into the Afghanistan War in 2001. The Canadian experience with trauma after 2001 was particularly instructive in what it revealed about the contingencies of medical categories and the importance of culture in determining the relevance of medical diagnoses. Throughout the early twenty-first century, trauma remained a contentious issue for physicians and military reformers, and caused continuing public debates about Canada's national identity and role in international affairs. Behind those debates lay the traumatized veteran, a figure who once again demonstrated the importance of socio-economic factors in a soldier's road to recovery. Veterans' experiences showcase the consistent role of trauma as a prism through which to view contemporary social norms, medical knowledge, and cultural anxieties. Despite all of the changes over the one-hundred-year period covered, the final chapter highlights trauma's ongoing existence – both as a clinical entity, and as a metaphor for the nation's struggles to reconcile its national identity and military accomplishments with the traumatic experiences of those serving on its behalf.

While choosing to explore an entire century, I have focused greater attention on the post-Cold War period, due in large part to a dearth of books published on this era. The period is, to a significant degree, a history still untold. Nevertheless, to describe the evolution of Canadian military trauma after the Cold War it is necessary to provide the subject's longer history and the myriad links that exist between conceptualizations of trauma in 1914 and a century later. Thus the first three chapters, encompassing mainly the First World War, Second World War, and Vietnam War, should be viewed as the first part of a larger story, and a necessary one for understanding the development of Canadian military culture and societal views of mental illness. This section relies more heavily on secondary sources and the scholarly work conducted on First and Second World War experiences with shell shock and battle exhaustion. The book's second half, beginning with chapter 4, covers the post-1991 peacekeeping era and leads up to the return of Canadian troops from Afghanistan in 2014. Chapters 4, 5, and 6 are based almost entirely on primary source analysis, and provide a fuller account of how trauma has been viewed by Canadian soldiers themselves, as well as how medical and popular discussions interact with, shape, and are shaped by military trauma.

In bringing together the history of trauma in the Canadian military across unique periods in the nation's development, this book relies on a diverse array of sources. For tracing medical trends and changes to theory and practice, I have relied heavily on the *Canadian Medical Association Journal*. As a mainstream journal of Canadian medical practices and ideas, and one that has been continuously published across the timeframe of this book, the *Journal* proved crucial for tracking how and when Canadian physicians discussed trauma, as well as when such discussions faded into relative obscurity throughout the twentieth century.

Other medical journals, such as the *Canadian Journal of Psychiatry*, were similarly useful for providing comparisons and contrasts between medical and cultural representations of trauma, as well as how and *when* trauma became a subject of significant interest for Canadian researchers.

Newspapers add another layer of depth to historical discussions of trauma in Canada, and constitute one of the most important cultural sources drawn upon in this book. To capture national, popular narratives over a one-hundred-year period, I have relied extensively on two newspapers with lengthy publication records: one nationally circulated, the *Globe and Mail*, and the other circulated in Ontario, the *Toronto Star*. I have also utilized the *Ottawa Citizen* for its consistent (and early) coverage of military trauma in Canada after the Cold War, and, for an occasional non-Canadian perspective, *The New York Times*.

Canadian soldiers' memoirs and letters from conflicts across the twentieth century also proved useful for allowing a glimpse "from the trenches," and are sprinkled throughout the book. When possible, I supplemented their accounts with memoirs of Canadian and non-Canadian medical officers such as R.J. Manion and Lord Moran. This approach helps to compare and contrast the medical view with that of the frontline soldier.

The aforementioned Croatia Board of Inquiry documents constitute one of the book's most prominent primary sources and help to drive the narrative in the latter chapters. Trauma was the elephant in the room during many soldiers' testimonies of what went wrong in the Balkans in the early 1990s. Discussions of how the military dealt with overwhelming stress on both an individual and collective level provide an in-depth look at Canadian military culture and its approach to mental injuries during the 1990s. They also point to both continuity and change within the Canadian Forces. But most importantly, Board of Inquiry testimonies complement oral interviews with living Canadian peacekeepers who experienced harrowing post-Cold War peacekeeping missions first-hand. Their recollections create a fuller picture of the challenges that those with stress injuries faced after their return.

My aim, especially in the book's second half, has been to capture as authentically as possible veterans' lived experiences of trauma and how it affects them not just medically, but in their daily lives. In this regard, the most important primary source material was oral interviews with clients/members of the Operational Stress Injury Social Support (OSISS) program, a combined Veterans Affairs Canada and Department of National Defence peer-support program for soldiers and veterans with operational stress injuries such as PTSD.[66] In my search for the lived experiences of CAF members and veterans with psychological injuries, I was graciously put in contact with Peer Support Coordinators and other OSISS members by then-OSISS national program manager Major Carl Walsh.[67] Within twenty-four hours I received several phone calls and e-mails from members willing to speak. Over the next few months I conducted phone interviews with eight OSISS members of various ages and ranks, consisting of seven men and one woman from many provinces across Canada, such as Alberta, Ontario, Quebec, and Newfoundland and Labrador. Given the sensitive nature of the subject – something that precludes "cold calling" or e-mailing veterans out of the blue – my candidate pool was limited to the number of individuals who made first contact. In addition to the eight interviewees who completed discussions with me, several others initially expressed interest but either got cold feet on the arranged interview date or did not respond after initial correspondence. I later learned from those who chose to stay the course that this was a common occurrence when speaking with OSISS members, since many were concerned about the career implications of speaking with someone outside the military. It gradually became clear that a fear of discussing military matters with "outsiders" was still prevalent among many within the Canadian Forces, and that mental illness, despite increasing discussions within civilian and military circles, is still a largely taboo subject.

The majority of interviewees were peacekeeping veterans who participated in operations throughout the 1980s, 1990s, and early 2000s. There were also Afghanistan veterans, and a few who participated in both war and peacekeeping operations. Discussions usually lasted between one and two hours, and after some initial questions related to biographical information, generally became free-flowing conversations. Each interview began with a series of prepared questions, but I did not attempt to steer any interviewee toward a subject they were hesitant to discuss. I wished to avoid "triggering" any disturbing thoughts or recollections, and to avoid any perception that I was probing for voyeuristic purposes. Thus, I attempted to sense the interviewee's comfort level and adjust my questions accordingly. In most cases, I let the interviewee direct the conversation, though I tried to keep the discussion on military matters and military culture.

The interviews were moving, inspiring, and sometimes emotionally disturbing. In several instances the interviewee had to stop and collect him or herself, and relistening to the discussions for transcribing purposes turned out to be at times unexpectedly difficult. In an unflinching manner, several interviewees freely related traumatic and harrowing operational events. I was particularly moved by the effect that such experiences had on their subsequent lives, and the many years that some went without relating their experiences to anyone except their closest friends and family. A few suffered in silence for close to a decade, reaching the point of almost total collapse before finally seeking help. Some of their recollections, though graphic and disturbing, proved to be encapsulations of numerous recurring themes I wished to address. Thus, interview excerpts are reproduced at the beginning of several chapters to highlight the prominent issues faced by veterans with psychological injuries, and the challenges of bringing this history out into the open.

Interviewees' recollections proved to be a microcosm of larger narratives, and demonstrate the human story behind the medical, cultural, and political controversies. Readers should be warned: soldiers' reflections can be strikingly blunt, and in some cases the straightforward language they employed to describe traumatic events is in itself disturbing. Although I offered total anonymity to every interviewee, none wished it. Several instead expressed the hope that their uncensored and public story would prove helpful to other veterans afraid to come forward about their mental difficulties. Such testimonies represent a unique moment in Canadian history when some soldiers and veterans are willing to speak publicly about their personal battles – both with trauma itself, and with a military culture that emphasizes resiliency and toughness while shunning weakness. Prior to the 2000s, creating this book would have been next to impossible, since groups such as OSISS did not exist; and given the closed nature of military culture, particularly in the 1990s, it is highly unlikely that anyone would have been willing to relate their experiences to someone outside of the Forces. A few interviewees confirmed this conjecture's validity, and one told me I was lucky to find "the softest spot to push."[68] It remains to be seen whether or not this window will remain open to future researchers.

Listening to post-Cold War Canadian veterans' difficult emotional journeys reveals a line that runs backward through time, to the similar experiences of their counterparts who served during earlier conflicts and operations. Although much has changed in Canadian society and the Western world since 1914, traumatized veterans of the twenty-first century encounter many of the same dilemmas and are subject to many of the same socio-economic and cultural challenges as those who returned from the First and Second World Wars, such as social ostracism and difficulties obtaining a pension. Their stories represent a direct link to the past and highlight the importance of viewing such experiences not just as individual struggles, but also as the metaphorical struggles of the nation as it attempts to grapple with the collective trauma of war and the country's role in international politics. Although previous authors and documentarians have utilized interviews with veterans, and some have even highlighted trauma, the second part of this book expands on that approach by making veterans' recollections the pivot point around which its historical discussion of trauma revolves. This story listens to veterans and uses their thoughts as a way to reflect on how trauma is socially and philosophically *experienced*: essentially, how trauma affects one's social life and worldview, rather than just how it is diagnosed and viewed in medical terms. As one interviewee poignantly stated, despite physicians' best efforts to treat PTSD and other stress injuries, trauma sufferers do not live in their doctor's office, and the longer history of trauma points to the need to reassess medical approaches to the subject. One might even go so far as to argue that the consistent socio-economic difficulties Canadian veterans have faced over the past hundred years should inspire us to rethink whether "PTSD" is even the correct term to encapsulate trauma's multifarious socio-economic effects. By listening to individual and cultural experiences of trauma, historians can add to a growing understanding of PTSD and its antecedents as both medical entities *and* profoundly shattering social experiences. Canadian veterans are finally willing to speak candidly about the effects of war on both the psyche and the soul, and it is our duty to listen.

1

A Shocking Introduction to Trauma

There is a legitimate nervousness, named "shell shock." The real cases of this condition, when they are extreme, are sad to see. An officer or Tommy, who has previously been an excellent soldier, suddenly develops "nerves" to such an extent as to be uncontrollable. He trembles violently, his heart may be disorderly in rhythm, he has a terrified air, the slightest noise makes him jump and even occasionally run at top speed to a supposed place of safety. He is the personification of terror, at times crying out or weeping like a child.

> From the war memoir of Captain R.J. Manion,
> Canadian Army Medical Corps.
> See Manion, *A Surgeon in Arms*, 163.

I'd seen men twisting and writhing in their sleep after big battles, tortured by visions that held them on a rack, by screams and shouts and the sounds of fighting that still echoed in their ears, and I knew that years would not entirely remove such remembrances. Those images of war would be with us as long as memory remained, needing but a slight impetus to make many nights an ordeal of dread, haunting us like scuttling winged ghouls, obliterating the finer, saner sensibilities. It would be harder for us than any others in the competition of life, for all our constructive thinking would be marred by overshadowing visions and phantoms.

> Bird, *And We Go On*, 229.

Writing in the late twentieth century, historian of military psychiatry Hans Binneveld opined that "one can no longer imagine a battlefield without psychiatrists and psychologists."[1] Retrospectively, Binneveld's assessment of the now-inseparable link between the mental health profession and the military was somewhat prescient. The final decades of the twentieth century, particularly the 1980s and 1990s, saw the growth of a "culture of trauma" that made PTSD – a disorder defined by the American Psychiatric Association in 1980 – a hotly debated topic in military circles, medical journals, and newspapers across the Western world.[2] PTSD thus became a considerable concern for military leaders, as well as for the civilian governments they reported to. But such was not always the case. Throughout the twentieth century, psychological trauma oscillated between being a prominent subject and a focus solely for specialist medical researchers. It was major conflicts like the two world wars and the Vietnam War that catalyzed the permanent place of trauma in the public eye.[3] The conceptualization and dissemination of knowledge about trauma and combat-related psychological injuries were largely forged and reignited by the fires of war, and, in the case of peacekeeping nations like Canada, "military operations other than war."[4] This chapter briefly traces early discussions of mental trauma in the nineteenth century before moving on to consider how early paradigms of "traumatic neurosis" and "shell shock" were challenged and reshaped amidst the apocalyptic scenes of the First World War. It then discusses the battle between organic, physical theories of shell shock, and psychological ones, investigating how medical knowledge both supported and clashed with military needs and culture. It concludes with a discussion of the role of physicians in postwar pension questions, and examines how prevailing notions of masculinity mixed with medical knowledge in determinations of whether or not a shell-shocked veteran was worthy of a disability pension.

RAILWAY SPINE AND EARLY THEORIES OF PSYCHOLOGICAL TRAUMA

Historians have discovered documented links between combat and intense psychological duress as far back as the seventeenth century, and the mental effects of battle on combatants were recognized even during biblical times.[5] Commenting on the timelessness of war's impact on the human psyche, military historian Richard Gabriel affirmed that, "If it were possible to transport a military psychiatrist back to the times of the Roman and Greek armies, there is little he would find in dealing with combat shock with which he was not already familiar."[6] Nevertheless, despite ancient peoples' familiarity with war's stresses, it was only quite recently, with the rise of professionalized medicine and modern technology, that psychological trauma was systematically studied. In their edited collection on the history of trauma, historians Mark Micale and Paul Lerner argued that in the period from 1870 to 1930, psychological trauma "acquired the status of a disease entity with a technical terminology, theories of causation, a classification, and therapeutic systems as well as medico-legal standing and governmental recognition."[7] Trauma's newly acquired status derived in part from the fact that modernity brought with it unprecedented assaults on both the body and mind, but it also crucially corresponded with organized medicine's first systematic study of how those assaults affected the human psyche.[8] The rise of psychiatry, neurology, psychology, and other allied disciplines coincided with, and was constitutive of, medical and cultural engagement with psychological trauma on a hitherto unprecedented scale.[9]

Medical theories about psychological trauma began with mid- and late-Victorian physicians' curiosity about the unique types of injuries that occurred when humans broke centuries-old rates of velocity and spatial boundaries.[10] In the case of early railways, one of the quintessential inventions of the modern age, a significant number of accidents resulted in "railway spine," "railway brain," or "traumatic neurosis," an amorphous set of diagnoses that often involved an individual's delayed stress response to the original traumatic event.[11] In his 1866 publication, *On Railway and Other Injuries of the Nervous System*, John Eric Erichsen, British surgeon and professor at University College Hospital in London, described seven cases of railway spine. Patients' mental difficulties confused physicians, particularly since Erichsen's original hypothesis was that a concussive force led to chronic inflammation of the spinal cord, producing a general disturbance of the nervous system. Mystifyingly, some patients appeared physically cured, but their psychological difficulties persisted. Detailing the case of a "Mr. R.," a patient seen fifteen months after his accident, Erichsen's notes stated that Mr R. was "unable to transact any business since the injury. Is troubled with frightful dreams. Starts and wakes up in terror, not knowing where he is. Has become irritable, and can neither bear light nor noise."[12] The fact that no damage had been done to the patient's spinal cord rendered Erichsen's organic explanation of the phenomenon untenable.[13] By the 1870s a number of physicians inter-

ested in psychological medicine and the puzzling nature of cases like
Mr R.'s began discussing the concept of psychological trauma, thus
applying the concept of "trauma" to what had previously been utilized
for strictly physical injuries.[14] During the 1880s, Erichsen's organic
explanation was challenged by other physicians, such as London surgeon Herbert Page, who argued that intense fright alone could
account for patients' symptoms and "traumatic hysteria."[15]

The debate over psychological trauma and its effects occurred on
both sides of the Atlantic. In an early Canadian example, during an
1898 meeting of the Association of Railway Surgeons in Toronto, a
solicitor named Mr B.B. Osler (former prosecuting counsel against
Métis leader Louis Riel and brother of medical authority Sir William
Osler) spoke to a group of Canadian and American physicians about
"'railway spine' or traumatic hysteria, which causes so much trouble to
railway surgeons and to lawyers."[16] Osler, like numerous future investigators, stated that "the subjective nature of the symptoms made the
subject very difficult," and that "doctors rarely agreed" when assessing
railway spine cases.[17] Thus, the railway accident and its mental effects
became an important and formative aspect of the history of trauma: it
was the first time that such phenomena were systematically researched
and discussed in medical circles.[18] Railway spine created a new awareness of the ability of traumatic experiences to provoke a series of physical and psychological symptoms. It also supported beliefs that modern life contained traumas of a previously unseen nature.[19] Railway
accidents metaphorically represented the rapid, uncontrollable, and
sometimes shattering impact of modern technology on the human
mind.[20] As a medical *cause célèbre* during the late nineteenth century,
railway spine laid the groundwork for future trauma debates. Thus,
when physicians encountered "shell shock" during the First World
War, they understood that despite pretensions of modern progress,
human beings were still inherently fragile and helpless against technology's darker, destructive side.

OVER THE TOP

Although railway spine brought trauma under the lens of modern
medicine, it was shell shock during the First World War that propelled
psychological trauma into the spotlight and attracted attention from
soldiers, civilians, and governments in addition to physicians. The

nature and scale of the weaponry, the manner in which it was utilized, and the generally appalling conditions during the First World War affected men's minds in diverse ways. Several months after the outbreak of war, in December 1914 the War Office in London received reports that an alarming number of soldiers from the British Expeditionary Force were being evacuated with "nervous and mental shock."[21] According to those reports, 3–4 per cent of all ranks were being returned to Britain due to "nerves" and other forms of mental breakdown.[22] Given the vicissitudes of what became a long and hard-fought war, every soldier counted, and as such, the British attempted to contain the problem. By early 1915 Charles Myers, MD, a Cambridge University psychologist and officer in the Royal Army Medical Corps, was tasked with reporting on an increasing number of "shell shock" sufferers.[23] Having seen his first British shell shock patient in November 1914, he was fascinated by its manifestations and keen to investigate further.[24] As a "Specialist in Nervous Shock" and later "Consulting Psychologist to the British Armies in France," his goal was to discover how to treat the numerous men ostensibly suffering from the thunderous impact of enemy shells.[25]

Historian Ben Shephard argued that shell shock was "an early example of a common modern phenomenon: a medical debate, hedged with scientific qualifications, taken up by public opinion and the media in an oversimplified way." He continued: "The early medical model of shell-shock, dominated by the image of the shell itself – a violent, concussive *deus ex machina*, which arrived from out of the heavens and left the soldier a shattered, gibbering wreck, his nerves destroyed and his special senses, like eyesight and hearing, impaired – imbedded itself, in a crude and oversimplified way, in the public imagination."[26] Much like how stress and PTSD in the late twentieth century became identified with Vietnam jungle warfare, shell shock, presumed to originate from exposure to the concussive power of artillery barrages, became an iconic medical disorder of the First World War – an image that persists in the public consciousness across much of the Western world today.[27]

Public sympathy toward shell shock in Britain and the rest of the Empire partially stemmed from frequent newspaper reporting, which by 1917 created the impression that shell shock was a normal and frequent consequence of war.[28] A 1918 *Globe* article certainly helped contribute to such an impression: while reporting on a Boston Smith

College course for women to assist in treating shell shock sufferers, it exaggeratedly proclaimed that in Canada, "90 per cent of returned soldiers suffer from some nervous disorder."[29] Nevertheless, sympathy and popular understandings went against military necessities and a military culture that did not tolerate weakness. Army attitudes to mental disorder were interwoven with traditional masculine principles of honour, stoicism, self-control, and camaraderie.[30] Mental disorder was linked with weakness, effeminacy, and cowardice, and viewed as something "treatable" by disciplinary actions.[31] Officially at least, it was only the abnormal man who was frightened or repulsed by the sights, sounds, and actions of battle.[32] But at the same time that the British military applied a simplistic, unofficial, "sick, well, wounded, or mad" approach to assessing soldiers' health, military physicians faced the reality that the war produced large numbers of soldiers who broke down in battle with illnesses that slipped between the cracks of crude categories.[33] Unable to fully grasp or classify the numerous types of troubled soldiers they encountered, doctors at the front sometimes resorted to reductive or idiosyncratic labels such as "Mental" or "Insane," and even unusual terms like "GOK," an initialism for "God Only Knows."[34]

Military physicians were in the unenviable position of having to "invert normal civilian practice and go to great lengths to deny that a soldier was sick" as a means of preventing military "wastage," while still tenuously clinging to their other duty – treating the wounded and ill.[35] Canadian surgeon Robert James Manion, a medical officer, Military Cross winner at Vimy Ridge, and later Conservative MP, provided an in-depth view of life in the trenches in his 1918 memoir, *A Surgeon in Arms*. He recalled frequently being visited by officers before battle and informed of individual soldiers' "cold feet," to prevent such soldiers from obtaining a medical reprieve under the pretense of illness.[36] Since many early cases of shell shock were evacuated back to England, with most never returning to the battlefront, the military became concerned about the degree to which knowledge of the term shell shock and its vagueness allowed malingerers – those feigning illness to avoid duty – to seek an honourable exit.[37]

Based on his experiences as a medical officer during the First World War, British physician Lord Moran stated in his 1945 account of war's psychological effects that "when the name shell-shock was coined the number of men leaving the trenches with no bodily wound leapt up.

The pressure of opinion in the battalion – the idea stronger than fear – was eased by giving fear a respectable name ... The resolve to stay with the battalion had been weakened, the conscience was relaxed, the path out of danger was made easy."[38] Put simply, shell shock's amorphous symptoms and the confusion about its causes allowed fearful soldiers to escape along with the genuinely ill. Colin Russel, a Canadian neurologist and later head of the neuropsychiatric ward of the Granville Canadian Special Hospital, Ramsgate, in England, summed up the situation in a 1919 article in the *Journal of Abnormal Psychology*: "Owing chiefly to the fact that these [shell shock and other] conditions were not fully recognized in the beginning, many cases were evacuated to England which would not otherwise have been, and the depletion of manpower in the front line from this cause became a very serious item."[39] In the summer of 1916 during the Battle of the Somme – one of the bloodiest battles in history – shell shock grew to "epidemic proportions."[40] As experts came into contact with a greater number of cases, it became clear that "shell shock" served far more as an evocative symbol of modern warfare, and in some instances as a symbol of fear, than as an accurate description of what was troubling many soldiers.

By June 1916, the first authoritative study of shell shock was published by Harold Wiltshire, an experienced London physician who saw over 150 cases and compared notes with military doctors at the front. He argued that in most cases patients showed little or no physical damage. The problem's root, he believed, was psychological.[41] He pointed to a "psychic shock" as the cause of many men's symptoms, providing one example of a soldier who was traumatized after clearing away the remains of a group of men killed by shellfire.[42] Presciently, Wiltshire also noted the ability of the mind to repress sights and emotions it was unable to fathom, an ability discussed at great length after the war and throughout the rest of the century in relation to trauma.[43] Charles Myers, who helped popularize the term "shell shock" in 1915 in the British medical journal *The Lancet*, now realized the reality of war trauma was far more complex; by 1916, with other experts like Wiltshire, Myers attempted to relabel shell shock and its manifestations "war neuroses" or "functional nervous disorders."[44] Their rebranding reflected a shifting medical consensus about the perceived psychological cause of many shell shock cases, and an attempt to preserve medical authority over such matters. At the command level, renaming shell shock highlighted the partnership between medical experts and military authorities to keep shell shock out of the hands (or more accurately, the minds) of rank-and-file soldiers. Replacing shell shock with the more esoteric terms "neuroses" and "nervous disorders" was a way to prevent soldiers from arriving at their own diagnosis and to ensure that stigmas about mental disorder kept them in line.

The Canadian Expeditionary Force (CEF), which totalled over 600,000 members during the First World War, also had between 9,600 and 15,000 soldiers diagnosed with war-related psychological injuries.[45] Faced with such numbers, the Canadian Army established two neurological hospitals at Granville and Buxton, England, in 1915–16.[46] Historian Tom Brown demonstrated that, similarly to the situation within the British Army, shell shock became a battleground on which Canadian physicians vied with each other as well as with the exigencies of war and military culture. Psychiatry was a "divided profession" on the eve of war. Somaticists, who believed that mental and nervous disorders were the product of physical lesions, contended with followers of Sigmund Freud and other prominent neurologists, psychologists, and psychiatrists, who argued such disorders were not brain diseases, but disorders of the mind originating in the psyche.[47] Robert Manion, mentioned earlier, believed that shell shock's root cause was "the subjection of the nervous system to a strain which it is unable to withstand, making it collapse instead of resiliently rebounding."[48] Such a collapse could be brought about by "the effects of severe shelling; by being buried by an explosion of shell or mine; or by the killing beside the sufferer of a companion."[49] Regardless of their theoretical stance, though, Canadian Army physicians were not free from contemporary value judgements about cowardly behaviour, nor from their prime directive: to return as many soldiers as possible to battle.

Many doctors did not consider shell shock a legitimate war injury. Instead, they believed the shell-shocked soldier "suffered from a lack of moral courage, a failure of the will, [and] a loss of self-control."[50] Manion, an exception to the rule, deemed shell shock "a legitimate nervousness," and something which in the extreme was "pitiable to observe."[51] But when assessing a soldier reporting mental or physical injuries, a medical officer's loyalty was first and foremost to the army.

Although the individual patient was of paramount concern to a physician in peacetime, in war it was necessary to "look at disease and physical non-effectiveness from a collective point of view."[52] It was for this reason that Manion, while reviewing a group of sick troops, once overheard a disgruntled soldier mutter that "one never gets a fair deal from a military doctor."[53] Distinguished Canadian physician Sir Andrew Macphail, an early editor of the *Canadian Medical Association Journal* and Vimy Ridge veteran, stated that shell shock was at its core a display of "childishness and femininity," adding that "against such there is no remedy."[54] He was less than sympathetic in his assertion that "hysteria is the most epidemical of all diseases, and too obvious special facilities for treatment [during the war] encouraged its development."[55] Macphail's belief, shared amongst most medical officers and civilian physicians, demonstrated the link contemporary doctors made between the hysteria-like symptoms of shell shock and hysteria's long history as a disorder deemed predominantly feminine.[56] For the soldier who had "his wind up" or simply wanted out, though, a shell shock diagnosis provided a legitimate way to exit the conflict. Thus shell shock constituted a serious issue for military authorities and governments, both ultimately concerned with victory. In *The Anatomy of Courage*, Lord Moran described the weariness and fear that pervaded the ranks by 1917 as "no longer a private anxiety, it had become a public menace."[57]

It is difficult to make generalizations about the frontline soldier's precise understanding of shell shock. Nonetheless, it is evident that many subscribed to the commonly held view that shell shock was caused by physical effects incurred during shellfire, as demonstrated by letters written during the war. Private Sydney Brightman of the Pioneer Corps wrote in November 1916 that although he initially believed "shell shock and 'cold feet' were much about the same thing," after seeing men killed by shell concussions without being directly hit, it seemed feasible to him that "some fellow will get such a shock that although it will not kill them, it will render them unfit for any more military service."[58] Likewise, Robert Shortreed from Guelph, Ontario, a member of the 12th Canadian Siege Battery, wrote to his mother in December 1917 that he was "Sorry to hear that Alf Morrans [sic] son is so bad," explaining that "it is what is called Shell Shock and results from being close to an exploded shell." He clarified that "Some cases of course are not as bad as others and any man having it is not sent back to France. In the shell which landed behind our dugout recently one man was Shell-shocked."[59]

Such letters show the connection that soldiers and physicians made between shellfire and its effect on the "nerves." Lord Moran concisely summarized the link, describing stress's effect as analogous to withdrawing from a bank account: "The call on the [man's] bank might be only the daily drain of the trenches, or it might be a sudden draft [e.g., a shell explosion] which threatened to close the account."[60] In this analogy, when the account balance reached zero, nervous breakdown occurred. Moran considered high explosives to be the "acid test of a man in the trenches," with soldiers' reactions teaching them "things about ourselves we had not known till then."[61] George Tripp from Huttonville, Ontario, who served with the 19th Battalion and was killed in May 1917, wrote to his friend Lola Passmore during a recuperation period after heavy shelling at the Somme in October 1916. In his letter, he noted that the battalion had recently experienced two "strenuous" spells in the trenches, one of which proved to be too much for a comrade, whose "nerves gave way," causing him to be "sent out [diagnosed with] shell shock."[62] Alexander Matier, an American-born veteran of the Spanish-American War who enlisted with the Canadian Expeditionary Force in 1915, wrote to his Aunt Lil from a Winnipeg convalescent hospital in January 1918 that, on top of having a leg paralyzed below the knee (treated with massage therapy and galvanic electricity), he had also developed "a slight dose of shell shock" a year prior.[63] He explained that "to this day [I] have spells, but the Surgeons tell me I will get over it entirely in time, as I have a good strong nerve system."[64] Belief in the ability of "nerves" to bounce back after intense physical and psychological duress, implying as it did that the associated condition was transient, did much to contribute to postwar arguments that veterans' enduring psychological problems were self-induced.[65]

Soldiers' wartime writing also shows that, like physicians and the public, they approached shell shock with an ambivalent mixture of sympathy and abhorrence, in much the same manner that mental illness in general was viewed within civilian society. Alfred Andrews from Qu'Appelle, Saskatchewan, a lawyer who enlisted in 1914, wrote in a May 1915 diary entry about volunteering to take an injured comrade out of the frontline. He reported that while walking the wounded man out, another soldier "suffering from shell shock" came along, ostensibly after being granted rest and recuperation. But shell-shocked or not, the man was still expected to do his duty; Andrews matter-of-factly stated that he "had to put the boots" to the man "to get him to do any work."[66] By contrast, in July 1916, Charles Richardson of Grenfell, Saskatchewan wrote from North Evington War Hospital in Leicester, England that it was "really pitiful" to see three patients there with shell shock.[67] William Bell from Innisfree, Alberta wrote in a similarly sympathetic tone to his sister in March 1917, advising her against discussing the war with a family friend heavily affected by war service: "Well you say Loyld [sic] East look[s] 10 year[s] older and gets 20 and feels 30 and he want[s] to forget it[.] I don't blame him a bit[.] For goodness sake don't ask him any questions about the war [and] where about was he wound[ed] anyway or was he shell shocke[d]."[68]

Soldiers' reactions to comrades and officers afflicted with shell shock demonstrated the sharp line drawn between those who had seemingly "earned" the attribution and those who had not, as well as the fine line between courage and cowardice. Thomas Leduc from Cache Creek, British Columbia drew close attention to those distinctions in a July 1917 letter discussing fellow officers he saw during a hospital visit in France.[69] After sympathetically describing one major who was "suffering principally from shell shock" and would not be rejoining the battalion, he referenced two other officers who "wont [sic] ever show their faces near this battalion again."[70] One can surmise that the two men in question, a captain and a major, had failed to remain stoic in the face of battle and proven a poor example to their men. Leduc was stern in his judgement that "a man or officer who gets shell shock has all my sympathies for that may come to any one at any time[,] but I despise a coward."[71] Like Leduc, military authorities were just as concerned with ensuring that officers and rank-and-file troops were aware that shell shock was not to be used as a mask for cold feet or cowardice.

By mid-1917, with the war's outcome still in doubt, Commander of the British Army Sir Douglas Haig forbade the use of the term "shell shock" in speech, in any reports, or on medical documents, except in cases classified by the officer commanding the special hospital. In place of "shell shock" doctors were to use "Not Yet Diagnosed – Nervous (NYDN)," a term that prevented soldiers from self-diagnosis and, at least officially, removed shell shock as a recognized war wound.[72] Haig's order reflected not only concerns about manpower, but also the reality that, as neurologist Colin Russel reported, many soldiers

were diagnosed with shell shock despite never actually seeing the battlefront.[73] Although physicians attempted to help officers "sort out
the shirkers from the heroes" and provided medical backing for the
military's stance on shell shock, it was evident by the end of the war
that psychological medicine could neither unequivocally explain and
categorize psychological trauma, nor prevent some (whether physicians or patients) from applying "shell shock" as they saw fit.[74] Once
the proverbial genie was out of the bottle, it proved difficult to put
back. In spite of authorities' attempts, the term remained in circula-
tion by both physicians and soldiers throughout the rest of the war
and beyond, becoming in one sense a medical condition, and in
another sense a metaphor for the physical, spiritual, and mental traumas of the Great War.[75] Shell shock's resonance also supported Paul
Fussell's appraisal of the war's ability to stimulate a shift in consciousness.[76] In a similar manner to how soldier-authors during the
Great War utilized literary traditions to rationalize the war's horrors,
shell shock symbolized a physical, mental, and societal attempt to
explain the Great War's effect on the collective psyche. Essentially,
shell shock became a medical ailment for some, and an explanatory
device for others.

SHOCKING LEGACIES

Shell shock's prominent appearance during the First World War was
a turning point in the history of psychological trauma. Abram Kardiner, an American psychoanalyst who saw over 1,000 patients with
war-related "neurotic disturbances" in the 1920s, wrote in his seminal
1941 work, *The Traumatic Neuroses of War*: "The neuroses incidental to
the great war made the world neurosis-minded. They were studied
with more care than at any time previously, and the literature is ency-
clopedic."[77] The most salient issues: the need to define "war neuroses";
sorting out the legitimately injured from the "effeminate" and malingerers, not just for battle but also for pension purposes; reconciling
military needs with the reality that modern warfare was inherently
traumatic for participants; and the role of the press in bringing psychological injuries to public consciousness. These remained common
themes throughout the twentieth century.

Regardless of physicians' ostensible success or failure during the
war, both psychiatry and psychology were visibly strengthened by

their wartime service. In Canada, as elsewhere, psychiatry was enhanced by its newfound need for services outside of the asylum, the profession's traditionally sole locus of practice.[78] The discipline emerged from the First World War with "a new-found sense of professional identity and self-worth, its status and prestige greatly enhanced in the public mind."[79] It was, historian Tom Brown noted, no coincidence that the Canadian National Committee for Mental Hygiene (CNCMH), the forerunner of the Canadian Mental Health Association, was formed in 1918.[80] After the Great War, psychiatrists and neurologists played a leading role in deciding many of the issues noted above, namely defining war neuroses, aiding governments in pension decisions, and modifying programs for mentally ill veterans. Leaders of the fledgling Canadian mental health field took steps to ensure that their position was secured and enlarged. One of the first aims listed for the newly formed CNCMH was "War Work," specifically both "psychiatric examination of recruits" and "adequate care of returned soldiers suffering from mental disabilities."[81] A February 1918 article on the CNCMH's formation in the home of a Mrs Dunlap highlighted the committee's ambitious aims: "[the study of] problems of mental health, nervous and mental disorders, mental deficiency, epilepsy, inebriety, and the mental factors involved in crime, prostitution, pauperism, immigration and the like."[82] Among the many luminaries present at the meeting were: Dr C.K. Clarke, dean of medicine and professor of psychiatry at the University of Toronto; Clifford Beers, founder of the American National Committee for Mental Hygiene; Dr E.A. Bott, later head of the Psychology Department at the University of Toronto and specialist in aviation psychology for the Royal Canadian Air Force in the Second World War; and the aforementioned Great War neurologist and shell shock expert, Colonel Colin Russel.[83] Top officials in the postwar mental health professions had a strong connection to the military. For many it proved to be a training ground for testing out new ideas and gaining credibility as experts on a wide range of non-military issues.

POLITICS, MANLINESS, AND PENSIONS

While the mental health professions benefitted from the war's stimulation of academic interest in the mind, the frontline soldier's experience with shell shock became an individual and collective trauma planted deeply enough that forgetting the war's darker side was often impossible. For those lucky enough to escape death or serious physical injury, there were the lingering effects of witnessing carnage and destruction on an unprecedented scale. The work of shell-shocked poets – Brits such as Wilfred Owen and Siegfried Sassoon, and Canadians such as John McCrae, whose "In Flanders Fields" was inspired by the death of McCrae's comrade Alexis Helmer – were testaments to a war that haunted many of its participants for the rest of their days.[84] Canadian author Will Bird wrote about his harrowing experiences as a soldier in the trenches in his 1930 memoir, *And We Go On*. Considered by military historian Jonathan Vance to be one of the two best accounts of the Great War produced by Canadian soldiers, *And We Go On* described several cases of shell shock and the effects that battles like Passchendaele had on men's minds.[85] Bird felt that "the courage that kept a man in his place in those terrible late November days at Passchendaele was the straining of the soul, the last limit of human pluck," and that "every man who had endured Passchendaele would never be the same again, [and] was more or less a stranger to himself."[86] Bird also recalled that after Passchendaele he twice woke in the middle of the night and "found a man on his hands and knees, gazing about him, wakened by the horrors of his own mind, unable to comprehend that at last the Salient stench had left his nostrils."[87] It is doubtful that such powerful memories were easily forgotten upon returning to civilian life.

Even civilians were fascinated by shell shock and attempted to distill its essence in print, a trend exemplified in the interwar period by the character Septimus Warren Smith in Virginia Woolf's 1925 novel, *Mrs Dalloway*. In the book, Smith, a First World War veteran suffering from shell shock, commits suicide after experiencing postwar hallucinations and receiving the news that he is to be involuntarily committed to an asylum.[88] Though fictional, Smith's story was representative of the ghosts that haunted numerous veterans after their return home. Cultural depictions of veterans' lingering trauma played an important role in helping postwar societies come to terms with the Great War's immense destruction and sense of loss. Crucially, they also underpinned political discussions about the veteran's role in postwar society. Books like *Mrs Dalloway* highlighted that for many men, the war's end only signified the beginning of the "second battle" – which included reintegration into civil society and the fight for financial compensation. For those whose minds were temporarily or permanently affected by the war, that battle was immensely more difficult.

The Great War produced thousands of veterans who returned physically and mentally wounded, and the question of what constituted a legitimate injury was a thorny issue after the 1918 Armistice. In Canada, as in other combatant nations, the return of wounded soldiers put a great strain on the already fragile socio-economic order. Unlike in previous wars, such as the Second Anglo-Boer War, when disease killed more soldiers than combat, the Great War was unique because the majority of sick and wounded troops returned home alive.[89] The sheer scale of returning men compounded a problem that existed because "pensions, bounty, [and] kindred issues hardly rippled the surface before 1914."[90] Nevertheless, as early as 1915, Canadian officials outlined a program for retraining and rehabilitating soldiers, first through the Military Hospitals Commission (MHC) and, by October of that year, the Military Hospitals and Convalescent Homes Commission (MHCHC).[91] The Commission, later absorbed by the Department of Soldiers' Civil Reestablishment (DSCR), provided medical care, vocational training, and occupational therapy. The goal was veterans' future independence and employability: a purported win-win for both parties.

The DSCR program was quite progressive, especially for an age when most relief and employment support was conducted at the municipal level and through private charities.[92] The DSCR not only broke new ground in vocational education but also aided in "fostering a more enlightened approach to disability."[93] In December 1918 the government also instituted a one-time war service gratuity payment, to help honourably discharged and able-bodied men re-establish themselves in civilian life. The amount each man received was based on duration and location of service, and marital status.[94] Rounding out the major assistance was the 1917 passing of the Act to Assist Returned Soldiers in Settling upon the Land and to Increase Agricultural Production. The Act created a Soldier Settlement Board, reserved government land for settlers, provided loans for agricultural endeavours, and created an instruction program to teach veterans how to successfully homestead. Like other federal measures, the Act allowed "the government to help ex-servicemen help themselves."[95] In all cases, the government's goal was to encourage individual industry and wean both able-bodied and wounded soldiers off federal assistance.

Although a large number of men benefitted from the various assistance programs, in 1919, the year the Pension Act received royal assent, Canada still had 42,932 disability pensioners. Twenty years later, their number had grown to 80,104.[96] In a testament to how tricky and controversial the pension question was, the Act required *sixteen* amendments between the end of the First World War and beginning of the Second.[97] The total value of disability pensions in 1919 and 1939 amounted to $7 million and $30 million respectively, or $154 million and $624 million when adjusted for inflation.[98] Those figures, which do not even include dependent pensions, were a great financial burden on the federal government. Between the world wars, the cost of veterans programming and pensions was second only to servicing the national debt.[99] Such assistance proved to be a heavily politicized issue throughout the interwar period, especially since contemporaries both hoped and expected that most veterans' injuries would improve with time.[100]

Federal officials attempted to steer a path between Britain's conservative approach toward veterans' pensions, and the "pension evil" that followed the end of the American Civil War just over fifty years prior. In the former case, Canadians visiting Britain before 1914 remembered veterans begging on street corners, while in the United States a more liberal approach to pensions had led to many abuses. So-called "deathbed marriages" and a proliferation of claims agents and pension attorneys looking to make their fortunes by exploiting loopholes in the system (supposedly on behalf of their clients) meant that by 1914, one-fifth of US federal spending was earmarked for veterans' pensions.[101] The Canadian government aimed to avoid both outcomes. The MHC's creation and its future incarnations represented an eclectic approach that attempted to balance veterans' needs, and the nation's obligation to them, against a desire to save money wherever possible. Keeping pension costs down (especially once the Depression took hold), and ensuring the public treasury was protected, meant taking a firm stance on the question of deserving and undeserving veterans. Unfortunately for numerous men, the ostensibly objective approach of pension officials and advising physicians was often coloured by contemporary moral judgements about masculinity and a prevailing doctrine of industry and adaptability. Canada was far from European battlefields. Although Canadians read about the horrors of trench warfare and witnessed its aftermath first-hand when seeing physically shattered soldiers on the streets of Toronto and Edmonton, many still viewed veterans who were unable to gain or retain employment as evidence of the traditional "fecklessness of soldiers."[102] Their attitude reflected historical middle-class views of the traditional soldier: a working-class man, usually of criminal temperament, who in Prime Minister Sir John A. Macdonald's opinion was only skilled at hunting, drinking, and chasing women.[103]

During the interwar period, when an ostensibly injured veteran appeared before a pension board, officials' biggest single concern was "attributability" – that is, whether or not the injury was attributable to war service.[104] If a man's injury was deemed attributable to service, his pension amount was assessed according to level of disability and military rank. The 1919 Pension Act created a scale that allowed officials to (seemingly) objectively determine a man's "percentage" of disability according to twenty classes, with class twenty – 5 to 9 per cent per cent disabled – constituting the lowest.[105] A class one, totally disabled veteran from the rank and file was entitled to $600, a figure fixed by Parliament as necessary in order to keep a disabled man who was unable to earn in "decent comfort."[106] His class twenty counterpart was granted $30.[107] Those who were considered less than 5 per cent disabled and did not fit on the scale were given a one-time payment of $100. Pensions could be granted in perpetuity, but in most cases were temporary, lasting only a few months or a year.[108]

The term "disability" was understood by officials to mean the degree to which an injury had reduced a man's "capacity for ordinary employment."[109] Thus, according to Lieutenant-Colonel J.L. Biggar of the Canadian Army Medical Corps, a man was "not pensioned because he has lost his eyes, but because, having lost his eyes, he cannot see."[110] In a fitting example, a Private Poirier was granted a $240 (class thirteen, 40 per cent disabled) pension for the loss of an eye in action.[111] One key problem with the disability scale, as noted by Biggar, was that it could not "be so elaborated as to lay down the specific percentage for each variation of disability resulting from every disease and injury."[112] What this meant in practice was that a man's injuries could be assessed and assigned to different pension classes depending on a board's subjective determinations of how disabled his injury made him. A man's current or previous occupation played a role in decisions about how much the disability in question affected his earning potential. Subjectivity was an even greater factor when a man's pre-existing health condition(s) complicated the board's ability to determine how much of his predicament was *actually* caused by war service.

The Great War produced a multitude of different diseases and injuries, and as such, pensions were granted for a wide array of general, circulatory, respiratory, and gastrointestinal issues, not to mention injuries involving gunshot wounds and amputations.[113] Mental illness produced another, less easily defined category, since there were myriad ways in which a damaged mind could hinder a man's ability to stay gainfully employed. Throughout the early 1920s and beyond, the pension system and the philosophy underpinning it helped concentrate pensioners at the low end of the scale; attributability was one of the ways in which this was accomplished.[114] While on the surface a seemingly simple question, the open-ended interpretation of attributability led down many paths. In their 1987 work, *Winning the Second Battle*, historians Desmond Morton and Glenn Wright succinctly stated the issue's intricacies: "Disability might be an objective medical question; how far the disability was 'attributable' to service was a matter of almost metaphysical complexity."[115] Visibly disabled soldiers who lost a limb or suffered gunshot wounds could, with experience, be quickly assessed and classified on the pension scale, but many injuries were not as easily pigeonholed.[116] As but one example, Morton and Wright cited soldiers who contracted syphilis overseas. Pension officials questioned, perhaps rightly, whether or not soldiers could attribute venereal disease to war service.[117]

Both throughout and following the Great War, mental illness even more than physical injuries constituted a troublesome category for the Commission and its later forms, the Department of Soldiers' Civil Reestablishment (DSCR) and the Department of Pensions and National Health (DPNH). That trouble was partially due to soldiers returning with lingering, war-related trauma, and partially to lax enlistment standards that allowed "obviously insane" recruits to sign up for overseas service.[118] While the provincial and federal governments argued over the cost and responsibility of sending them to an asylum, the public and veterans' associations objected to such measures, believing that veterans driven to chronic mental illness deserved more than overcrowded, neglectful, and stigmatizing mental institutions.[119] In the case of shell-shocked soldiers, anger over sending them to mix with incurable civilian patients, many of whom were at that time suffering from senility or chronic schizophrenia, eventually convinced the Commission to utilize a former mental hospital in Cobourg, Ontario as a centre for shell shock sufferers. The irony of housing veterans in a former civilian asylum and employing traditional asylum methods was lost on Commission officials.[120] At Cobourg, the treatment regimen ranged from benign therapy like sports and recreation to more intensive measures such as electroshock, utilized to help "will" the veteran back to good health.[121] Public sympathy and advocacy by groups including the Great War Veterans Association (one of the forerunners of the Royal Canadian Legion) helped ensure that there were places for the severely affected, but the compensation issue was much more complicated.

Military historians Terry Copp and Mark Humphries aptly summed up the Canadian interwar pension situation for shell shock sufferers, indicating that the pension issue "made sure that the debate over the aetiology [cause] of shell shock remained at the front and centre of the [medico-legal] discourse. After all, if shell shock was due to bursting shells or noxious gases, surely a soldier's disability was attributable to war. If it were due to some innate weakness of character or defect in biology, on the other hand, the state would be spared a significant burden."[122] Limited medical knowledge and a desire to control costs combined to ensure that physicians and pension officials fell back on heredity judgements and/or character flaws to deny "attributability."[123] They essentially explained shell shock victims' inability to engage in a productive postwar life as self-induced malingering.[124] Russel, the CEF's chief shell shock specialist, believed that shell-shocked soldiers willed themselves to sickness. By providing pensions, he believed the government only encouraged their inappropriate behaviour and their continued dependence on the state.[125] That belief allowed officials to reduce pension costs and, in their minds, renew veterans' desire for gainful employment.[126] Physicians commonly viewed their encounter with shell-shocked men as a symbolic battle in which the doctor must be victorious.[127] Essentially, "whether doctors took them seriously or dismissed them as cowardly malingerers, the consequences were virtually identical": no pension or only temporary relief.[128] Physicians did acknowledge that some severely affected veterans could never be employed or care for themselves again. For that category they recommended asylum committal. The remainder were left to convince pension officials that their inability to properly reintegrate was a result of war trauma rather than their own innate, personal flaws.

At a societal level, pension-seeking for wartime trauma was in and of itself viewed by many as a transgression of social norms, namely masculine codes that required men to be "aggressive, self-reliant, and unemotional."[129] Mark Humphries's research with Canadian veterans' pension documents showed that even soldiers whose diagnosis had verified them as "real men" in wartime were often refused state assistance in the postwar period.[130] Crudely stated, the reason, beyond cold economic concerns, was that "real men did not break down, nor did they allow their emotions to interfere with their manly duty as breadwinners and providers."[131] Constructed in this manner, the Board of Pension Commissioners responsible for granting and reviewing pension claims utilized ostensibly objective medical science to bolster beliefs that "shell shock," "neurasthenia," and other categories of psychological illness were the result of character defects, most often of a hereditary or dispositional nature.

The board's approach drew not just on medicine and psychology, but also on longstanding lay perceptions and constructions of manliness. Educational historian Mark Moss's 2001 work on the mid-nineteenth and early twentieth century education of young boys in Ontario – a province that produced almost half of CEF's volunteers – revealed that a host of secular organizations such as the YMCA, Boy Scouts, patriotic clubs, libraries, and schools instilled in young boys a belief that the ultimate test of manliness was war.[132] In a society undergoing vast socio-economic changes, war was "an antidote to the crisis of masculinity, the fear of being perceived as effeminate, the plague of luxury and materialism, [and] the changes brought about by industrialism and the feminization of society."[133] Viewed against this backdrop, doctors' hesitancy about legitimizing war trauma was both an expression and reinforcement of societal norms. Put simply, to be unduly affected after the war's end was to fail as a man. Physicians were ultimately concerned with perpetuating social norms, protecting the socio-economic order, and ensuring their own continued place as experts in pension questions.[134] It must be said that regardless of intent, their assessments were based more on professional interests and predominant middle-class beliefs than objective medical science.[135]

One of the unfortunate results of government and medicine's partnership in the interwar period was that "thousands of legitimately traumatized veterans were left uncompensated by the state and were constructed as inferior, feminized men."[136] Thousands of others, in the words of military historian Tim Cook, "fell through the cracks," left suffering from "damaged minds and shattered spirits."[137] While psychologically injured veterans' losses were measurable in denied compensation, the rejection and humiliation they received at the hands of pension officials and physicians was less tangible. Throughout the interwar period, the number of veterans manifesting psychological problems increased, particularly as the Great Depression set in. Many were confined in public asylums across the country, leaving them suffering in silence amongst other patients, and forcing their families to contend with the socio-economic difficulties of losing a father, husband, brother, or son. The rest, haunted by war but uncompensated in peacetime, were granted "the renewed privilege of fending for themselves in a business-like, profit-driven society."[138]

When shell shock pensions *were* awarded, they were often only granted for six months to a year, ameliorating their recipient's financial troubles for just a brief duration.[139] In terms of numbers, there were on record in 1934 a total of 4,021 temporary and 155 permanent pensions for "nervous system" injuries.[140] As noted by Terry Copp and Mark Humphries, though, most of the 155 permanent pensioners were probably committed to provincial asylums.[141] Humphries's research demonstrated that in the midst of the Depression, from 1931 to 1936, the amount of successful pension claims for shell shock and related conditions decreased from 694 to 148.[142] In the interwar years, state physicians did not look kindly on either hospitalization or payments for shell-shocked veterans. Men like Colin Russel and his colleague, Captain C.B. Farrar, viewed hospitals as something that "encouraged men to escape work as they had escaped danger," while the "flat and final" payment of $500 that some men received was "deliberately punitive" and deemed a "'moral prosthesis' for a weak will."[143] In the spirit of the times, "each discharge or denial of a claim" was deemed a "corrective victory" for the state.[144]

It must be acknowledged that for the majority of returned soldiers, life after demobilization resumed with previous or new employment, and eventually fell into a stable rhythm.[145] But for the thousands of psychologically affected veterans, postwar life provided a continuous challenge made all the more difficult by lingering wartime memories. Here, the quotation from Will Bird at the beginning of this chapter is worth repeating: "It would be harder for us [veterans] than any others in the competition of life, for all our constructive thinking would be marred by overshadowing visions and phantoms."[146]

The First World War brought trauma to the forefront of military, medical, and public consciousness in an unprecedented manner. Those who bore psychological war wounds – individual soldiers – were the most affected. A mixture of socio-economic conservatism and postwar anxieties, fuelled by the Depression, ensured that Canadian veterans were provided with a firm message from government and physicians that the best cure for their ills was a "brisk immersion in civilian life."[147] Pension officials and physicians were, Morton and Wright argued, "men of their time, as convinced of the virtues of economic individualism as they were of scientific expertise. For able-bodied veterans, they believed, a swift transition to civilian self-sufficiency and their breadwinner role was the best way to remove the vestiges of soldierly dependency. Even for the disabled, the transition must be as swift as possible."[148] Colloquially stated, contemporaries believed that an age-old "pull yourself up by your bootstraps" mentality and a return to their role as breadwinners would sort out veterans' problems.

Shell-shocked veterans, the "worst off" of those seeking pensions, had a difficult road, as their unseen injuries caused physicians and much of the lay public to designate them shirkers, malingerers, and inferior men.[149] In an era far removed from the standard double-income family of the twenty-first century, an early twentieth-century man was often the sole family breadwinner, meaning that his competence as a father and husband was intimately tied to his ability to provide.[150] A veteran without this ability was not only viewed as having a weak character, but also deemed a failed specimen of masculinity. Rigid standards of male behaviour and comportment, including a strong work ethic and willpower, were seen as crucial for maintaining the social order.[151] Nervousness, exemplified in the shell-shocked veteran, was deemed the behaviour of "weak and womanly men" and viewed as a threat to society.[152] The "nervous" man was a "principal foe of manliness" throughout the early twentieth century and beyond.[153]

The Canadian public's response to psychologically troubled veterans also demonstrated a distinct desire to focus on the noble ideas for which the war had been fought, rather than the inability of some veterans to purge its traumas from their minds. Although many citizens were familiar with the "ruined veteran" seen in postwar life and literature, that man had no place in the "myth" of the war, or the national project to praise the dead and get on with living.[154] The situation was similar in Europe, where, as cultural historian Modris Eksteins affirmed, "'Lest we forget' was intoned on every conceivable occasion, but forget was exactly what everyone wanted to do."[155] The memory and glory of those who had made the ultimate sacrifice were raised to new, often intensely religious heights in postwar Canadian society, but that did not mean "the survivor should be pitied," nor did it mean that ruined veterans should be viewed as anything other than "the exceptions who proved the rule" about the war's noble purpose.[156] As poetically expressed by Canadian historian Jonathan Vance, "The soldier could not have been coarsened by the war because the cause was righteous: it was unthinkable that the twentieth-century crusader could have been transformed into an animal or an empty shell by fighting God's battles in Flanders."[157]

In short, the traumatized veteran struggled for his place in the post-1918 Canadian social order. Physicians and researchers studying "war neuroses," on the other hand, greatly benefitted from the war, establishing themselves as the go-to experts on psychiatric/psychological illness, despite the evident lack of progression in definition or "cure." With the emphasis placed on veterans' heredity, predisposition, and character, the examination of individual case histories became invaluable for pension officials to separate the deserving from undeserving. Physicians were the natural experts for that task. For historians of trauma, the most pertinent legacies were the issues that shell shock framed for future decades: the perceived causes of, and medical debates over, trauma; the medico-psychological community's role in defining such debates; the socio-economic considerations tied to traumatized soldiers, such as pensions and treatments, both of which became a public concern; and lastly, challenges to views of the ideal soldier and ideal man which trauma brought to light.

Another particularly controversial legacy of the Great War was the execution of 306 British and Commonwealth soldiers for desertion, cowardice, and other offences from 1914 to 1918.[158] Some of those men are now believed to have suffered from shell shock or what would today be termed combat stress or PTSD. In 1992–93, a movement was begun by British member of Parliament Andrew MacKinlay to obtain retrospective pardons for all those executed, but MacKinlay was rebuffed by Prime Minister John Major on the grounds that doing so would be rewriting history. The thrust of Major's argument was that shell shock was known to medical men during the First World War; his implication being that if men were innocent and indeed shell-shocked, medical knowledge should have prevented their execution.[159] Such arguments seem spurious given the abundant evidence that there was no single, uniform understanding or approach to shell shock among officers and their medical staff, nor was it always easy to spot the difference between "cold feet," cowardice, and shell shock. Nevertheless, the fight to obtain pardons for executed soldiers raised important questions about how to interpret controversial historical decisions in light of current understandings.

On the other side of the Atlantic, in 2001, the twenty-three Canadian soldiers executed for desertion and cowardice during the Great War had their names added to the First World War Book of Remembrance in the Memorial Chamber of the Peace Tower on Parliament Hill in Ottawa.[160] That gesture allowed the federal government to avoid being accused of rewriting history, while still recognizing that the men in question died while serving their country. It was a stereotypically Canadian attempt at compromise. In 2006, the British government eventually pardoned the 306 executed men, including the twenty-three Canadians, but the decision was not without controversy. Cliff Chadderton, chairman of Canada's National Council of Veterans Associations, argued that despite the executions seeming brutal by twenty-first century standards, "I think it's wrong to pardon them, because they deserved what they got."[161] Historian Desmond Morton opined that the British decision amounted to "self indulgent" revisionist history, conducted to provide a "golden glow" to the unpalatable aspects of victory, including the need to guard against desertion.[162] Caught up in that unsavoury history and in perennial debates about heroism, cowardice, sacrifice, and duty, shell shock still proved a controversial issue almost a century after the war's end.

But in 1919, amidst the aftermath of Allied victory and the psychological need to move on after so much death and destruction, those debates were a luxury left to the future. As the interwar period progressed and the Great Depression deepened in the 1930s, the Canadian public's focus was on basic necessities such as food and employment. As veterans needed more, civilians wanted to give less. Many now looked askance at those deemed shirkers, believing that numerous pensions had been granted to fraudsters and the undeserving.[163]

Economic struggles bred, in the words of Morton and Wright, "a sour, selfish mood."[164] In 1932, the government of Conservative Prime Minister R.B. Bennett even came close to issuing a "blue book" listing pensioners' names and addresses, as well as the benefits they received. The purpose was to discover potential fraud through the encouragement of communal surveillance. Only strong protests stopped the plan from coming to fruition.[165] The government saved money in other ways, though, including by making pension payments subject to income tax.[166] With many destitute veterans complaining about their plight and receiving a patchwork of relief from municipal authorities and the Department of Pensions and National Health, the Bennett government created an enlarged body – the Canadian Pension Commission (CPC) – to bring order to the chaos. In 1933, the CPC took over responsibility for veterans' pension adjudication, and retained that role until 1995.

The Great Depression exacerbated already intense debates over how much the public owed to veterans, and whether the country was failing to live up to that debt. The CPC battled "heavy weather" throughout the 1930s from veterans frustrated by denied claims and by the CPC's conservative interpretation of pension legislation.[167] Many felt that the CPC took an "overly bureaucratic and high-handed approach" to pension claims, and despite the creation of a Federal Appeal Board for those whose claims were denied, controversies continued right up to the beginning of the Second World War.[168] Battling the turmoil of high unemployment, government austerity, and lingering wartime demons, numerous shell-shocked veterans sought pensions they never received.[169] Whether in the asylum or struggling in civilian life, many simply faded into the background of a tenuous socio-economic order. It took another war to bring discussions of trauma back into the public spotlight.

2

Battle Exhaustion and Medical Movements

The question at issue is of some consequence in war. If a man is rested in time will he have another summer of high achievement, or if that is only a forlorn hope is it more sensible to cut losses? To put it differently, can a good fellow who is showing signs of wear and tear come back?

Moran, *The Anatomy of Courage*, 77.

As an intellectual successor to shell shock, the term "battle exhaustion" was a further refinement of psychiatrists' and psychologists' attempts to explain how and why certain men broke down in battle, and especially why some were permanently unfit for frontline duty thereafter. Of particular interest in this chapter are the theories and treatment approaches employed by psychiatrists to counteract "combat neurosis" during and after the Second World War. Their thoughts and techniques were in many ways a reflection of an evolving psychiatric profession that was still nonetheless tied to prevailing notions of masculinity and manhood. As in the aftermath of the First World War, such notions combined with new beliefs in psychodynamic theories to once again produce a pension system that denied numerous veterans long-term pensions for psychological disorders. This chapter also concisely explores psychiatry during the Korean War before turning to examine how the Second World War and physicians' encounters with battle exhaustion stimulated an increased interest in psychiatric care outside of the asylum, and an expansion of mental health initiatives in civil society. It concludes on the eve of the Vietnam War: a war that Canada did not fight in, but one that nevertheless had far-reaching effects on the conceptualization of war trauma throughout the late twentieth century.

When the Allied nations entered the Second World War, they had to re-establish many of the techniques used in "forward" psychiatry toward the end of the Great War.[1] Forward psychiatry involves the placement of psychiatrists at or close to the front, and the treatment of soldiers close to the front line, rather than at hospitals far behind the line or out of country. It relies on three principles: proximity to battle, immediacy, and expectation of recovery, known as the PIE method or system. During the enormous demobilization that took place after 1918, the relationship between psychiatrists and the military had largely disintegrated and had to be rebuilt.[2] War neurosis, or "battle exhaustion" as shell shock was rebranded in 1943, was initially dismissed as a significant concern in the Second World War, partly because combat in 1939–40 was swift and decisive, leaving little time to set up organized structures for dealing with mental casualties.[3] Anthropologist Allan Young characterized the classification of war neuroses in the Second World War as "too confusing to be properly interpreted by historians" and without a "Rosetta stone" to provide clear translation.[4] Likewise, in his 2007 essay on battle exhaustion in the Canadian Army during the Second World War, former CAF reservist and Afghanistan War veteran Ryan Flavelle opined, "Battle exhaustion is an easy condition to be sympathetic to, but a much more difficult one to understand."[5] Historians have long been challenged by the term's vague nature as well as the manner in which, like shell shock, battle exhaustion provided a blanket diagnosis for numerous manifestations of anxiety. Nevertheless, generalizations can be made. While during the early stages of the First World War shell shock was deemed the result of physical factors, by the Second World War the "pendulum had swung almost entirely in the other direction."[6] In 1939, most physicians believed war neuroses originated in the mind – that they were "psychogenic."[7]

As in the First World War, most military officers tried to reject psychological experts' integration within the military hierarchy. Their rationale was by then well-established: whatever the chosen term, psychiatrically sanctioned war neurosis provided soldiers with an alternative to fighting, and was a potential escape hatch for cowards.[8] Resistance was also partly based on a social-psychological and sociological approach to human behaviour that developed between the wars and placed importance on strong leadership and primary group relationships – in the military's case, a strong *esprit de corps*.[9]

Military officers believed that a strongly led and tightly knit group was less likely to break in combat, thus preventing psychological breakdowns as well. That approach also had medical backing. Influential medical journals like *The Lancet* promoted the idea that a man's constitution and connection to the unit were paramount in determining his likelihood of cracking during or after combat.[10] But in spite of military leaders' misgivings, the long, intermittent, and brutal nature of the Second World War meant that psychiatrists and psychologists were eventually perceived as a necessary part of casualty prevention and management.[11]

A few researchers noticed early in the war that trauma was again becoming a focal point of discussion. An American psychoanalyst and Freud devotee, Abram Kardiner, stated in his 1941 work *The Traumatic Neuroses of War* that, with regards to manifestations of war neurosis in soldiers of the Second World War, "the symptomatology [symptom profile] of this syndrome is no different today than it was during the last war."[12] Like numerous colleagues, Kardiner believed that modern war "introduced certain conditions conducive to neuroses in those so predisposed."[13] His research and work with traumatized soldiers convinced him that in every war there were soldiers who suffered long-term psychological effects. He was unequivocal in his statement that "one of the certainties with which a warring nation must contend is that at the termination of the conflict there will be a considerable number of problems dealing with those soldiers who return more or less damaged."[14] For psychiatrists and psychologists the debate still hinged on whether trauma's persistence in some soldiers was due to predisposition, which by 1939 was largely associated with life history and upbringing, or whether every man had a breaking point regardless of his perceived character.

Despite its prescience, Kardiner's book went largely unnoticed for three more decades.[15] In the military milieu, the potentially troublesome nature of trauma was downplayed by medical officers and leaders who believed that well-trained units minimized mental breakdowns, even in sustained bouts of combat.[16] If breakdowns did occur, soldiers were to be treated close to the front. These treatments included rest, an immediate medical response to the trauma, reassurance from physicians about a soldier's prognosis, and a firm message about his duty to return to combat. That method, developed during the second half of the First World War, became known as the PIE system (i.e., *proximity* of treatment to the battlefield, *immediacy* of response, and *expectancy* of recovery and a rapid return to the unit).[17] PIE was used with some success in the later stages of the First World War, again in the Second World War, and is still a generally accepted system in use by militaries in the twenty-first century.[18] Under such a system, army officers believed no specialists were needed, except for serious cases that could be treated in distant neuropsychiatric hospital units.[19] For the military, what mattered most was, as always, preserving manpower. Psychiatrists and other mental health professionals were disruptive to this goal because they removed men who, in officers' eyes, simply needed a quick rest and firm pat on the back. Even Winston Churchill was skeptical of wartime psychiatry, believing that psychiatrists were a burden on the army and that their work was capable of descending into "charlatanry."[20]

A RUDE AWAKENING

At Dunkirk in May 1940, the British became the first Commonwealth nation to feel the full brunt of war, and the psychological effects on surviving soldiers provided clues that even seemingly "normal" and well-trained individuals could break under intense pressure. Pushed by the Germans back to the French port, 250,000 British Expeditionary Force troops waited for evacuation while enduring sleeplessness, shelling, and bombing by German Stuka dive bombers. The effects on men's psyches were evident: one soldier proclaiming that he was Mahatma Gandhi, and another remaining absolutely still while protecting an imaginary basket of eggs, were just a few examples of troops who had reached their breaking point.[21] Dunkirk tested the assumption that no forward psychiatrists were needed. It also poked holes in the view that combat breakdowns were attributable to a soldier's weak disposition.[22]

On 6 July 1940, William Sargant and Eliot Slater, two civilian physicians working for the Sutton Emergency Hospital in London, published a report on the treatment of military war neuroses seen after Dunkirk.[23] In it, they made an important distinction between "acute shell shock," seen after Dunkirk in many seemingly normal men, and neuroses seen in soldiers during the Phony War from September 1939 to May 1940, when Allied soldiers faced German forces along the Western Front but did not experience any major battles. Sargant and

Slater's study generated interesting insights. First, they recognized that under enough physical and mental strain, including witnessing the deaths of their comrades, even men with solid work records, high intelligence, and normal personalities could "crack." Second, they noted that even with regard to intense anxiety states, the symptoms were usually of a short duration. Lastly, they wrote that the longer soldiers' symptoms were allowed to persist without treatment, the greater the chance that their thoughts and behaviour patterns became ingrained.[24] Sargant and Slater's treatment plan involved inducing a hypnotic state in patients with the widely used sedative sodium amytal, after which they attempted a "recovery of amnesia," a "reinforcement of suggestion," and "the relief of hysterical symptoms."[25] Psychiatrists believed that this method helped the patient relive and work through the repressed traumatic events – a process called abreaction – while also preventing the nervous system from incurring further stress. In a publication several decades later, Sargant expressed his belief that Dunkirk demonstrated the folly of trying to quickly "patch up" soldiers and send them into battle again, given that battle was what caused their breakdowns in the first place. Citing the First World War, he pointed out that even the threat of being executed for cowardice was not enough to prevent breakdown in soldiers under intense and continuous stress.[26]

It was not until a few years after Dunkirk, during the battles in the Middle East and North Africa, that the British Army was forced to acknowledge that a number of men were breaking down due to what they believed was fatigue and nervous exhaustion.[27] British Army consultant psychiatrist G.W.B. James, a veteran of the Somme and Passchendaele, encountered a situation when he arrived in 1940 that reminded him of the early First World War. He was dismayed to find no "modern" program for psychiatric casualties, and felt that army physicians "had no conception of breakdown in war and its treatments, though many of them had served in the 1914–18 war."[28] By 1942, when forward psychiatry was finally put in place, he was certain that there were limits to what a soldier could endure. Convinced by his examination of fifty psychiatric casualties in July 1942 that much of the problem stemmed from the physical toll of modern warfare (and especially the desert) on a soldier, he changed the term "Not Yet Diagnosed – Nervous (NYDN)" to "physical exhaustion," and then to "battle exhaustion." Similar to how shell shock captured the shattering effect of shells on soldiers' bodies and minds during the First World War, battle exhaustion encapsulated and symbolized the physically and mentally exhausting effects of the Second World War on infantrymen.[29]

Although the British Army came to accept the reality of battle exhaustion and other forms of mental breakdown among troops, it did so very grudgingly, assigning battlefield psychiatry a low priority throughout the war. As but one example, among General (later Field Marshal) Bernard Montgomery's staff, there was a prevailing belief that psychiatry was something akin to witchcraft.[30] Thus, for the war's duration – despite occasions such as in July 1944 when infanteers in Montgomery's 21st Army Group suffered a 25 per cent battle exhaustion casualty rate – military leaders continued to attribute mental breakdowns to swings in morale from a long, tough campaign, rather than to the nature of combat.[31] There was certainly a link between the duration and intensity of battle, troops' experience level, and the number of battle exhaustion diagnoses, but the military had a desire to downplay numbers. In a testament to the resilience of the human mind and spirit, most symptoms of trauma, as predicted by Sargant, were relatively short in duration; or so it seemed.

Military leaders' optimism about battle exhaustion rates also reflected another development of the interwar and early Second World War years. While psychiatrists were busy digesting the lessons of the First World War during the post-1918 period, psychologists were equally busy researching human behaviour, and more importantly in a military context, developing tests to screen out those "predisposed" to breakdown. Simply put, while psychiatrists focused on emotional and behavioural pathology, psychologists claimed expertise on normalcy and personality development.[32] Given an adherence by numerous psychologists to the hypothesis that breakdowns could be accurately predicted by personal and family histories as well as deviant behaviours like drug use, they affirmed that with proper testing most of the "unfit" men could be weeded out before induction. That approach, in theory, saved the military time and money on training "neurotic" men, and lowered the incidence of mental breakdown in combat. The problem with such a belief, though, was that it conflated two different issues: mental disorder stemming from stress, and mental disorder stemming from perceived deficiency.[33] A seemingly normal man breaking down because he "had enough," or because he was exposed to traumatizing events, was different in kind from an individual cracking because of a pre-existing, latent mental disorder that rendered him less able to cope with mental duress. Sargant and Slater's distinction between "acute shell shock" and "neurosis" was an important one, since it made clear that many men who had broken down during the Phony War despite the lack of combat were not in the same category as those who had been unable to continue because of trauma. Unfortunately, it was easy to confuse the two, and researchers were limited in their ability to neatly categorize the myriad ways in which mental capacity and behaviour expressed themselves.

Both the British and Canadian armies rejected intelligence testing and psychiatric assessment for recruits at the beginning of the war.[34] Each nation went in its own direction, but they shared some general beliefs and trends. Physicians took away from the First World War the lesson that a rigorous selection process was necessary, due to the number of ostensible "misfit" men who made it into uniform. But putting measures into place to prevent a similar recurrence was a mammoth task. The questions, such as what criteria should be used to assess a man's fortitude for service, and whether that assessment should be made by an army officer, military physician, or a civilian psychologist, were thorny.[35] Military leaders at first preferred the safest option for bringing in the highest number of troops, which was no formal intelligence testing or psychiatric screening at all.[36] In the Canadian case, the decision to forego screening measures was a reflection of the medical profession's attitude toward psychiatry and psychology. The majority of civilian and military doctors believed that well-trained physicians, particularly those with previous war service, could evaluate a soldier's character and fortitude just as effectively as specialists.[37] Dr John Griffin, long-time Canadian Mental Health Association president and consultant to high-ranking psychiatrist Brock Chisholm during the war, stated that "the medical profession, including those in Canadian Medical Corps ... seemed even anti-psychiatric in attitude."[38] Thus, when the Canadian military first entered the war, leaders believed that their own selection process, which consisted of a very informal screening which inadvertently put men with physical disabilities into uniform, was sufficient.[39]

The British Army initially approached personnel screening with similar attitudes, and it was the first to see the consequences. After Dunkirk, the British implemented a testing and screening program with the help of psychiatrists and psychologists, partly in response to criticism from publications like *The Lancet*, which claimed that more men were breaking down from pre-existing neurotic disorders than from combat – an obvious indicator that the Army's ad hoc screening method was ineffective.[40] Psychiatrists in particular gained traction within the British Army between 1940 and 1942, "advising on a range of issues that went well beyond usual definitions of psychiatry."[41] They were even allowed to create their own medical division at Whitehall. Nevertheless, the power of commanders on the ground meant that throughout the war psychiatric casualties were dealt with inconsistently, in a manner largely dependent on officers' whims.[42] Psychiatrists were, in practice, never entirely welcomed in any Allied army. Perhaps the most infamous symbolic – and literal – rejection of psychiatric casualties came from American lieutenant-general George S. Patton Jr, who in 1943 slapped one mentally affected soldier with his glove, calling him a "goddamned coward." One week later he threatened another with his pistol and punched the man in the head.[43] Patton's frustration partially stemmed from the "wastage" that occurred during the Sicily campaign that year, and his actions exemplified a reticence among military leaders to acknowledge the reality of mental casualties, despite mounting evidence in both world wars.[44]

In Canada, psychological testing gained ground in 1941 when Minister of National Defence J.L. Ralston took an interest in the potential benefits of intelligence and aptitude measurement. By the Second World War psychology and intelligence testing had attained a foothold in Canadian schools and social welfare institutions, in part because of its relationship with the mental hygiene movement and the Canadian National Committee for Mental Hygiene throughout the 1920s and 1930s.[45] The profession's forays into the war effort were a reflection of its incipient growth and influence. E.A. Bott, chair of the Department of Psychology at the University of Toronto and president of the newly formed Canadian Psychological Association, went to Britain to consult with the Canadian Army overseas and report on British research.[46] Bott later joined the Royal Canadian Air Force, and his studies on Canadian aircrew, told in great detail in historian Allan English's 1996 book *The Cream of the Crop*, came to similar conclusions as numerous army psychiatrists: given enough cumulative stress, any man would break, and treating men away from the battlefront turned most "curable" patients into chronic cases.[47] Psychological testing was given its biggest boost when the charismatic and larger-than-life colonel and psychiatrist George Brock Chisholm was put in charge of a new directorate of personnel selection in 1941.[48]

The directorate was established to create a comprehensive system of personnel selection. Its goals were to classify all Army personnel; identify potential officer material; identify those of higher intelligence; uncover so-called neurotics; and weed out men deemed to be of lower intelligence. The directorate's aims mirrored several initiatives in civilian circles, and clearly expressed psychologists' expanding ambitions.[49] Though a psychiatrist, Chisholm espoused many "neo-Freudian theories of sexuality," and as an adherent of the mental hygiene movement he saw psychology's value in preventing "mental weaklings" from entering the Army.[50] Chisholm's plan was not without controversy, however, and it revealed professional jockeying between psychologists and other mental health professionals. Colin Russel, the shell shock expert, was then consulting neuropsychiatrist to the Royal Canadian Army Medical Corps (RCAMC) and believed that the number of men referred for psychiatric examination based on their psychological test results was excessive.[51] It was Russel's opinion that psychologists were better suited to identifying and reassigning men who, based on perceived capabilities, were being misused by the Army. Put another way, he intimated that psychologists were out of their depth.[52] Somewhat chastened by his Great War experiences, Russel was convinced that attempting to identify potential neurotics through psychological testing was a fruitless endeavour.[53]

Nonetheless, the support that psychological testing received from Chisholm and Ottawa meant that in 1942 personnel selection officers were given a daunting task: conduct a psychological examination and psychiatric history of all Canadian troops overseas, covering family, school, employment, and other factors such as sexual adjustment.[54] Chisholm, who was no stranger to controversy, believed that an undue feminine influence during childhood rearing was a prime reason for men being unfit for military service. In two speeches on 11 February 1944 given before the Rotary Club and Welfare Council of Toronto, he affirmed: "Too many women are bringing up too many boys on women's values."[55] He argued that women were "not oriented toward society. They are oriented toward men." That orientation, which in his estimation led to coddled, feminine men with a weak sense of communal obligation, made women a liability, particularly in wartime. Thus weakening the influence of mothers over men was the best strategy for helping recruits adjust to army life.[56] Given women's extensive involvement in the war effort, Chisholm's opinions unsurprisingly caused a "furor stirred in women's circles," many of whom felt he had denigrated their contributions.[57] The fallout led Defence Minister Ralston to make a "clarification" in the House of Commons on Chisholm's behalf. After being asked by Member of Parliament A.G. Ross from St Paul, Alberta to verify the accuracy of Chisholm's remarks, Ralston read a statement prepared by Chisholm himself. In it, Chisholm assured Parliament that his comments referred to women in "developing tribes" and had been taken out of context by reporters. He affirmed that in modern times, "in warfare as in peace – women generally are an enormous asset to society."[58] Chisholm did not clarify his comment that too many women were bringing up boys on "women's values," but the controversy nevertheless died down after Ralston's reading.

In a *Globe and Mail* article covering the controversy several days later, the author defended Chisholm's view, stating, "The records of this war indicate that, emotionally and psychologically, many young Canadians went into uniform badly equipped for war."[59] Echoing Chisholm's earlier statements, the author continued: "It has been pretty well established by the psychiatrists, in their search for weaknesses which develop in later life, that some men are the victim of a 'mother complex.'"[60] The result was that "today cases of war neurosis are treated according to the basic causes, often present in the individual from early childhood."[61] Evidently, Chisholm's theories of childhood development and women's influence on a soldier's psychological profile had supporters among the lay public. Statements about the negative influence of overbearing mothers helped relocate the blame for war-related mental disorder from traumatic wartime events to individual failings, and, at a societal level, to the women who predisposed men to failed masculinity.[62] Thus, in the mood of optimism about the "progress in the 20 years between the two wars," Chisholm and his supporters decided to proceed with psychological testing and a combing of soldiers' life histories, to ferret out those who bore the mark of excess femininity and mental weakness.[63]

In practice, though, many psychologists and psychiatrists were tolerant of difference and exercised circumspection about the varying degrees of masculinity, harbouring suspicions about the connection between men's subjectively assessed masculinity and its use as a prediction of combat performance. As the war continued, it became clear that ostensibly "feminine" men often performed well in combat, and conversely, "masculine" men sometimes failed that test. Historian Paul Jackson's work on homosexuality in the Canadian military during the Second World War demonstrated that throughout the war (particularly in 1944 and beyond as frontline manpower became a concern), psychiatrists often looked the other way, even when faced with openly homosexual or otherwise "effeminate" recruits. Likewise, homosexuals who had been tested in battle and proved themselves good soldiers were often spared medical discharge, even when their homosexuality became known to physicians and was no longer just an open secret within their unit.[64] Despite official policies that were hostile to homosexual men and women within the military, homosexuals were usually deemed too valuable to the war effort to be considered a problem unless their behaviour was regarded as particularly egregious or it became a scandal for officers and higher authorities.[65] Psychiatrists' handling of homosexuality was a reminder that assessments of a man's character, especially those involving judgements about masculinity and femininity, were fluid, and the way a soldier performed in battle and his value to the unit were the prime factors in whether or not his "femininity" became a problem for authorities.[66]

Nevertheless, when Chisholm was appointed director general of Medical Services in 1942, and later deputy minister of health, it was clear that his star was on the rise, and with it his views. In 1943, personnel selection officers were ready to "reclassify" and re-examine the entire Canadian Army overseas, but the plan was scuttled when the tides of war sent the 1st Canadian Division to the Mediterranean and other units became focused on training for Operation Overlord, the future D-Day landings.[67]

Ottawa and the Canadian military were not oblivious to psychological trauma and psychiatric casualties prior to Canada's engagement in combat operations.[68] Only five months into the war, in January 1940, Ottawa announced the planned establishment of a neurological hospital behind the front lines in France, the "spearhead of a scientific drive to reduce the heavy toll taken by nervous disorders in wartime."[69] Covered by *The Globe and Mail*, the hospital was to include several prominent Toronto and Montreal doctors and nurses and be headed by Colin Russel, then neurological consultant to the Medical Services and professor of neurology at McGill. It was designed to treat both brain injuries and nervous disorders.[70] Medical authorities believed that the hospital would be "an important factor in reducing postwar pension costs."[71] Reflecting perceptions both of advances made since the Great War and of neuropsychiatry's role as preventive medicine, the authorities affirmed that "men suffering from various types of hysteria who in the last war spent months and even years in hospitals will this time be discharged fully fit for duty in a matter of days."[72] The *Globe* article's author, R.A. Farquharson, cited the example of a neurological hospital for Canadian troops in England set up toward the end of the First World War, noting that 71 per cent of cases were able to return to full duty in six months. Similar results were expected by Ottawa in 1940.[73] Reinforcing the primacy of early treatment in ensuring recovery, the article summarized the specialist's crucial role in that process: it was "to give the patient a new philosophy to overcome his troubles before something, which doesn't exist physically, succeeds in making a physical wreck of a man."[74]

For Russel, the "secret of psychotherapy" and cure for battle exhaustion was a "mental contest resulting in the victory of the physician."[75] As was so often the case in both world wars, unforeseen events altered the army's best laid plans, and several months later the German Blitzkrieg swept the Allied forces off the European continent. Russel and his staff, who arrived in Britain just as the Dunkirk evacuation was taking place, were rerouted from the planned French hospital to a spacious mansion near Basingstoke in Hampshire, England. The 200 bed hospital they established there became known as No. 1 Neurological and Neurosurgical Hospital, or simply Basingstoke.[76] Colloquially, many troops referred to Russel, his colleagues, and the hospital itself as "No. 1 Nuts."[77] The hospital's original structure as a mobile unit accompanying the army was changed, and they instead found themselves treating civilian victims of the Blitz, Dunkirk evacuees, and reckless Canadian soldiers injured (and psychologically affected) by the numerous motorbike accidents that occurred during the nighttime blackout. Those early experiences, many with civilians and soldiers who had not seen combat, convinced Russel and his staff that their belief in the predisposition hypothesis of neuroses was correct.[78] If men broke down without seeing battle, it stood to reason that the cause of their illness must stem from "constitutional predisposition."

Although Canadian combat units in Europe saw little action until the Sicily campaign in 1943, their gruelling battles in the Mediterranean and Western Europe after D-Day caused many troops to end

up mental casualties, in spite of initial optimism among military leaders and medical men. During the Italian campaign alone, the Canadian Army suffered 5,020 neuropsychiatric casualties, out of a total of
25,090 casualties.[79] Canadian author Farley Mowat, a second lieutenant in the Hastings and Prince Edward Regiment, wrote an
account of the "Hasty P's" in his 1955 book *The Regiment*, and later his
1979 memoir *And No Birds Sang*.[80] In *The Regiment*, Mowat described
witnessing his comrades being visibly affected after a particularly
tough battle against German troops during the Moro River Campaign in mid-December 1943. He wrote: "These men were beyond
pride, beyond praise, beyond condemnation. They were empty of all
emotions and knew nothing except for a stupefying weariness. The
medical officers had a term for individuals who had reached the end
of their tether. They called it 'battle exhaustion' and it was a polite
term that meant 'burned out.'"[81] Subsequent to one particularly sav-
age battle, after tallying the regimental deaths, Mowat lamented,
"Physically the exhaustion of the Regiment was just short of total ...
Spiritually, the wastage had been even greater."[82]

   Within Mowat's books there were numerous examples of traumatic events and their effects, including watching a tank officer struggle
to pull himself from a burning tank turret and failing as the flames
consumed him.[83] In another passage Mowat discussed terror's effect
on a soldier who took refuge in a nearby house to escape enemy
shells: "Under the stairs was a human being, but not human in its
abject terror. It was a soldier, crouched hard against the wall, and
weeping bitterly and piercingly into cupped hands."[84] He laconically
reported the reaction of combat-hardened soldiers familiar with such
terror, affirming that "they, too, did not forget."[85] Perhaps most evocative was Mowat's description of a thirty-five-year-old stretcher-bearer
who broke under the strain of battle. Amidst the nighttime explosion
of mortar bombs, Mowat caught sight of the man: "Stark naked, he
was striding through the cordite stench with his head held high and
his arms swinging ... He was singing 'Home on the Range' at the top
of his lungs. The Worm That Never Dies [fear] had taken him."[86] In
the days that followed, Mowat noted that ambulance jeeps were constantly on the move, and for the first time since the regiment had
gone to war, "they also carried casualties who bore no visible
wounds."[87] He also wrote of how he was warned about psychological
casualties in a letter from his father, a First World War veteran, who

called them "the most unfortunate ones" who "had their spiritual feet knocked out from under them." With a mixture of pity and anger, Mowat's father told him that "the beer halls and gutters are still full of such poor bastards from my war, and nobody understands or cares what happened to them."[88] Mowat, like his father, witnessed the creation of more "poor bastards."

LESSONS SLOWLY LEARNED

Like the poets and novelists of the First World War, Mowat captured the spirit of a war that, despite its occasional lighter side (he was keen to note the humorous moments), left an indelible imprint on participants' minds. As with its allies, the Canadian Army entered combat in 1943 poorly prepared to deal with battle exhaustion, regardless of its experiences during the First World War.[89] Terminology was also chaotic before 1943 and carried pseudo-scientific connotations. Many men were labelled "psychopathic personality, inadequate," "grossly inadequate personality," or "inadequate with added battle neurosis," before battle exhaustion became the preferred diagnosis.[90] Rather than being a watershed moment in the way that psychological trauma and casualties were understood, the official medical history of the Second World War stated that the same diagnostic and treatment methods of 1914 to 1918 were retrieved and slightly advanced.[91] In fact, when the 1st Canadian Infantry Division went to action in Sicily in 1943, its preparation for mental casualties consisted of one psychiatrist.[92] What was unique about the Second World War was that psychiatrists were, when present, more closely attached to the division, and their relationship with the administrative authorities was tighter.[93]

Taking their cue from the British, in October 1943 the assistant director of Medical Services, acting on the advice of neuropsychiatrists, issued instructions that all suspected neuropsychiatric cases be labelled with the temporary diagnosis of "exhaustion" (eventually "battle exhaustion") until seen by a specialist.[94] That decision was made because the term "carried no stigma," and because it "suggested an innocuous curable condition to the casualty himself rather than frightening him with psychiatric terminology or making him think he suffered from some mental illness of a serious and disabling nature."[95] Authorities and psychiatrists were keen to avoid another "shell shock" epidemic. The "exhaustion" label allowed a soldier honourable escape from the battlefield while also suggesting that his condition was transient instead of permanent, since "exhaustion" implied a state of weariness reversible by rest.[96] The term had the added bonus of preventing medical officers ignorant of battlefield psychiatry from mistakenly diagnosing soldiers who were suffering from other maladies as psychiatric cases.[97] Nevertheless, the recorded occurrence of malarial soldiers being accidentally labelled as neuropsychiatric cases demonstrated, among other things, that the multifarious nature of psychological trauma could easily be confused with something rather different by non-specialists.[98]

As with the First World War, it is difficult to appraise psychiatrists' professional success during the Canadian campaigns of 1943 to 1945. In his retrospective survey of Canadian military psychiatry in the Mediterranean theatre, A.M. Doyle, a psychiatrist attached to the 1st Canadian Division during the war, described his role as being one of a traveller. He saw few psychiatric casualties in the early stages of the Sicily campaign, but as fighting intensified on mainland Italy in December 1943 – during the same battles Mowat experienced – he recounted that in one twenty-four hour period he saw "57 patients and still did not keep abreast of the deluxe."[99] Doyle, for his part, stuck to his guns that most cases were predisposed to neuropsychiatric disorder and "should have been weeded out as unfit for combat duty long before they got into action."[100] Doyle's view, reflecting beliefs in psychological predisposition and the need for more rigorous personnel screening, was echoed in May 1943 by RCAMC District Psychiatrist Major D.G. McKerracher, who similarly opined that "experience has shown that these newly revealed psychiatric disorders invariably existed, at least potentially, before the individual was inducted into the army."[101] In spite of the consensus by the end of the war that any man, "normal" or not, had his breaking point, Doyle and McKerracher still believed that "most of our mistakes have been in the direction of trying to keep too many inadequate or neurotic people in positions of stress that they cannot endure."[102]

Also clear from Doyle's account was that psychiatrists were still unwanted participants. He commented that although the Sicily campaign was unsatisfactory, he had "at least been 'accepted' when he was given command of a company of #9 Canadian Field Ambulance to take them on the assault upon Italy at Reggio."[103] Many officers and physicians still felt that psychiatrists allowed too many men to shirk

patriotism that German prisoners of war were kept "like tourists" in the cottage getaway region of Muskoka, Ontario, while Canadians "shell shocked, [and] driven crazy with the awful sights they have seen and experienced" were lodged in a hospital no better "than a flophouse."[117] In another instance, Mrs Jimmie Smith angrily described how the army returned her son to combat despite his evident psychological difficulties. The young man was accidentally blown into the air on D-Day by Allied planes and saw his friends killed. He suffered from shell shock, but shortly after the event she received word that "he was out of the hospital and back in the lines."[118] She quoted a letter from the young man, in which he mourned, "Mom, the way I feel right now, I will never be any good for army or civilian life."[119] Such letters reflected a gradual shift in public attitudes regarding the care of wounded soldiers and veterans. Mothers, many of whose husbands had fought through the First World War, and who had witnessed its effects on physically and psychologically affected veterans first-hand, were "no longer content meekly to take back their boys as shattered hopeless parcels dumped on their doorsteps," and instead often "demanded them back good as new."[120]

From the war's beginning, Prime Minister Mackenzie King and the Liberal government were quick to address returning veterans' needs. On the advice of Canadian Pension Commission chairman Harold French, himself a Great War amputee, the King government established a committee on demobilization and rehabilitation in 1940 to create a program for returning veterans.[121] By December 1940, several subcommittees were exploring a number of salient issues, including "neuropsychiatric cases."[122] Under what became the General Advisory Committee on Demobilization and Rehabilitation, the federal government broke from past practices, creating a system of rehabilitation benefits for everyone who served overseas (men and women inclusive).[123] Returning military personnel, cared for after 1944 by the newly created Department of Veterans Affairs (DVA), were provided with a range of statutes, orders, and regulations, all of which came to be known from 1945 on as the Veterans Charter.[124]

Measures included, among other things, a year's free medical care following discharge, student loans, and training courses for ex-servicewomen.[125] The Charter had many long-reaching effects, such as a rise in university enrollment, an increased understanding and treatment of disability, and the creation of "big government." Nevertheless, while the Veterans Charter was a "nation building experience," it was, like all social programs, a product of its time and place. The Charter and its principles were still rooted in traditional attitudes that deemed a strong work ethic, ambition, and independent financial means to be the proper goals of every man.[126] The program made a break with the past in much of its practice, but the ideology behind it was essentially conservative. The Charter's goal was above all else to utilize short-term programs and costs to prevent veterans' long-term dependency on the state.[127] As with the interwar period, psychologically injured veterans unable to work or retain employment were once again judged to be undeserving of pensions.

After the war psychiatrists repeated their advice about granting pensions to "neurotic" veterans. Despite the profession's skepticism toward personnel selection systems and admittedly chastened knowledge of war neuroses, those deemed experts nonetheless felt certain enough in their theories to deny mentally ill veterans compensation using a similar justification as their interwar counterparts.[128] In Canada, care of neurotic veterans was given to the DVA. In turn, the DVA's Division of Treatment Services appointed Dr Travis Dancey as adviser in psychiatry, making him one of the key officials behind DVA policy.[129] Dancey began his career at the Verdun Protestant Hospital for the Insane in Montreal, served overseas at No. 1 Neurological Hospital, and later became head of the No. 1 Canadian Exhaustion Unit in late 1944.[130] In the final months of the war, he treated hundreds of battle exhaustion cases using physical therapies and hypnosis.[131]

Notwithstanding his experimentation with physical therapies, Dancey was a firm adherent to the psychodynamic (life-history) approach to mental illness. As such, he subscribed to the concept of "secondary gain," something he defined à la Freud as "the psychological and sociological advantages obtainable through being ill."[132] In a similar manner to Russel and many Great War physicians, Dancey and his Second World War colleagues saw pensions as detrimental to neurotic veterans' recovery. Psychiatrists believed that neuroses stemmed from childhood and upbringing, *not* from war trauma. Thus any anxieties from the war were expected to disappear with time. If symptoms persisted, a physician need only look to how the trauma symptoms were utilized to cover up the ostensibly original traumas from early life.

To understand how Dancey conceptualized the physician's role in pension questions, it is worth quoting his comparison between neurosis and physical illness at length. In 1957, Dancey and a colleague, G.J. Sarwer-Foner, both employed at Queen Mary Veterans Hospital in Montreal, wrote an article for the *Canadian Medical Association Journal* which discussed the persistent problem of the "secondary gain patient."[133] The authors unequivocally stated the unique character of the pension issue, which by then was also a widely discussed topic in the civilian context, as it related to neurosis:

One might say that the subject of a neurosis is looked upon in a different way from other sick people. This may be true, but physicians should not be guilty of assisting the patient to remain ill through the payment of a monthly sum of money. It may well be that some people are penalized by this policy, but it must be kept in mind that this over-all policy is much more productive of good mental health than the opposite scheme would be.[134]

Dancey and Sarwer-Foner's rather utilitarian approach was self-evident. In the battle between patient and physician, the latter must always prevail, even if his Hippocratic tendencies urged him otherwise. Some patients might be harmed by this approach, they acknowledged, but most would benefit; the alternative, which was dependence, unemployment, and continued sickness, was far worse. Their view was not a radical one, having been elucidated by others before, during, and after the interwar period. Abram Kardiner claimed in 1941 that "the demand for and the dependency upon compensation is an essential and unconsciously determined defense mechanism and cannot be considered a prime factor [in secondary gain], although it is often an obstinate source of resistance in treatment and rehabilitation."[135] Throughout the postwar years, Dancey compiled Great War psychiatric research conducted in the same vein to reinforce his position. He also consulted and engaged in correspondence with those of a like mind, including Dr J.P.S. Cathcart, chief neuropsychiatrist of the DVA.[136] Their view of neurosis pensions both fit with and reflected a conservative government program, namely the Veterans Charter, which had the ultimate aim of encouraging work and reducing veterans' dependency on the state. For all of their good intentions, Dancey and Sarwer-Foner's characterization of neuroses placed a medically endorsed stamp on any denial of compensation for those suffering from chronic war trauma.

Dancey and his colleagues' view was more striking because it went against increasing evidence of cases involving "normal" men who suffered from war trauma and did not recover with time, as expected. In an August 1947 article in the *Canadian Medical Association Journal*, Major R.M. Billings, Captain F.C.R. Chalke, and Captain L. Shortt, all from the Royal Canadian Army Medical Corps, published a follow-up study of fifty-five veterans diagnosed with battle exhaustion during the war.[137] They discovered that even six months after being discharged, the men reported a wide range of persistent maladies, including: "nervousness and restlessness," "depression, hostility, seclusiveness, shyness," "battle dreams," "startle reaction," "insomnia," and "psychosomatic disturbances."[138] Their study bore out the impression that "psychiatric disturbances precipitated by the severe mental trauma of warfare are not entirely benign, and that physical and mental symptoms persist into civilian life."[139] Presciently, they inferred that they were "dealing with men whose difficulties and treatment-needs were increasing rather than decreasing, difficulties which may have future social implications, and treatment-needs which will have to be met eventually."[140] Perhaps indicative of the social climate and stigma toward mental illness was the fact that only 25 per cent of those deemed in need of treatment had sought medical advice by the time of follow-up.[141] Until the 1960s, most mental health services were provided in large, custodial, overcrowded psychiatric hospitals. That situation did little to foster positive views toward mental illness or discussions of psychological difficulties.[142] Moreover, despite the commonplace nature of battle exhaustion diagnoses in the later war years, a laissez-faire attitude toward the socio-economic order encouraged veterans to fight through problems and avoid dependency on the government.[143]

Thus, after 1945 an "uneasy compromise between psychodynamic doctrine and the empirical evidence of veterans suffering from war-related chronic neurosis" developed in Canada.[144] The original post-1945 program for demobilizing veterans was supposed to include treatment only for conditions that arose up to one year after service. Nevertheless, the persistence of war-related neuroses among some veterans, and the delayed manifestation of others, forced the DVA to consider other approaches.[145] Hence, while Dancey and Canadian Pension Commission officials worked to ensure that their compensation was minimal, the eventual alternative for chronic neurosis patients was hospital and therapeutic treatments. After consulting a 1943 American Psychiatric Association (APA) report on pensions and considering "those methods employed in other [presumably Commonwealth] countries," the DVA decided to offer treatment to any veteran with a neurosis "regardless of his time or place of service or of his income provided it was felt that his symptoms could be expected to fade after a brief period of therapy."[146] For psychiatrists (and historians of psychiatry), that program, which included the option of outpatient treatment, provided, among other things, the first clue that psychiatric care was possible outside of the mental hospital.[147] Dancey and his colleagues were nonetheless careful to ensure that "dangers inherent in other schemes" were prevented, which meant that "no financial allowances were permitted either to the patient or to his family."[148] Dancey was characteristically blunt: "Although this may create hardships, it does minimize any desire that a veteran may have to remain more or less permanently in hospital." An added outcome of that approach was that it created "a state of affairs where his family will urge him to return to work as soon as possible."[149] Under this system, chronic "neurotics" were encouraged to seek treatment rather than pensions. Simultaneously, a socio-economic milieu developed which prodded those outside the hospital to return to their prescribed, manly duties as family breadwinners.

At a 1950 meeting of the APA, Dancey discussed the ostensible successes of the DVA's modified program. He declared that 420 veterans had received treatment under the new "classification" from 1 January 1948 to 31 December 1949.[150] That number corresponded to roughly 20 per cent of all general hospital psychiatric cases under treatment at the time. He affirmed that DVA district psychiatrists held the opinion that a "definite benefit" was noticeable in approximately 75 per cent of cases. In a testament to the prevailing and enduring spirit of a pull-up-your-bootstraps work ethic, one of the main criteria for judging treatment success was the patient's ability to return to work; the other was the patient remaining symptom-free for three months to one year.[151] As an example of the work being undertaken, Dancey reported on the Montreal system. At Queen Mary Veterans Hospital, a group of resident physicians enrolled in the McGill psychiatry course and other, part-time psychiatrists (who held private practices) utilized "analytically oriented psychotherapy" as the chief treatment method. In line with current practices, they also utilized "aids" such as insulin therapy and "diversional therapy," the goal of the latter being to ensure that every patient was fully occupied during waking hours.[152] In 1946, Veterans Minister Ian Mackenzie (described by Tim Cook as a "cheerful scallywag" and "bon vivant who had an affinity for fast cars and strong drink") boasted that Montreal's St Anne's Hospital had good reason to hope for a 75 per cent success rate by treating "psychotics" with "electric shock therapy and insulin and sub-insulin shock."[153] According to Mackenzie, the same treatments were also effective for neurotics.[154]

A March 1947 *Globe and Mail* article on neurosis therapy at Westminster Hospital in London, Ontario provided a more complete picture of what the DVA program entailed.[155] There, doctors focused on promoting "Self," "Job," "Home," "Friends," and "Religion" to a group of "young victims of neurosis" and other psychologically troubled veterans.[156] Westminster provided care to 700 veterans of both world wars suffering from "neurosis" or "psychosis," and the *Globe and Mail* glowingly reported that treatment consisted of "much more than drugs and psychotherapy." Patients were divided into three groups: neurosis patients, "parole" patients (who had suffered from psychosis but were deemed to be "cured of a psychosis sufficiently"), and "psychotic patients" in closed wards under orderly supervision. The article noted the presence of grand pianos in multiple sun rooms, and patients' artwork hanging on the walls. Patients also benefitted from occupational therapy shops, where they worked at hand looms, carpenters' benches, and potters' wheels. Their tooled leather was so well-crafted that it apparently aroused "the acquisitive instincts of feminine visitors."[157] In addition, a significant degree of co-operation with the University of Western Ontario allowed patients to tour the university's observatory, natural science collection, and museum. The author reported that during the previous Christmas season, 450 men from both closed and open hospital wards had been treated to a university Follies song-and-dance production. He happily concluded that "there wasn't a single 'incident.'"[158]

It is difficult for historians to appraise the relative success or failure of the DVA approach in terms of veterans "cured," though it was evident that at least some remained ill and did not seek hospital treatment. Most men simply carried on as best they could, with many using the timeless method of alcohol to cope with troubling memories. Decades later a Second World War veteran at Toronto's Sunnybrook hospital stated that, "You were viewed as weak if you couldn't handle it ... In the culture of the time, you didn't talk about it."[159] For his part, Dancey confidently claimed that there was a "universal opinion" among district psychiatrists that the modified program for neurotic veterans should be preserved, with minor alterations.[160] He concluded by pointing to the "wider ramifications" of the pension question, particularly since the veterans' pension program was part of a "rapidly developing interest" in social security for the non-veteran "man in industry."[161] Regardless of Dancey and his colleagues' views on the compensation question, pressure from veterans across the country who were unresponsive to the treatments on offer slowly eroded psychiatrists' ability to completely prevent pension-granting.[162] Moreover, the Assessment and Rehabilitation Unit of the DVA, through which neurosis pensions were granted, allowed a "backdoor route" for those who had been denied compensation by the Canadian Pension Commission. Dancey was firmly opposed to any system that granted veterans a second pathway for obtaining a pension. Ultimately, the alternative route was not heavily utilized, but in Dancey's estimation this was only due to limited publicity and the complexity of the appeal process.[163]

Dancey continued writing even in 1970 to campaign against pensions for what he then termed "socio-psychological disability." He deplored the conditions whereby war veterans avoided work and forced their spouses to earn in order to keep their meagre pension. The result was detrimental to the family because "the husband then does the housework and there is a significant degree of reversal of role, with its deleterious results."[164] With more than a hint of paternalism, Dancey cautioned against blaming the veteran, contending that a pensioned veteran was to be viewed as "a victim of circumstances and perhaps rather fortunate in being able to obtain a marginal income, in spite of its emasculating qualities."[165] The real problem, in his estimation, was the clinical physician, who was considered the "weakest link" and often demonstrated "sheer ignorance" of the patient's "psychodynamics."[166] For Dancey the pension issue was primarily a medical one, but his characterization of the interaction between illness and socio-economic questions was clearly influenced by contemporary gender norms. Thus the "uneasy compromise" between psychiatric doctrine and war-related neurosis persisted.

The DVA's post-1945 reliance on psychiatrists, a relationship that expanded throughout the postwar years, represented "a more general trend ... in which the dictates of masculinity were medicalized."[167] Although the federal government's approach to psychologically injured veterans evolved during the 1918–45 period, there was more continuity than change. The same "masculine codes" of self-reliance and stoicism that permeated post-1918 society were also evident after the Second World War.[168] Pension-seeking was still construed as an "unmanly" activity, since pensions for war-related neuroses promoted dependence and prevented men from pursuing their ostensibly natural role as breadwinners. Psychiatrists like Dancey were absolute in their linking of idleness and illness. Men were deemed "better" or "cured" largely based on their attempt to return to their traditional manly vocations.

Hence there was what cultural historian Christopher Dummitt called an "awkward overlap between the state's emphasis on the ideals of liberal self-sufficiency and manly breadwinning" with regard to the treatment of disabled veterans, especially those with troubled minds.[169] The common mission of the federal government and psychiatrists was to literally and figuratively get men back into working condition. In Veterans Minister Mackenzie's words, the aim was to return neurotic war veterans to society "as normal, useful citizens."[170] A veteran's mental state mattered only if it hindered gainful employment, a situation which disrupted the family unit and society.[171] Nevertheless, like their physically disabled counterparts, men traumatized by war felt entitled to compensation. Some in Canadian society agreed. The author of a January 1948 *Globe and Mail* article noted that although DVA physicians argued against pensions for neurotics, "some believe it [the policy] is obsolete and should be amended, [and] an ex-serviceman suffering from neurosis is entitled to [a] pension, just as if he had lost an arm."[172] By denying the legitimacy of that claim, the psychiatrist represented for many veterans the "worst agent of the modern state."[173]

Moreover, by diagnosing and describing veterans' mental states, behaviour, and upbringing, psychiatrists "trod on the territory of manliness, secreting negative attitudes toward mental illness into this domain that the veterans considered sacrosanct."[174] At a time when psychiatry was going through an "expansive period of professionalization" which extended the borders of medical knowledge into the socio-economic domain, psychiatrists' explicit "medicalization of manhood" codified and reinforced masculine norms.[175] Put simply, to work was to be a healthy, proper man; to be a pensioned neurotic was the inverse state of health and manliness, since it left a man primarily in the home and dependent, which was a naturally feminine state. There was little separation of medical knowledge and socio-economic norms. Like their First World War comrades, psychologically injured veterans of the Second World War faced an inherently unequal relationship with psychiatrists in both pension hearings and the hospital. A psychiatrist's judgement of their mental state and behaviour affected not only pension eligibility, but a man's personal and home life as well. As demonstrated by Dummitt's research on Shaughnessy Hospital in Vancouver, the process was in and of itself painful and disturbing for many men. Their life history, behaviour, work ethic, and subjectively assessed manliness were all simultaneously placed on trial.[176]

KOREA

Just as 1918 brought about a dismantling of the psychiatric services created by militaries during the Great War, demobilization after 1945 caused "a rapid and remarkably complete collapse of the elaborate psychiatric system developed by the medical services of the Commonwealth armies."[177] Most psychiatrists, having served their country, were keen to quickly resume interrupted careers.[178] Military psychiatrists returned to "an uncertain future," with prominent men obtaining university-affiliated hospital appointments and their less eminent colleagues resuming careers in provincial mental hospitals.[179] The army lost interest in psychiatry, and after 1945 the few psychiatrists who remained were once again placed in a screening role, an apparent act of amnesia regarding the lessons learned during the war about screening's effectiveness.[180] Consequently, when Canadians went to fight in the Korean War as part of the British Commonwealth Forces Korea in 1951, their one forward psychiatrist initially represented the only psychiatric specialist in the 1st Commonwealth Division.

As with the two world wars, what began as a relatively lax policy on battle exhaustion gave way to a system resembling forward psychiatry in August 1951.[181] Psychiatric casualty rates, like in the Second World War, were worst during intense fighting or prolonged artillery bombardments.[182] For Canadians, the fact that many battles were "counted in hours rather than days or weeks" meant that battle exhaustion was, according to Korean War historian Brent Byron Watson, "comparatively rare."[183] In the "battle of Hill 355," responsible for the largest proportion of neuropsychiatric casualties, battle exhaustion still accounted for less than 1 per cent of total casualties incurred by the 1st Battalion of the Royal Canadian Regiment.[184] Watson argued that, given the degree of deficiencies in training and equipment, it was "astonishing" that more Canadian soldiers did not succumb to battle exhaustion throughout the conflict.[185]

In most major respects, psychiatry during the Korean War was akin to the previous war: the preferred diagnostic term was still battle exhaustion, and one of the best therapies for it was still considered motivation – namely the "expectancy" principle.[186] Mild cases were sent back to duty almost immediately, while more severe cases were evacuated to the field dressing station, sedated, and provided with short-term psychotherapy. The majority of exhaustion cases were eventually returned to their units, though more seriously affected soldiers were placed in support units or sent back to Canada.[187] Upon their return from Korea, Canadian veterans with psychiatric problems were provided with the same treatment programs as their Second World War comrades and encountered many of the same difficulties and dilemmas.

As the Cold War set in during the late 1940s and early 1950s, the Canadian government began a re-expansion of its defence capabilities. From 1949 to 1953 the number of Regulars increased from 47,000 to 104,000, and the Canadians established a long-term commitment to European defence against communist encroachment.[188] Canadian military communities and bases remained in Germany for another forty years, with CFB Lahr in southern Germany being the last to close in August 1994. Nevertheless, after Korea, with the military's loss of interest in psychiatry and Canadian soldiers no longer engaged in large-scale combat, veterans' mental health discussions were once again relegated to psychiatric hospitals and beer halls.

THE SPOILS OF WAR

While veterans' mental health was less of a prominent issue than it had been during and immediately after the two world wars, psychiatric services were nonetheless on the rise. That trend reflected a burgeoning professionalization of Canadian psychiatry that began with the Great War. In the CMHA's 1963 national appraisal of Canadian psychiatric services, titled *More for the Mind*, they acknowledged the galvanizing effect that the First World War had on psychiatry. Contrasting that effect with the pessimism toward the treatment of mental illness in the early twentieth century, they stated: "Realization that a rational and even scientific psychological treatment of mental illness was possible [sic] began only when the thousands of World War I shell shock casualties demonstrated dramatically that everyone has his breaking point, everyone is vulnerable to psychological, social and physical stress."[189] In the first decade of the twentieth century, psychiatrists were mainly employed in asylums and had little respect among their medical colleagues, being considered "just a step, if that, above the spa-doctors and the homeopaths."[190] After the Great War, psychiatrists and other mental health professionals, such as neurologists, became the de facto experts on shell shock and its myriad presentations. Their professional prestige rose accordingly. Historians have been somewhat more circumspect about the Great War's legacy for Canadian psychiatry. Tom Brown has pointed out that the Great War led to the beginning of psychiatry's foray into purposes outside of its essential mission, and that the "Therapeutic State," a system in which medicine and the state collaborated to control putatively deviant thoughts and actions, was "first forged in the crucible of the Great War."[191] The First World War initiated the spread of wartime psychiatric ideas into medical and civilian culture, and paved the way for psychiatrists to be called upon again in the next war.

The Second World War and Canadian physicians' experiences with battle exhaustion generated even more confidence within the Canadian psychiatric profession, and they were a key factor in the profession's expansion after 1945.[192] The succumbing of many soldiers to war-related traumas reified the idea that "mental-health problems could befall normal individuals," setting the stage for the growth of the mental health industry.[193] In his 2001 assessment of the postwar period, editor of the *Canadian Journal of Psychiatry* Quentin Rae-Grant wrote that 1950 was "marked by an aura of optimism derived from the experience of the need for, and value and recognition of, psychiatry during World War II."[194] Psychiatric manifestations during the Second World War were responsible for renewing interest in psychiatric disorders and treatments after decades of pessimism stemming from overcrowded asylums and few effective remedies for mental ailments.[195] Numerous physicians who learned psychiatric theories and techniques during the war became eminent leaders in the post-1945 field. They brought their war experience into civilian practice, shaping Canadian psychiatry in the process.[196]

To appreciate the Second World War's impact on the mental health profession, one need only survey the author list of *More for the Mind*. F.C.R. Chalke, medical officer during the war and postwar researcher on battle exhaustion, became the chair of the University of Ottawa's Department of Psychiatry, one of the founders of the Canadian Psychiatric Association, and editor of the *Canadian Psychiatric Association Journal* (now the *Canadian Journal of Psychiatry*) from 1956 to 1972. John (Jack) D. Griffin was a colonel in the Canadian Army and worked under Brock Chisholm during the Second World War, later developing psychiatric rehabilitation programs for ex-servicemen and women, and among many other accomplishments, became the general director of the CMHA from 1951 to 1971. B.H. McNeel served as Officer Commanding of the 2nd Canadian Corps Exhaustion Unit in Normandy. He was later appointed as adviser to the deputy director of Medical Services and became chief of the Mental Health Branch of the Ontario Department of Health.[197] All three men had significant experience with wartime mental disorders, and specifically battle exhaustion, during the Second World War. They all went on to have long and influential careers in psychiatry and psychiatric policies after the war.

The war was also responsible for stimulating the CMHA's growth and the creation of distinctly Canadian psychiatric institutions, most notably the CPA. Until 1951 many Canadian psychiatrists were APA members, attending meetings south of the border, keeping up with developments through professional journals, private correspondence, and face-to-face discussions at symposiums.[198] The "magnitude of the psychiatric disorders facing veterans and their families after the war" drove home Canada's relative unpreparedness, as well as psychiatrists' inability to lobby as a national body.[199] Canadian psychiatrists also acknowledged that despite collegiality with their American neighbours, the APA could not effectively lobby the Canadian government. Consequently, intermittent discussions began in the mid-1940s to create a Canadian association, culminating in the 1951 establishment of the CPA.[200] The CPA, along with the CMHA, became one of the leading Canadian institutions for encouraging public and government interest in psychiatric issues, and helped in establishing a professional identity for Canadian psychiatrists.

In 1950, the Canadian National Committee for Mental Hygiene became the Canadian Mental Health Association. Throughout the decade, the CMHA developed provincial divisions and local branches across Canada. One of the CMHA's main goals was to increase public interest in mental illness and health. That task was accomplished largely through developing volunteer programs in psychiatric hospitals, creating information and referral services, and consistently lobbying the federal government on mental-illness related issues.[201] To put it concisely, "scientific and professional opinion was marshalled in support of better methods of treatment and care."[202] The CMHA also helped create a National Mental Health Research Fund to provide money for young researchers interested in mental illness and mental health – areas which had hitherto received little funding or curiosity from medical students, in large part due to psychiatry's low status among their peers.[203] The CMHA acknowledged that words reflected the prevailing spirit of the times, and fought to have contemporary legal and public language changed to abolish terms such as "idiot," "imbecile," and "lunatic."[204] CMHA general director John Griffin and his colleagues lamented that even the medical profession was often reluctant to accept mental illness as a group of diseases that deserved an investment of professional time, research, and money.[205]

The CMHA's efforts coincided with the 1948 National Health Grants Program introduced by the Mackenzie King government and Paul Martin Sr, minister of National Health and Welfare. The program included a Mental Health Grant to aid provinces in developing and improving facilities for the mentally ill.[206] The great mobilization of medical and ancillary personnel into the Canadian Army during the Second World War created a situation in which many overcrowded mental hospitals were severely understaffed, leading to deteriorating conditions into the late 1940s.[207] The Mental Health Grant not only helped to reverse that trend, but over the next ten years fuelled the creation of new buildings, the opening of clinics, an increase in staff numbers, and according to Griffin et al., a "new professional interest in mental health and illness."[208]

The Second World War and war-related mental disorders nonetheless illuminated some of psychiatry's most evident shortcomings, perhaps the best example of which was the lack of any standardized set of diagnostic criteria or definitions for mental disorders. Although psychiatrists devised names and rough symptom criteria for major psychiatric disorders like schizophrenia, combat created psychiatric manifestations quite different from the "insanity" experienced in asylums.[209] Many affected soldiers were just "normal" men who had broken under the psychological strain of war.[210] As in the First World War, before psychiatrists settled on "battle exhaustion," reactions to stress and anxiety were given many varying and idiosyncratic names.[211] During wartime, military hierarchies could impose a standardization of terms, such as battle exhaustion; but in a civilian context psychiatrists were free to use any terms they wished. Moreover, since most of the existing manuals were influenced by decades of asylum practice – a milieu where patients suffered from chronic mental illnesses like dementia and schizophrenia – they did not reflect what many patients presented after 1945.[212] Van Nostrand's lament about the situation once again seemed accurate: "the nomenclature of psychiatric disease has no uniformity, and many of the terms have no precise meaning, except to the persons using them."[213]

The manifestations of trauma and other psychological disturbances, as well as the absence of any standard manual or system, resulted in a proliferation of terms and ideas that by the late 1940s amounted to "chaos."[214] The American Psychiatric Association responded by creating a standard manual to bring order to that chaos. In 1948 a naming committee laboured over an all-encompassing and national classificatory system, the result being the 1952 publication of the first *Diagnostic and Statistical Manual of Mental Disorders*, or DSM-I.[215] DSM-I was a striking example of how the Second World War influenced civilian psychiatry across North America: it was a modified form of the US Army's War Department Technical Bulletin, Medical 203 (known as Medical 203 for short), created in 1943 by a committee chaired by Brigadier-General William C. Menninger, an influential psychiatrist serving in the Office of the Surgeon General.[216]

Medical 203 codified the psychodynamic bent of numerous APA practitioners. Heavily influenced by Swiss-American psychiatrist Adolf Meyer, the first psychiatrist-in-chief of the Johns Hopkins Hospital in Baltimore, in addition to Freudian theories, Medical 203 and DSM-I both characterized mental disorders as "reactions" of the individual to emotional states brought on by life events and circumstances.[217] Meyer, who coined the term "psychobiology" to describe his approach, emphasized the importance of researching all biological, psychological, and social events pertinent to a patient's case history.[218] Reflecting its Freudian-Meyerian spirit, Medical 203 saw combat exhaustion as "often transient in character" when promptly treated, but something which might progress into "one of the established neurotic reactions" if left unchecked.[219] The authors viewed combat exhaustion as a predominantly transient phenomenon, thus making it a "temporary diagnosis" until a more "definitive diagnosis" – that is, the "real" disorder related to the patient's life-history – could be established.[220] In DSM-I, combat exhaustion was replaced by "Gross Stress Reaction (GSR)," and categorized as one of the "Transient Situational Personality Disorders," but DSM-I nonetheless copied almost word for word the language and characterization of Medical 203.[221] As with combat exhaustion, GSR was an appropriate diagnosis if the individual had been exposed to "severe physical demands or extreme emotional stress," but DSM-I went a step further by stating that this reaction could occur not only in combat, but also "in civilian catastrophe (Fire, Earthquake, Explosion, Etc.)."[222] The broadly conceived approach taken by both documents illuminated a shift in the "institutional geography" of North American psychiatry as more psychiatrists in the postwar period moved into private practice, and hospital and community psychiatrists brought with them a synthesis of Meyer and Freud's ideas.[223] Although DSM-I was less widely read than the manual's future editions, it was an important document for enshrining psychiatry's predominant approach for the following few decades. And, while it is difficult to gauge the extent to which psychiatrists actually consulted DSM-I in their daily practice, the spread of the psychodynamic approach was apparent in a 1959–60 survey by the American Group for the Advancement of Psychiatry (GAP), which reported that eighty-eight out of ninety-three US and Canadian medical schools taught psychodynamics.[224]

Between 1945 and the late 1960s, North American psychiatry, and in particular academic psychiatry, was also dominated by psychoanalysis, an approach popularized by the teachings of Freud and his followers. Psychoanalysis aimed at, among other things, finding the root of present psychological difficulties in childhood events.[225] Even at McGill University's Allan Memorial Institute, where the influence of biologically-oriented researchers like Heinz Lehmann and Ewen Cameron was pronounced, psychoanalysis was still represented; according to Dr Thomas Ban, the milieu was one where every type of psychiatric approach, psychoanalysis included, was represented.[226] That period, which medical historian Edward Shorter termed the "psychoanalytic hiatus" in psychiatry, was characterized by a brief era during the mid-twentieth century when "middle-class society became enraptured of the notion that psychological problems arose as a result of unconscious conflicts over long-past events, especially those of a sexual nature."[227] Psychiatrists embraced this approach because it helped them to escape the dreary and stultifying nature of large mental hospitals, allowing them to seek community hospital employment or private practice opportunities.[228] One effect of that movement was that for a few decades psychoanalysis and psychotherapy became synonymous, with psychiatrists at the forefront despite the fact that neither practice *necessarily* required medical expertise or even a medical degree. There was some truth in Shorter's argument that psychiatrists medicalized the psychoanalytic approach because it helped to "exclude psychologists, psychiatric social workers, and other competitors from the newly discovered fountain of riches," but their motivation went beyond financial matters.[229] Psychoanalysis, with its ostensible ability to explain the mind's complexities and individual motivations, "filled a vacuum" that earlier heredity-based theories left after their dissipation.[230]

In Canada, Brock Chisholm's rapid rise as director general of Medical Services for the army in 1942 and appointment as the first deputy minister of Health in 1944 ensured that he disseminated the psychodynamic approach to a generation of Canadian psychiatrists both during and after the war.[231] Although Canadian psychiatrists were less influenced in the postwar period by Freud and Meyer than their American colleagues, the psychodynamic influence on Canadian practitioners remained significant, particularly on those who went to war. Echoing Brock Chisholm's wartime speeches, in January 1947 John Griffin, Chisholm's consultant psychiatrist in wartime, told the Forest Hill Home and School Association in Toronto that during the war "it was common to find vigorous, healthy young men who – as a result of inhibiting crippling dependence on their mothers – were incapable of participating in the defense of their country." Once again stressing the importance of letting boys be boys, Griffin asserted that "the over-solicitous parent and mother who pampers, dominates and controls her son interferes with his mature development into young manhood."[232] Griffin believed that parents must take their lesson from the army, with its capacity for instilling traditional masculine virtues.

Like Chisholm, Griffin affirmed that a boy whose "basic boyness" was not lauded and encouraged by his mother would become laden with guilt, fear, and perceived inferiorities, making him far less adaptable to difficult situations – including wartime stresses – later in life.[233] B.H. McNeel, a co-author of *More for the Mind* and chief of the Mental Health Branch of the Ontario Department of Health in the 1960s, stated like Chisholm and Griffin that a possessive mother was "often a contributing factor" to her child's mental difficulties.[234] Thus, influential Canadian psychiatrists treated their war service and experience with war-related mental disorders as confirmation that, as gender historian Christopher Grieg put it, mothers converted "'normal' boys into emasculated boys who lacked the necessary amount of masculinity to engage successfully in military combat."[235]

In postwar Canada, men like Chisholm, Dancey, Griffin, and Mc-Neel became defenders of traditional masculinity, and attempted to defeat gender anxieties brought on by altered postwar labour and gender relations. They used putatively objective psychiatric knowledge to reassert a traditional, "normal" masculinity prevalent earlier in the century. While during the war their quest was largely confined to propping up anxious soldiers and reminding them of their duty to the country, after 1945 numerous physicians carried on that mission, becoming stalwart advocates of a fearless and stoic masculine ideal. As they did with pension questions, psychiatrists utilized medical knowledge to affirm the legitimacy and primacy of their mission.[236] Boys, like their fathers, needed to be taught to be "rational, physically and emotionally self-controlled and disciplined, upright and moral, loyal, and obedient."[237] Chisholm and others preached that such values had already been taught by the military. War had schooled them in the connection between prewar coddling and postwar neuroses that came not from the trauma of battle, but from faulty, effeminate parenting.

Psychiatrists returning from war brought back novel ideas about treatment approaches. Those who saw battle exhaustion first-hand, and, for better or worse, sent many psychologically affected soldiers back into combat, believed that environmental stresses played a key role in mental illness. From that inference it was a short step to the belief that in a civilian setting early treatment outside of the asylum could also produce positive results.[238] Given that most psychiatrists had trained and been employed before the war in large mental hospitals, where patients often languished for decades, the potential of early psychiatric treatment to head off chronic illness and eliminate the need for prolonged institutionalization was groundbreaking.[239] Put simply, "the success in returning to active duty servicemen who experienced psychological problems renewed a spirit of therapeutic optimism and activism, which was carried back into civilian life after the war."[240]

In Canada, that confidence intersected with Chisholm's and other influential psychiatrists' enterprise to "rouse the Canadian public to an awareness of the problems of mental health."[241] Just as the Group for the Advancement of Psychiatry (formed in 1946 under the stewardship of American Brigadier-General William Menninger) aimed to make psychiatry an important part of the postwar shaping of American society, Chisholm, his allies, and the CMHA in particular were keen to position social psychiatry at the vanguard of a new Canadian social order.[242] One of the CMHA's key aims was for mental illness to be "dealt with in precisely the same organizational, administrative and professional framework as physical illness."[243] The association's successes throughout the early postwar period included designating the first week of May Mental Health Week, beginning in 1951. Local branches across the country used that week to raise awareness of mental illness through public visitation of mental hospitals, school poster and essay contests, and press articles.[244] Amidst great socio-economic changes over the next few decades, the Canadian psychiatric profession remained deeply involved in treating mental illness in the community and in local hospitals, as well as spearheading campaigns to de-stigmatize mental illness and gain a foothold for psychiatric services in publicly funded health insurance legislation. Thus, while in 1963 Griffin and his *More for the Mind* co-authors lamented that the federal Hospital Insurance and Diagnostic Services Act of 1957 specifically excluded mental hospital patients from the benefits given to psychiatric patients in general hospitals, in 1966 they saw the fruits of their labour enshrined in the Medical Care Act, which provided funding for all psychiatric hospitals and did not discriminate between physical and mental illness.[245]

Concurrently, as "social" psychiatrists strove to ensure a more equal treatment for mentally ill patients and psychoanalysts in private practice treated less severe mental illnesses and "neuroses," in another important site – the laboratory – researchers in the 1940s and 1950s were at work on experiments to ameliorate and classify mental illness through the drug-induced alteration of brain chemistry. During a time when, for example, Montreal's Verdun Protestant Hospital had 1,600 psychiatric patients and only a few physicians, researchers such as Heinz Lehmann undertook experiments to mitigate the symptoms of schizophrenia and other major mental illnesses.[246] Although most of those experiments came to naught, in 1953 Lehmann introduced a new antipsychotic drug – chlorpromazine – that seemed to miraculously ameliorate the psychotic symptoms of chronic schizophrenia.[247] Lehmann quickly introduced English-speaking North America to chlorpromazine, and in doing so heralded "the era of psychopharmacology." That moment was "a turning point in the history of psychiatry."[248] Beyond the alleviation of psychotic symptoms in schizophrenia, depression, and mania, chlorpromazine and future drugs had the societal effect of accelerating deinstitutionalization – the downsizing or closing of large psychiatric hospitals across the country. Many patients previously unable to live outside the walls of the hospital became free to live independently.[249] On a professional level, biological psychiatry, an approach characterized by the idea that major psychiatric illnesses were the result of disordered brain chemistry and development, was given a renewed confidence. Slowly but surely, the biological orientation overtook psychoanalysis/psychodynamics as the dominant conceptualization and treatment of mental illness later in the century.[250]

In the meantime, the 1960s became "the high-water mark of the psychoanalytic movement."[251] The most influential chairs of psychiatric departments across North America were trained psychoanalysts, and psychiatrists trained in analysis even began talking about treating mental illnesses as serious as schizophrenia.[252] The spread of psychodynamic psychiatry and Freudian ideas could also be seen in the DSM's second edition (DSM-II), released in 1968, which replaced most of the

Meyerian "reactions" in *DSM-I* with Freudian "neuroses."[253] As with *DSM-I*, the second edition characterized many disorders as the result of underlying psychological conflicts, and like its predecessor, the diagnostic criteria it provided remained vague.[254] *DSM-II* also made a significant break with its earlier edition in that Gross Stress Reaction, which had encapsulated psychiatrists' experiences with war trauma, was eliminated, or, seen another way, reclassified and placed under the umbrella term "Adjustment Reaction to Adult Life (ARTAL)."[255] Instead of a full analysis and description, the manual provided just three short examples of ARTAL, one of which simply stated: "Fear associated with military combat and manifested by trembling, running and hiding."[256] Such a simplistic description hardly scratched the surface of the multifarious symptoms observed by psychiatrists over the previous half century. The manual's appendices provided a list of other stressful events connected to it, such as railway accidents, but made no attempt to explain how the events specifically related to the symptoms.[257] Thus, *DSM-II* "contained no specific listing for a psychiatric disorder produced by combat."[258]

Scholars interested in the *DSM*'s evolution have viewed the elimination of GSR from the second edition in various ways. Psychologist John Wilson, who examined the historical evolution of PTSD diagnostic criteria across the twentieth century, opined that the simplicity and inadequacy of the examples used in *DSM-II* to describe ARTAL gave "pause to inquire as to why there was not a more adequate and complete delineation of the various types of trauma; their common effects on psychological functioning and the known clinical features associated with such stressful life experiences."[259] Perhaps even more puzzling, he wrote, was why despite the occurrence of many traumatic events such as the Korean and Vietnam wars in the period between 1952 (publication of *DSM-I*) and 1968 (publication of *DSM-II*), GSR was not retained or enlarged. Ben Shephard explained this omission by noting that in the mid-1960s "few psychiatrists with first-hand experience of warfare were still around," but there was more to it than that. After all, throughout the 1960s there were studies published in prominent journals such as the *American Journal of Psychiatry* and *Archives of General Psychiatry* on the persistence of "stress reaction" among combat veterans, so it was not true that psychiatrists were no longer aware of, or disinterested in, war trauma.[260]

By 1965, when the DSM-II was in its planning and editing stages, American troops had already entered the Vietnam War. Their early experiences there from 1965 to 1967, when the rate of psychiatric breakdown among soldiers was only about five out of every thousand troops (compared with about fifty at the beginning of the Korean War), convinced military psychiatrists that they "appeared to have licked the problem."[261] Unlike during previous wars, the Americans immediately provided each battalion with medical personnel trained in psychiatric disorders, and assigned psychiatrists to infantry divisions.[262] Shephard concisely summed up the situation: "There was [during Vietnam] military psychiatry from the start, not from the point where things began to go wrong."[263] The Americans' early implementation of forward psychiatry appeared to prevent an epidemic of psychiatric casualties, as had occurred during the First and Second World Wars. Their ostensible success was confirmed by the 1970 book *Men, Stress, And Vietnam* by psychiatrist Peter Bourne, a team member of the Walter Reed Army Institute of Research and a Vietnam veteran.[264] Bourne attributed the initially low rate of breakdown among American troops to the implementation of forward psychiatry, which featured empirically grounded ideas of war neurosis.[265] Bourne was so confident in early successes that he thought there was "reason to be optimistic that psychiatric casualties need never again become a major cause of attrition in the United States military in a combat zone."[266] The lack of wartime experience among DSM-II editors, combined with the early successful treatment of war neuroses in Vietnam, convinced them that there was no need to focus on or retain GSR.[267]

The psychodynamic leaning of many practitioners was a likely factor in this decision. As with the Second World War, numerous psychiatrists believed that Vietnam veterans haunted by their war experiences suffered from a neurosis or psychosis that originated prior to combat.[268] Despite decades of evidence to the contrary, they affirmed that any persistence of war-related psychological problems could be explained by underlying conflicts within the individual which stemmed from earlier life events. With years of distance between the end of the Korean War in 1953 and the Vietnam War in the 1960s – years in which veterans' issues became less prominent – psychiatrists became convinced their model was accurate. But changes in the Vietnam War's course, and an increasing number of American veterans reporting psychiatric problems in the early 1970s, coincided with sweeping changes in psychiatric research and thinking to set both psychiatry and trauma on a different trajectory by the end of the decade. As Ben Shephard put it:

> More than any other war in the twentieth century, Vietnam redefined the social role of psychiatry and society's perception of mental health. Five years after the fall of Saigon, a new psychiatric term was devised, tailored to the needs of veterans. Psychiatric counselling was made available on an unparalleled scale, paid for by the United States government. Even more significantly, Vietnam helped to create a new 'consciousness of trauma' in Western society.[269]

3

Vietnam, Trauma, and Recognition

Perhaps wars weren't won any more. Maybe they went on forever.
Hemingway, *A Farewell to Arms*, 118.

Then ... the vets began to insist upon dealing with immediate psychological struggles, which were considerable, having to do with relationships to those around them, with their changing sense of masculinity, and with their conflicts with the society to which they returned.
Lifton, *Witness to an Extreme Century*, 187.

As the Vietnam War drew to a close, the rise of veterans' groups such as Vietnam Veterans Against the War (VVAW) reflected a troubled social milieu in the United States. Given the war's unpopularity and the difficulties numerous veterans had readjusting to civilian life, war-related psychological problems once again became a subject of discussion. Veterans of earlier wars had returned home by ship with their unit; but many soldiers abruptly returned from Vietnam on a plane by themselves. That change gave returning men less time to mentally decompress and readjust to life as a civilian, and few or no comrades with whom to vent about their experiences. It was a culture shock, to say the least. Moreover, unlike their Second World War counterparts, troops came home to protests and civilian disgust at their participation, as well as difficulties finding employment.[1] One prominent sign of trouble was the 30 April 1971 shooting death of African-American Dwight "Skip" Johnson, a Medal of Honor recipient killed in Detroit by a grocery store owner during an attempted robbery.[2]

A month later, a three-part *New York Times* special series on Johnson (published in Canada by the *Globe and Mail*) attempted to explain how "a Medal of Honor winner ended up dead in a holdup."[3] Johnson, like myriad soldiers in many wars, was haunted at night by his wartime memories. He was especially troubled by a face-to-face encounter with a North Vietnamese soldier whom he shot and killed at point-blank range, only managing to avoid death because the other man's AK-47 – drawn and ready before his – misfired.[4] Stan Enders, a gunner in Johnson's tank on the morning of 14 January 1968, recalled Johnson saving a friend from a burning tank nearby. Unfortunately, he was forced to watch the machine explode with the rest of his comrades inside after its artillery shells ignited within. Johnson, Enders remembered, "just sort of cracked up" and went into a berserker rage, hunting down all Vietnamese in the area with a pistol and submachine gun. He killed a number of them until running out of ammunition, and then used his machine gun stock to bludgeon another. Still frenzied, Johnson next tried to kill several Vietnamese prisoners rounded up after the battle. Enders recalled that it took "three men and three shots of morphine to hold Dwight down."[5] Johnson was taken away in a straitjacket and released from hospital the next day. His Vietnam tour was over. He was given the Medal of Honor for bravery by President Lyndon Johnson at the White House ten months later, in November 1968.

Conflicted about his wartime deeds, Johnson mostly kept silent about his tour. A friend recalled him being "all jumpy and nervous" and having to "be doing something all the time."[6] One of his cousins remembered him bringing back a series of coloured slides "of dead people." A US Army psychiatrist later wrote that Johnson suffered from "depression caused by post-Vietnam adjustment problem."[7] He became increasingly disillusioned about his heroism and the divided nation he had returned to, and confided to his psychiatrist that he had recurring bad dreams and "entertained a lot of moral judgements as to what had happened at Dakto [the aforementioned battle]." Johnson also experienced guilt about his survival and wondered if he was sane, asking his psychiatrist: "What would happen if I lost control of myself in Detroit and behaved the way I did in Vietnam?"[8] It seems that he never could square in his mind the fact that he was officially a hero, but had received that appellation for actions which included taking several human lives.

Johnson was eventually committed to a US Army hospital in Phoenixville, Pennsylvania, but after a short stay in March 1971 he used a three-day pass to abscond back to Detroit. The final year of his life was marked by increasing debts and isolation from others. On the evening of 30 April 1971, he visited his wife, who was in the hospital to have an infected cyst removed. Before leaving, he joked with her, asking if she was going to give him "a little kiss goodbye." Then he asked his family for a ride, claiming he needed to pick up money from someone who owed him. He rode with his mother, stepfather, and a friend to a predominantly white neighbourhood of Detroit, and asked them to stop. After leaving the car, he walked down the street and out of sight. His family became nervous when thirty minutes went by without his return. At about 11:45 p.m., a police car appeared and two officers drew pistols on them, demanding to know the reason for their presence. After replying that they were waiting for Dwight Johnson, they were told by the officers that he was "[dead] on the floor of a grocery store around the corner."[9] His mother later wondered whether "Skip tired of this life and needed someone else to pull the trigger."[10]

Johnson's case was an extreme but nonetheless representative example of the importance of both medical and socio-economic concerns for returning soldiers. He returned traumatized and haunted by his wartime experiences; he also believed Vietnam had irrevocably changed him. The war's polarizing effect on American society also contributed to a sense that his actions were for naught.[11] Unlike soldiers of the First and Second World Wars, Johnson could cite no definitive cause to alleviate his guilt, nor could he necessarily expect a warm reception from civilians, despite the official praises he received. Johnson and his comrades "were not given victory parades and church services; did not receive absolution. Because the war seemed to them to have no meaning, the killing was doubly sinful."[12] On a societal level, the shock of a Medal of Honor winner dying during a grocery store robbery, and the media coverage it received, put veterans' issues on the map and once again raised public consciousness of war-related trauma.[13] Johnson's case was discussed in numerous newspapers and academic journals, and a play about his life was viewed around the United States and on television.[14]

This chapter explores the historical events leading up to the creation of the psychiatric term "post-traumatic stress disorder." It first briefly looks at the Vietnam War's effect on American society and veterans, particularly highlighting the connection between disaffected veterans, radical psychiatrists, and a divided social milieu. The chapter also examines the vast changes that occurred in American psychiatry during the 1970s as the profession shed its heavy reliance on Freudian psychology and moved towards targeted, "biological" psychiatry. Those changes coincided with the campaign by veterans and radical psychiatrists to define and enshrine a trauma disorder in the *Diagnostic and Statistical Manual of Mental Disorder*'s third edition. Their ultimate success, which led to post-traumatic stress disorder being defined and included in DSM-III in 1980, was a revolutionary moment in psychiatry and psychiatric history. For the first time the American Psychiatric Association's official manual, its bible, included a definition and description of trauma's effects that legitimated long-term psychiatric symptoms stemming from outside of the sufferer, removing the blame from "over-mothering" and other previous scapegoats. Importantly, the new term also united civilian and military trauma, essentially universalizing the condition and opening up multiple avenues for research and discussion among clinicians and the lay public. The effect was the creation of what Ben Shephard pejoratively called a "culture of trauma" throughout the Western world.[15] This chapter's final section looks at the reception of the PTSD concept in Britain and Canada during the 1980s. Despite the fact that civilian researchers were initially uninterested in PTSD and dismissed it as a largely American-specific, Vietnam War-related syndrome, after Britain won the Falklands War, cases of PTSD among British vets forced a public debate among military leaders, politicians, and the public. In Canada, a country that did not participate in any wars in the 1980s, PTSD was initially discussed only rarely, in specialist medical journals. But by the 1990s, the end of the Cold War and numerous Canadian peacekeeping operations would change all that.

PSYCHIATRY, POLITICS, AND THE WAR THAT NEVER ENDED

One year after Dwight Johnson's death on 6 May 1972, *The New York Times* published an article about Vietnam veterans' struggles by Chaim Shatan, a radical psychiatrist and co-director of the psychoanalytic training clinic at New York University's Graduate Department of Psychology.[16] Shatan's article was based on the veterans' "group rap" sessions that he and other antiwar colleagues had organized in New York, and the "commonly shared concerns" that emerged.[17] The meetings began two years earlier in 1970 through the combined efforts of Shatan, vvaw president Jan Crumb, and Shatan's colleague Robert Jay Lifton, a former Korean War Air Force psychiatrist who wrote about Japanese survivors of the Hiroshima bombing.[18] Crumb sought out Shatan and Lifton because their careers "combined professional knowledge with antiwar advocacy."[19] Veterans attended the meetings because of a distrust of "establishment" psychiatric services, and also because their postwar disturbances "manifested themselves too late to prove the 'service connection' required for Veterans Administration [va] treatment." In the *Times*, Shatan listed a number of basic themes revealed during the sessions, including guilty feelings "for those killed and maimed on both sides"; feelings of being scapegoated and victimized, first by "inadequate" va treatment and benefits, and then by society for using and betraying them; rage stemming from "the awareness of being duped and manipulated"; feelings of brutalization after being "chewed up in the Vietnam war machine" and "spit out unfeeling"; alienation from their feelings and other people; and doubt about their "continued ability to love others."[20]

Robert Lifton noticed common effects among civilian and military trauma survivors, especially "intense expressions of psychic numbing."[21] But there were also ongoing and spontaneous moments of terror. Shatan's article described individual cases of Vietnam veterans, such as "Steve," who eighteen months after discharge from Marine combat duty still suffered "unpredictable episodes of terror and disorientation," even in familiar places like Times Square. Since the veterans' shared concerns did not fit "any standard diagnostic label," Shatan wrote that "we refer to them loosely as the post-Vietnam syndrome." The sum total effect of the syndrome was "impacted grief," in which "an encapsulated, never-ending past deprives the present of meaning."[22] Those group sessions further revealed that numerous veterans were dealing not just with war trauma, but a "changing sense of masculinity."[23] Session participants often discussed the "John Wayne thing" and society's emphasis on traditional "macho emotions" – feelings which were stoked by the military, and which often led to violent inclinations even once out of uniform.[24] Lifton recalled one particularly emotional session when a veteran described killing a Viet Cong soldier with a knife. The man expressed moral ambivalence about his actions, feeling sorry for killing another human being but failing to understand his regret, since it was in the line of duty, and because "John Wayne never felt sorry."[25] Such emotional quandaries reflected Vietnam veterans' desire to achieve a moral equilibrium amidst conflicting feelings about their own bravery, masculinity, and sense of duty, all set against the backdrop of a deeply fractured American society.

Like shell shock before it, post-Vietnam syndrome was an ambiguous but evocative term that metaphorically captured the troubles of many "lonely" soldiers, who, as during their time in Vietnam, were "unable to see their enemies," but nonetheless felt anonymous and haunting threats.[26] Politically, the term also became "a frightening buzz word among clinicians and journalists" and a "thinly veiled position of opposition to the war."[27] Despite the term's use in popular discourse, though, even within the Veterans Administration the nomenclature for classifying and treating patients with war-related trauma remained largely idiosyncratic.[28] Shatan and his colleagues, especially Lifton, were influenced by a growing literature about Holocaust survivors.[29] Along with veterans' advocacy, psychiatric work with post-Holocaust and other "survivor" groups "created a new professional model: the psychiatrist as patients' advocate, helping a group of wronged victims to win reparation. Their work also popularized the idea of a general, loosely-defined 'syndrome' among a group of patients, made the idea of delayed emotional after-effects of trauma respectable, and put guilt, particularly survivor guilt, on the agenda."[30] For critics of Shatan and his colleagues' advocacy on behalf of veterans and other trauma victims, the key legacy of the new "syndrome" was a shift in understandings of victimhood. The term and its meaning placed much greater emphasis on victimhood than endurance, making even those veterans who had perpetrated atrocities into victims of their own actions.[31]

By the mid-1970s, Shatan, Lifton, and VVAW were still fighting to persuade the APA to revise their nomenclature and acknowledge veterans' psychiatric problems.[32] Shatan was dismayed about the disappearance of a combat-stress diagnosis in DSM-II, and his 1972 Times article was part of a long campaign to ensure that the situation was reversed.[33] For his part, Lifton attacked both the APA and military psychiatry, particularly the latter for the primacy it placed on conserving the army's fighting strength at the expense of the individual soldier.[34] Lifton and Shatan's advocacy efforts also made them radical vis-à-vis their colleagues, their vocal antiwar stance placing them outside the psychiatric mainstream. Lifton recalled in his 2011 memoir that "psychiatrists like Hy [Chaim] Shatan and myself were also experiencing war-related alienation from American society ... the rap groups, which functioned outside ordinary channels, were a product of this shared alienation."[35] After establishing links with the National Council of Churches and various universities and publication outlets across the United States, they helped to form the National Veterans Resource Project, a group created to convince mainstream psychiatrists and the APA to recognize post-Vietnam syndrome.[36]

Fortuitously, in the same period the APA was also under attack by gay rights activists for the inclusion of homosexuality as a "disorder" in *DSM-II*.[37] In December 1973, 20,000 APA psychiatrists voted on the heated issue, with 58 per cent approving revisions to *DSM-II*.[38] Homosexuality as such was recategorized as a "sexual orientation disturbance" instead of a disorder, and the manual's architects decided that homosexuality would only be considered a disorder if the individual in question experienced distressful feelings about their sexual orientation.[39] With just one referendum the APA reversed a century-old position on homosexuality. In the short term, the revision slightly relieved pressure on the APA, which was fighting several battles at once. The long-term effect, however, was bluntly but accurately stated by Edward Shorter: "Once it became known how easily the APA's Nomenclature Committee had given way on homosexuality, it was clear that the psychiatrists could be rolled."[40] The homosexuality controversy demonstrated that socio-political pressure could be exerted on the APA to obtain the addition, alteration, or deletion of psychiatric syndromes from the *DSM*. Shatan and Lifton's quest to gain mainstream psychiatric recognition for post-Vietnam syndrome repeated a similar pattern as the homosexuality controversy, and their well-intentioned efforts exposed psychiatric classification as a process that was not always purely "objective."

In June 1974, *Psychiatric News* reported that a new *DSM* – *DSM-III* – was in the works.[41] Around that time, the head of the *DSM-III* task force, Robert Spitzer, stated during a phone call that "no change" was planned with regard to combat-stress disorders. Surprised and angered after hearing about Spitzer's decision through word-of-mouth channels, Shatan and Lifton met to discuss a future plan of attack.[42] The decision was made to apply public pressure through a radio station in New York City. They arranged an all-day broadcast about Vietnam veterans, and were quite successful, with many listeners phoning in to discuss the issue.[43] Next, they arranged a meeting with Spitzer at the APA's annual convention in 1975. At the convention, Spitzer challenged Shatan and his colleagues to refute arguments against classifying Vietnam veterans' problems separately. Shatan once again took the lead, organizing a working group to research the issue and gather evidence. The group came up with the term "post-combat disorder," but as time went on, and after consulting Holocaust literature, the group began to conceptualize the syndrome they envisioned as a more general disorder affecting both civilian survivors and combatants.[44] Spitzer, still somewhat skeptical, nevertheless appointed a Committee on Reactive Disorders to proceed with research and report to the *DSM-III* task force. Spitzer assigned the committee to work with Shatan and Lifton to justify and develop a diagnosis.[45]

Shatan's group received a significant intellectual boost when Mardi Horowitz joined the fight. Horowitz was a professor of psychiatry at the Langley Porter Neuropsychiatric Institute at the University of California, San Francisco, and was in the process of putting together a book about the effects of stress on the mind. The final product, his landmark 1976 work *Stress Response Syndromes*, presented an overarching theory of the cognitive and emotional responses to stress – traumatic stress in particular. The book discussed the thorny nature of enduring stress-related psychological difficulties, stating: "The crucial issue concerns the existence, nature, and etiological [causal] importance of general stress response tendencies as contrasted with idiosyncratic or person-specific types of variation in response to stress."[46] In spite of the evident difficulties in sorting cause from effect and general from specific, and the absence of something like Gross Stress Reaction in *DSM-II*, Horowitz boldly predicted that *DSM-III* would "probably take cognizance of such issues as will be discussed here, and return a stress response entity to the official list of diagnoses."[47] Horowitz's work signalled a significant break from the past. It affirmed that with regard to long-term stress syndromes, the issue of "how much is predisposition and how much is the effect of immediate stress is hard to elucidate because every syndrome will be composed of both sources of influence."[48] Such statements indicated that the intellectual ground was shifting: predisposition was no longer thought of as *the* deciding factor in the mind's long-term response to abnormally stressful events.

Stress Response Symptoms was an amalgamation of theories and works by Freud, Kardiner, and other Second World War authors, and Shatan and Lifton's more recent work with Vietnam veterans and Hiroshima survivors.[49] Horowitz utilized the vast literature available and surmised that there were eight common responses to highly stressful events: fear of repeating the event; shame over helplessness or emptiness; rage at the source; guilt or shame over aggressive impulses; fear of "aggressivity" toward others; survivor guilt; fear of identifying or merging with victims, that is, self-identifying as a victim, even when the reality was otherwise; and sadness in relation to loss, either of another person or symbolically of "the self."[50] Several of those responses later became enshrined as PTSD symptoms. Horowitz, who was a "tireless builder of intellectual structures," built a bridge between civilian trauma in events such as natural disasters, serious car accidents, or shipwrecks, and the trauma of combat soldiers.[51] He also created a coherent framework for important factors in chronic stress syndromes, including the concept of "phases of stress response." Horowitz used the literature of the Second World War, the Holocaust, and Vietnam to demonstrate that although such events produced incredible strain, there were "phases of response in which denial or intrusive symptoms and signs may predominate."[52] There was thus provision within his system for delayed symptoms – something observed in previous wars and their aftermath, but most often attributed to character weakness or neurosis rather than the mind's attempt to suppress traumatic experiences. With Horowitz's theories as a framework, Shatan's vague concept of post-Vietnam Syndrome was given intellectual support and academic credence.[53] *Stress Response Syndromes* became a classic work in the field of trauma studies.

Although resistance continued for another few years, by 1978 Shatan and his colleagues had gathered enough evidence to convince Spitzer and the other two members of the APA's Committee on Reactive Disorders to call a meeting and review the findings. In January 1978, Spitzer and the Committee finally acquiesced. They recommended a diagnosis under the label "post traumatic stress disorder," which appeared in the DSM's third edition.[54] No longer would emotional distress after combat be lumped under standard psychiatric syndromes of depression, alcoholism, or schizophrenia, and considered a product of the individual's maladaptive capacities owing to earlier life events.[55] Sociologist Wilbur Scott elucidated the socio-political dimension of Shatan and his colleagues' campaign: "PTSD is in DSM-III because a core of psychiatrists and veterans worked consciously and deliberately for years to put it there. They ultimately succeeded because they were better organized, more politically active, and enjoyed more lucky breaks than their opposition."[56] Once again, war proved a catalyst for altering psychiatric thought and practice.

The PTSD concept drew a decisive line in the sand. It was the first time that the presumed cause and persistence of stress disorders were relocated from the patient's life history to the trauma incurred during wartime (or, for civilians, during disasters or other traumatic events). The nomenclature was a key factor. "Post traumatic," meaning "after injury," made it clear that the disorder indicated a change in well-being *as a result of the trauma*, not because the trauma triggered emotional and psychological conflicts from earlier life, as was thought with neuroses.[57] The prime criterion for diagnosing PTSD was "the existence of a recognizable stressor [stressful event] that would evoke significant symptoms of distress in almost everyone."[58] That criterion was crucial because it acknowledged that a high magnitude of stress was enough to evoke psychological trauma in, precisely, "almost everyone," making PTSD symptoms normal rather than aberrant manifestations of psychiatric illness, even in the long term. Thus, the "uneasy compromise between [psychodynamic] doctrine and the empirical evidence of veterans suffering from war-related chronic neurosis" was finally shattered.[59] The APA's official recognition of PTSD was "a turning point, a major paradigm shift, in ideas about psychological trauma."[60] On a societal level, PTSD's enshrinement helped legitimize long-term psychological difficulties in Vietnam veterans and other trauma sufferers, and at least in principle, it made diagnosing trauma symptoms an objective matter.

PSYCHIATRIC ADVENTURES

Crucially, while traumatic stress and its effects were reformulated in the 1970s, another paradigm shift was in the making. The 1960s, which saw the high-water mark of the psychoanalytic movement as encapsulated in DSM-II, also saw the nascent rise of "biological psychiatry."[61] Beginning in the late 1960s and early 1970s, a small group of dedicated researchers from Washington University, St Louis, interested in brain chemistry, biology, and disease classification, formed a "counterrevolution" against Freudian psychoanalysis.[62] Psychodynamic theorists were largely uninterested in the classification of mental disorders. On the other side, the "St Louis group" and Robert Spitzer, head of the DSM-III task force, sought to make psychiatric diagnosis as accurate as possible in order to reflect what they presumed were biologically rooted diseases.[63] In 1972, John Feighner, a diagnostician at Washington University, published with his colleagues what became known as the "Feighner criteria," a list of diagnostic criteria for fourteen psychiatric illnesses.[64] As a testament to the intellectual shift occurring in the profession, Feighner's paper was the most-cited psychiatric paper of the 1970s.[65] Spitzer and a few colleagues refined Feighner's work into the "Research Diagnostic Criteria (RDC)," which for the first time attempted to use standard, fixed criteria for diagnosing mental disorders, instead of the clinical intuition of the past several decades.[66] Spitzer and his co-authors confidently wrote that "the data presented ... indicate high reliability for diagnostic judgements made using these criteria."[67]

Previously a psychiatrist was required to spend a significant amount of time with a patient to arrive at a diagnosis. Using fixed criteria (i.e., a patient must have symptoms A and B to have disorder C), that determination could be made in hours or minutes.[68] Moreover, once diagnoses were standardized, research could be focused and targeted, and clinicians could communicate across universities and countries, a difficult task when almost all disorders were thought to stem from individual patients' idiosyncrasies and life histories.[69] The RDC and its adherents' position went against "decades of neglect" with regard to diagnosis and classification (sometimes termed "nosology").[70] Writing shortly after DSM-III's release in 1980, psychiatrist Gerald Klerman, a specialist in depression and schizophrenia, argued that the DSM-III approach was a clean break from psychodynamic attitudes toward diagnosis.[71] He succinctly summarized the reason why most psychoanalysts ignored diagnosis and classification: "If all conditions [disorders] were indications for psychotherapy, then diagnosis and differential treatment were not necessary."[72] Stated another way, if psychoanalysis was always the prescribed treatment, the diagnosis was of secondary importance, or none at all. Luckily for Spitzer and like-minded colleagues, he was appointed head of the task force to revise DSM-II, and was keen to use the RDC during DSM-III's editorial process.[73]

Spitzer, who later wrote extensively on his role in DSM-III's creation, aimed to make the new edition a distinct reorientation of American psychiatry toward what has been called "descriptive psychiatry," and more importantly, toward basing psychiatric diagnoses on empirical data rather than individual case histories and clinical experience.[74] In contrast to DSM-II's editorial board, which consisted of many psychoanalytically-oriented members, the DSM-III task force was heavily "weighted against it [psychoanalysis]" and favoured the biological approach.[75] Spitzer was a deft politician, and carefully chose committee members whose research interests aligned with his own.[76] His goal was to produce, for the first time, a "science-driven document." Thus, as much as possible, Spitzer's task force used research evidence to verify and refine diagnoses placed in DSM-III.[77] In a signal even prior to its publication that DSM-III was a revolutionary document, the US National Institute of Mental Health (NIMH) sponsored a DSM-III trial run between 1977 and 1979, during which time 500 psychiatrists from many different centres used the new edition drafts to diagnose over 12,000 patients. After the diagnoses, psychiatrists were paired and their assessments were compared for consistency.[78] Such a large-scale diagnostic test had never been undertaken before. As a further testament to its landmark nature, upon its release in 1980 DSM-III was almost 500 pages long, with many pages containing long lists of diagnostic criteria. The new manual's bulk was a far cry from the first and second editions, which were 130 and 134 pages respectively.[79]

With DSM-III, Spitzer and his colleagues were also responding to serious pressures on their profession in the 1960s and 1970s. The first challenge related to pharmaceutical drugs and drug research. With the widespread use of drug therapies for psychiatric patients by the 1960s, diagnosis became a practical and sometimes crucial matter for both treatment and targeted research.[80] In addition, major sources of research money and funding for treatment, namely the NIMH and insurance companies, began to demand more reliable diagnoses, greater accountability, and evidence-based practice.[81] Under those conditions, numerous psychiatrists abandoned the psychoanalytical approach for the biological one. Consequently, "psychoanalysis lost its identification with psychiatric reform" and began to fall out of fashion.[82]

A second source of pressure came from a pair of studies within and outside the profession which displayed the woeful state of psychiatric diagnoses and a lack of diagnostic uniformity. One study was a 1970 NIMH-funded British and American study on the diagnosis of patients in London and New York City psychiatric hospitals. Focusing especially on schizophrenia, project psychiatrists interviewed and diagnosed 192 patients from New York and 174 from London shortly after admission. They concluded that there was an evident lack of consensus – in fact, major discrepancies – in how schizophrenia was appraised and diagnosed in each country. The discrepancies, according to the study's researchers, were "primarily a result of differences in the way the two groups of hospital psychiatrists diagnose patients," and not the result of any differing psychopathology exhibited by patients.[83] Essentially, psychiatric diagnostics failed to achieve a uniform or "scientific" standard.[84] The fact that two groups, albeit from different countries, could not reach a consensus on a major mental illness like schizophrenia, left the impression that psychiatrists were using idiosyncratic rather than empirical considerations when making their determinations.

The second and more troubling study was published in 1973 in the prominent journal *Science* under the title "On Being Sane in Insane Places." Psychologist David Rosenhan, professor at Stanford University, sent a group of healthy individuals to twelve psychiatric hospitals across the United States, each feigning symptoms of schizophrenia. Claiming to need treatment, the "pseudo-patients" were voluntarily admitted and subsequently reported their experiences within the institution. They also described their unsuccessful attempts to achieve release upon claiming they had recovered from their illness.[85] In all cases except one, the pseudo-patients were admitted, and once admitted, were forced to adopt a drug therapy regimen as a condition of their release. Rosenhan's test drew attention to the power of "labels" – that is, the power of diagnoses to "stick" and stigmatize, influencing patient and practitioner once given. The test also drew attention to the dehumanizing nature of large hospitals. But Rosenhan's most powerful intellectual indictment related to the continued use of psychiatric diagnoses despite their evident unreliability: "The facts of the matter are that we have known for a long time that diagnoses are often not useful or reliable, but we have nevertheless continued to use them."[86] He also delivered an even more scathing volley: "We now know that we cannot distinguish insanity from sanity."[87] On top of the embarrassment for psychiatrists, such studies also fuelled the "antipsychiatry" movement, a misnomer applied to a diverse group of thinkers that in the 1960s and 1970s published critiques whose common ground was that "psychiatric illness is not medical in nature but social, political, and legal."[88]

Spitzer, who directly responded to Rosenhan's study with his own 1976 article, was acutely aware of the popularity of criticizing diagnostic labels, but nonetheless affirmed that "when properly used, they have been shown to be of considerable value."[89] Spitzer's aims with DSM-III were, among other things, to defeat critics like Rosenhan and place psychiatry on a more scientific footing. Thus, when DSM-III was finally released in 1980, the anticipation, controversy, and immediate impact were evident in the number sold. Within six months of its publication, more people ordered DSM-III than all previous editions combined, even factoring in their thirty-plus reprints.[90] Whether critics or supporters, all noted that DSM-III signalled a new era in psychiatry; historians and others have agreed. Edward Shorter called it "an event of capital importance, not just for American but for world psychiatry, a turning of the page on psychodynamics, a redirection of the discipline toward a scientific course, a reembrace of the positivistic principles of the nineteenth century, [and] a denial of the antipsychiatric doctrine of the myth of mental illness."[91] Psychoanalyst Mitchell Wilson called the story of DSM-III "a story about the changing power base, as well as the changing knowledge base, within American psychiatry," noting how clinicians were replaced by biomedical researchers as the most influential voices in the field.[92] Psychopharmacologist and historian David Healy argued that DSM-III's popularity indicated "the importance that psychiatry had assumed in the popular mind."[93] And although they were both DSM-III critics, political scientist Rick Mayes and sociologist Allan Horwitz nonetheless pointed to its powerful impact, stating that "for the first time, psychiatrists, psychologists, social workers, and counselors had one common language to define mental disorders."[94]

POLITICS, TRAUMA, AND POPULAR PERCEPTIONS

By providing a common language and symptom profile to conceptualize PTSD, DSM-III contributed to the monumental growth of research into psychological trauma in the 1980s and beyond. In medical circles and the popular mind, PTSD created a common framework for how all humans responded to trauma, helping to reveal connections between war trauma and the myriad ways in which civilians were affected by harrowing events.[95] Psychiatrist and researcher into the socio-cultural underpinnings of PTSD Derek Summerfield stated that PTSD was "the flagship of this medicalized trauma discourse," a discourse which spread rapidly in the United States after 1980.[96] But the PTSD concept's osmosis into popular consciousness was uneven throughout the next few decades, and although it was immediately felt in the United States, PTSD was almost unheard of in Canada, a nation that in 1980 had not been at war for almost thirty years.

Although the idea of PTSD provided American Vietnam War veterans with symbolic and literal compensation for their psychological injuries and social alienation, the estimated 12,000 Canadians who fought with US forces in Vietnam had their postwar troubles go unnoticed by the Canadian public throughout the 1980s.[97] There were a few key reasons for their invisibility. Since Canada was officially a non-belligerent during the conflict, many Canadians viewed those who volunteered to fight as morally questionable mercenaries.[98] Others were outright hostile. Sensitive to Canada's role as a haven for American draft dodgers, horrified at the images brought to their living rooms through the relatively new medium of television, and attuned to antiwar sentiments across North America, they viewed Vietnam veterans as "baby killers."[99] Doug Clark, a freelance writer researching a book on Canadian Vietnam veterans in 1984, stated in a *Globe and Mail* article that there were "few charitable adjectives" used towards those who fought with the Americans.[100] In addition, the Royal Canadian Legion refused to grant Canadian Vietnam War veterans full membership and also denied them participation in Remembrance Day ceremonies.[101] Lastly, due to the murky number of Canadians in the war and their unpopular decision to participate, newspaper coverage was strikingly sparse. The net effect was that most men opted to stay out of the public eye, preferring to keep their war service, and subsequent troubles, secrets known only to their closest family and friends.[102] Canadian Vietnam veterans became in effect "Canada's unknown warriors."[103]

Despite their relatively furtive existence within Canadian society in the 1970s and beyond, there were glancing indications that Canadian Vietnam veterans were suffering like their American counterparts.[104] Doug Clark's article argued that in a few key respects Canadian veterans had a *more* difficult postwar adjustment, largely due to the "absence of a readily identifiable peer group and lack of competent medical help."[105] According to Clark, the roughly 20 per cent of Canadian veterans afflicted with various mental disorders (most commonly PTSD) were "further disadvantaged by a [Canadian] medical profession that either cannot or will not address itself to medical concerns judged legitimate by U.S. colleagues."[106] His article scathingly attacked not just the medical profession, but also the Canadian public, who had in the "finest Canadian tradition" denounced the Vietnam War and its veterans without acknowledging the profits accumulated by Canadian corporations manufacturing all varieties of war matériel for the United States, including the famous green berets and the infamously toxic defoliant Agent Orange.[107] Future critics of Canada's role in the Vietnam War agreed with Clark's assessment. Historian Ian McKay and journalist Jamie Swift wrote in their 2012 book *Warrior Nation* that although Canadians feigned innocence because of their non-combatant status, "the hard realities of Canadian involvement [in Vietnam], from arms sales to spying, were a good deal more sordid."[108]

In 1986, the *Toronto Star* published an article about Canadian Vietnam veterans and the "void" they returned to after their tours. Pointing to the differences between Canadian and American veterans, the author wrote that Canadians "were ignored" and "remained isolated, not even knowing each other."[109] One veteran reported having flashbacks of a terrified comrade's face even ten years after the war's end, something that caused him to "stay away from people." Others expressed strong feelings of alienation, particularly since the Canadian government did not provide aid and the US Department of Defense refused to admit that any Canadians participated in the war.[110] Alex Mills, nineteen years old when he volunteered to fight in Vietnam, lamented: "The experiences were brutal enough in the combat zones, but they seemed worse once we got home."[111] The article's author demonstrated the relative lack of knowledge about PTSD among the public in the 1980s when he identified the stress-related disorder that numerous Canadian veterans displayed not as PTSD, but as its former name: "post-Viet Nam syndrome."[112]

South of the border, in 1985 *The New York Times* spotlighted the plight of Canadian Vietnam veterans in a two-page article.[113] Drawing on several interviews, the article highlighted the socio-economic difficulties facing veterans, including limited access to benefits from the American government, none from the Canadian government, and being shunned by the Canadian public.[114] Veterans' anecdotal evidence pointed to the psychological troubles those men shouldered, including one veteran the article described as a "pill-popping former paratrooper who insisted on walking around Montreal armed."[115] Interviewees also drew attention to the dearth of knowledge among Canadian physicians about "post-Vietnam stress disorders that American doctors have begun to recognize."[116] One veteran laconically summed up the situation by saying that doctors in Canada "want to commit you or incarcerate you." Another spoke of contemplating suicide before finally checking himself into a hospital for assessment.[117] Tallying up the situation amongst his comrades, a Marine veteran – appropriately named Teddy Canadian – declared, "Some of these guys are still [psychologically] in Vietnam … They are in bad shape but they won't admit it."[118] Vern Murphy, spokesman for the Department of Veterans Affairs, bluntly declared that Canadian Vietnam veterans could not "be a burden on the Canadian taxpayer, because we weren't involved in it [the war]."[119] His comment displayed the distance that both the public and the federal government placed between themselves and the Vietnam War.[120] Unfortunately, fragmented but poignant testimony also showed the distance that Vietnam veterans placed between themselves and Canadian society.

Veterans' stories also raised the issue of the degree to which Canadian physicians ignored or dismissed veterans with PTSD symptoms. The answer, pieced together by examining Canadian medical publications in the 1980s and supporting works on PTSD outside of the United States, was that Canadian mental health professionals, save for a few researchers, were largely uninterested in PTSD or unaware of its existence. Colloquially speaking, PTSD was not a hot topic in Canada in the 1980s like it was in the United States. Joel Paris, prolific writer on psychiatric topics and editor of the *Canadian Journal of Psychiatry,* stated: "Everybody [psychiatrists] accepted PTSD as a diagnosis after 1980, but I can't think of anyone who studied it in those early years."[121] There were in fact no articles about PTSD in the *Canadian Medical Association Journal* during the 1980s. A 1985 editorial about Canadian physicians in the Second World War made passing references to battle exhaustion, but drew no links to postwar psychiatric problems and did not connect the term with later knowledge about PTSD.[122] Likewise, a 1987 article about Canadian prisoners of war from the Battle of Hong Kong in 1941 cited almost 200 veterans who developed "psychiatric problems as a result of their imprisonment," but the author made no mention of PTSD and never used the *DSM-III* concept of trauma.[123]

The *Canadian Journal of Psychiatry*, the CPA's official journal, made only two specific mentions of PTSD throughout the entire decade, including articles, editorials, and subscriber letters.[124] The first instance was a short 1985 article focusing on PTSD after car accidents, conducted by a group of researchers at the University of Toronto.[125] The second instance was a 1987 letter to the editor on "Management of Post Traumatic Stress Disorder and Ethnicity," which cited the case of a Vietnamese immigrant who was committed to a provincial psychiatric hospital after threatening his apartment caretaker with a knife.[126] Believing that communists from Vietnam were in Canada and plotting to kill him, the man also experienced recurring nightmares and appeared to be reliving traumatic moments from his past life. The article's author, somewhat aware of current trauma literature, noted that "the catastrophic effect of the Vietnam War may have influenced the emergence of the Post Traumatic Stress Disorder as a distinct syndrome."[127]

One lone researcher, Robert Stretch, a psychologist and US Army major, studied the Vietnam War's effects on Canadian personnel.[128] Stretch published three articles in 1990 and 1991 which examined the psychological and social adjustment of Canadian veterans who had served in combat and peacekeeping roles.[129] With regard to the former group, he concluded that not only did Canadian Vietnam veterans have "significantly greater rates of posttraumatic stress disorder" compared with US combat veterans, but part of their illness stemmed from "prolonged isolation from other Vietnam veterans, lack of recognition, and no readily available treatment for PTSD in Canada."[130] Presciently, Stretch's 1990 study of 121 Canadians who served in a peacekeeping role in Vietnam suggested that "one does not have to be a combatant to be traumatized by war," and that social support (or lack thereof) after returning home had a marked effect on the prevalence of PTSD.[131] All three of Stretch's articles pointed to the importance of social support for peacekeeping and combat missions. There was, however elusive, a crucial link between a participant's ability to connect his acts and experiences to a tangible, supported cause, and his mental health after service.[132]

The scarcity of research about PTSD and the health problems of Canadian Vietnam veterans were also related to another factor. Given the emergence of the PTSD concept as a result of the Vietnam War and its political aftermath, many experts initially felt it to be a disorder unique to that conflict and its veterans, rather than a universal phenomenon. Much like how shell shock and battle exhaustion became associated with the First and Second World Wars, PTSD became linked to the uniquely stressful experiences of Vietnam – a war often conducted in the jungle, where the enemy was an ephemeral, ghostly figure, rarely heard and even more rarely seen.[133] Building on this view, others attributed the Vietnam War's aftershocks to the polarizing effect of the conflict on American society, particularly since most veterans seemed to develop psychological difficulties at home as opposed to in theatre.[134] Taken together, it was easy for researchers in Canada and elsewhere to dismiss PTSD as a primarily American, Vietnam-specific phenomenon.

As a useful comparison, in the United Kingdom, like in Canada, PTSD had an initially slow entry into research circles and the public forum. A 1981 historical survey of trauma by Michael Trimble, researcher and lecturer in neuropsychiatry at the National Hospital for Nervous Diseases in London, utilized the historical concept of "post-traumatic neurosis" rather than "post traumatic stress disorder" in its title, and never specifically mentioned the latter concept throughout.[135] Trimble later commented that when he was writing his book, DSM-III had not yet been published, and at the time the book came out in 1981, PTSD, "concocted largely by political veterans was not within the general psychiatric community."[136] Trimble, as with numerous psychiatrists outside of the United States, believed PTSD to be a rebranding of "patterns" observed for hundreds of years, rather than a new and scientifically based disorder.[137] Thus, the PTSD concept was not granted immediate acceptance in Britain as it was in the United States.[138] Anecdotal evidence, as well as PTSD's absence from British psychiatric textbooks in the early to mid-1980s, also pointed to the disorder's slow and muted entry into British civilian psychiatric circles.[139] As it had in the United States, it would take another war for PTSD to become a front-page news item in the United Kingdom.

Between the end of the Korean War and the 1980s, Britain was involved in only one major military campaign – the Suez Crisis of 1956. Consequently, when the Falklands War began in April 1982, British Royal Navy psychiatrists were aware of PTSD but deemed it a disorder specific to American Vietnam War conscripts.[140] The Falklands War's short duration, as well as the great honours and recognition its participants received upon returning to the United Kingdom, helped create the impression that war-related mental disorders were a rare and insignificant problem.[141] Psychiatric casualties during the Falklands War were reported as being only 2 per cent of the total number of wounded, which was a far smaller figure than during past conflicts.[142] Nevertheless, in a similar pattern to the Vietnam War, several years after their return numerous British veterans reported service-related psychological problems.[143] While there was no consensus on the precise number of veterans with PTSD, comprehensive press coverage and widespread public interest in both the war and its consequences brought war-related mental disorder to the forefront in a manner unseen since the Second World War.[144]

As government officials did in past conflicts, the British Ministry of Defence (MOD) initially denied that PTSD or other psychiatric consequences were related to the war, and military physicians followed suit.[145] But by 1986, with public pressure growing after several news stories about suffering veterans, the MOD was forced to recognize PTSD as a disorder not limited to America. Nonetheless, in a testament to the strength of military culture and the traditional warrior ethos, British military physicians and officers were still divided on the issue, with some stubbornly viewing war-related trauma as an indication of a weak character, and one army college lecturer using the term "Compensation-itis" to describe PTSD.[146] Despite the relatively low number of Falklands War casualties, it became difficult for the ministry to maintain its position in the face of evidence that many men were witness to horrific scenes, such as one naval veteran injured by a bomb blast who returned below deck to find his best friend's mutilated body.[147] The MOD nevertheless maintained a hard stance on the issue, refusing to carry out a large survey of Falklands veterans for fear of opening the government to litigation from ex-servicemen claiming that the ministry failed in its "duty of care."[148]

By the 1990s numerous veterans went ahead regardless, suing the MOD for medical negligence on the grounds that inadequate care was given to detect and treat PTSD during and after the Falklands War.[149] Their litigation culminated in a 2003 High Court decision that rejected the claims of more than 2,000 military veterans from various wars that the MOD had failed in its duty of care.[150] The court's decision flew in the face of reports such as a 2002 article from *The Mail on Sunday*, which claimed that more Falklands veterans had committed suicide since 1982 than had died in combat.[151] One of the main factors on which the court's decision hinged was that during the early 1980s, British military authorities and psychiatrists believed that PTSD was a Vietnam-specific disorder. The judge ruled that "it was reasonable for the MOD to assume that this [PTSD] was due to factors specific to that war [Vietnam], or indeed not so much the war itself, but America's reaction to it."[152] The landmark trial highlighted that while the MOD was not obligated to provide a duty of care above and beyond that of any other employer, military authorities were now unable to deny the existence of war-related mental disorders or easily dismiss them as weakness of character.[153] The Falklands War, like Vietnam in America, brought war-related trauma into public consciousness in the United Kingdom. Although it differed from Vietnam in some key respects, such as the great public adulation and societal support given to Falklands veterans, much of the historical pattern was similar. After the Falklands, PTSD became a widely accepted consequence of war.[154] Moreover, the Falklands War, like future peacekeeping operations in Canada during the 1990s, helped create the impression that PTSD was not an American, Vietnam-specific disorder, but a universal reaction to trauma.

4

Peacekeeping, Politics, and Perceptions

It isn't Sesame Street out there.
Davis, *The Sharp End*, 205.

That [peacekeeping] is a bullshit word. In Cyprus, that was peacekeeping.
You've got a buffer zone, a demilitarized zone keeping warring factions at
bay. Bosnia-Herzegovina wasn't peacekeeping – or Croatia or Kosovo or
Somalia or Rwanda. None of those were peacekeeping missions. They're
war monitoring and you're in it, baby, you're right in the middle of it.
Wood, "Tom Martineau: Warrant Officer,"
in John Wood, *The Chance of War*, 183.

During his twenty years in the Canadian Armed Forces, from 1986
until retirement in 2006, Warrant Officer Andrew Godin bore witness
to historic changes in the nature of peacekeeping operations throughout the world.[1] As with numerous CAF members during the 1980s,
Godin's first overseas tour, as part of the long-established United
Nations Peacekeeping Force in Cyprus, was one of relative calm.[2]
Although there were occasional incidents, UN peacekeepers occupied
a well-established buffer zone – established in 1964 and extended in
1974 – between the opposing Greek and Turkish sides. They were generally able to carry out their duties without fear of injury or death.[3]
Many Canadian peacekeepers, Godin included, jokingly referred to
the mission as "Club Med," given the island's generally relaxed atmosphere and balmy climate.[4] Unfortunately, Cyprus proved ill-suited to
preparing peacekeepers for future operations. Testifying before the
Croatia Board of Inquiry in September 1999, Chief Warrant Officer
(ret.) M.B. McCarthy stated:

I have done four tours there, Cyprus killed us. Cyprus was the worst thing that has ever happened to us. Cyprus put NCOs [non-commissioned officers], not so much soldiers, but NCOs in a mind-set. Even though we were there for 20-some odd years and every-one knew it was a party and it was. Cyprus was a good time, a good tour. Seventy-four ('74) wasn't a good time, you know, but after that it was great. And some people, some NCOs went over, 'We are going to Yugoslavia. Another UN mission. More partying.' Things changed dramatically.[5]

Thus when Godin and the 4th Combat Engineer Regiment arrived in the former Yugoslavia in 1992 as part of the United Nations Pro-tection Force (UNPROFOR), the sights, sounds, and events he witnessed affected him long after his tour ended. He learned early on that in conflicts fuelled by ancient, ethnic hatreds, traditional ideas of respect for one's foe, and even the sanctity of human remains, meant little to the participants. In Croatia he saw a dead Serbian soldier "dragged through the streets like a dog" and thrown into a river "like a piece of garbage."[6] He recalled seeing numerous "floating, bloating bodies" that moved downriver and at first glance reminded him of swans.[7] On another occasion his unit came upon a local spa where the entire out-door pool was filled with the bodies of Serbians who had not heeded Croatian threats to leave. And in several instances Godin saw Croat and Serb combatants' skeletal remains on the side of the road, left to rot because they were in a sniper zone and no one from either side dared to risk being shot attempting a recovery.[8] Appraising his tour, Godin bluntly stated, "That's what you witnessed, that's what you saw."[9] Making the situation even more difficult to process was the fact that Godin and his comrades were unable to intervene in tragedies they witnessed because it was not part of their UN mandate – a man-date which in Croatia often made them "incidental bystanders at someone else's battle."[10] After relating the above events in an inter-view, Godin paused for a few moments and then quietly said, "Those are the things that eat away at you."[11]

Upon his return from Croatia and Bosnia in late 1992, Godin sensed that something was wrong when he experienced difficulty falling asleep, followed by nights filled with "massive nightmares."[12] He also felt increasingly jumpy and noticed that sudden noises jarred and unnerved him.[13] Unable to put a name to his troubles, he began drinking heavily in his off time to forget about his experiences. He carried on with his work. A few years later, Godin sat in a military classroom during a pre-screening prior to a Bosnia deployment while a "suit" – CAF slang for a civilian Department of National Defence worker – discussed PTSD symptoms. He checked off most of the symptoms in his head. Later, during a six-month training course, he made an appointment with a social worker from National Defence Headquarters (NDHQ) in Ottawa. He remembered sitting down and presenting his overseas experiences and subsequent psychological difficulties for "quite a few hours." He was nonetheless told afterward that things would get better with time, and until then to keep going on as usual.[14] So he did just that, returning to the former Yugoslavia two more times, first to Bosnia in 1996, and again to Kosovo and Macedonia in 1999–2000.

Godin likened his worsening mental situation to a bank vault: "What do you do with that stuff? You package it up and say to yourself, 'I'll deal with this later,' and you tuck it away in this bank vault, never to see the light of day again ... Because if you stop to think about it you're going to shut down ... And you won't be able to do your job ... Well, one day, your bank vault is full."[15] He knew his vault of traumatic experiences had reached its capacity when, one night during the Christmas season, he found himself contemplating how to drive his car off the Bank Street Bridge in Ottawa and make it look like an accident. The next day, he went to the National Defence Medical Centre and spoke with his doctor. After sitting down with a social worker, a psychologist, and finally a psychiatrist, he was diagnosed with PTSD in 2003, roughly ten years after his concerns began.

Godin's journey from health to illness, and his peacekeeping experiences, mirrored larger developments within the Department of National Defence (DND) and Canadian society during the 1990s. While Godin struggled with an individual, personal understanding of his psychological difficulties, at a macro level the CAF, DND, and Canadian public struggled with their own understanding and recognition of the traumatic effects of peacekeeping operations on soldiers. By the late 1990s, with cases of peacekeepers' trauma coming to light in military circles and the press, Canadians were for the first time exposed to what journalist Carol Off retrospectively called "Canadian post-traumatic stress disorder that comes from peacekeeping."[16] The Canadian experience was unique because unlike in Britain and the United States, it was not war per se, but "military operations other than war" that brought widespread attention to psychological trauma.[17] By the new millennium, peacekeepers' trauma had not only shattered many Canadian soldiers' minds; it had also challenged traditional myths and attitudes about mental illness and masculinity, and demonstrated that in many instances there was little peace involved in peacekeeping.

PEACEKEEPING – THE SUEZ CRISIS, A NOBEL PRIZE, AND NATIONAL IDENTITY

Three years after the end of the Korean War in 1956, the Suez Crisis erupted when Israel, Britain, and France invaded Egypt – a response, in the British case, to Egyptian President Gamal Abdel Nasser nationalizing the Suez Canal Company.[18] The tense months that followed after the United States, the Soviet Union, and Canada (among others) pressured the Israelis, French, and British to withdraw have been described as one of the death throes of the British Empire and some of the darkest hours after the Second World War.[19] Suez, metaphorically, was when "the [British] lion roared for the last time."[20] For Canada, though, Secretary of State for External Affairs Lester Pearson's prominent role in helping to defuse the situation and creating a United Nations Emergency Force (UNEF) to quell further violence led to a new Canadian specialty: peacekeeping.[21] The "Pearsonian" model of peacekeeping, in which neutral UN troops deployed to a buffer zone with the consent of conflicting parties to enforce a cease-fire, was the ideal, though not always standard, model for subsequent peacekeeping missions throughout the next several decades.[22] While Pearson's actions and rhetoric were criticized by some Canadians who felt he had betrayed the motherland with his critique of British actions during Suez, he was nonetheless internationally praised for his efforts during the crisis, and for his role became the first Canadian to receive a Nobel Peace Prize in 1957.[23] Gunnar Jahn, chairman of the Nobel award committee, stated during the ceremony that Pearson was "the man who contributed more than anyone else to save the world at that time."[24]

Pearson was rather humble about his achievements during his Nobel Lecture, praising both the UN and Secretary-General Dag Hammarskjold for the mission's success. He also expressed caution about expecting any long-term political successes or solutions, stating, "I do not exaggerate the significance of what has been done. There is no peace in the area [the Middle East]. There is no unanimity at the United Nations about the functions and future of this [UNEF] force."[25]

Nevertheless, the UN mission's success and the plaudits Pearson received convinced both Canadian politicians and the public that peacekeeping was a way for Canada to play an important role on the world stage.[26] Despite Canadians' pride in their country's efforts during the First and Second World Wars, in the half-century after the 1950s, participation in UN missions allowed Canadians to define themselves more by their ability to keep the peace than to wage wars.[27] For several decades after Pearson's UNEF mission, Canada contributed more soldiers to peacekeeping operations than any other nation in the world.[28]

As a middle power, peacekeeping allowed Canada to punch above its weight in international politics. It also symbolically contributed to a sense that Canada was, as Governor General Adrienne Clarkson later stated, a "peaceable kingdom."[29] By the late 1980s, 100,000 Canadian troops had been deployed to more than thirty peacekeeping missions under UN and non-UN authority.[30] It was Canadians' consistent willingness to engage in peacekeeping efforts that led Chief of the Defence Staff (CDS) General Paul Manson to affirm in 1988: "The image of a Canadian soldier wearing his blue [UN] beret, standing watch at some lonely outpost in a strife-torn land, is part of the modern Canadian mosaic, and a proud tradition."[31] Thus when the 1988 Nobel Peace Prize was awarded to UN peacekeepers, many Canadians felt that it was *their* prize – a notion reinforced by a Defence White Paper several years later that declared that more than thirty years after Pearson's Nobel win, "Canadians could once again take pride in their contribution to peace as the Nobel Peace Prize was awarded in recognition of the work of peacekeeping personnel."[32] The same paper reported that both Pearson's prize and the 1988 prize were important reflections of Canada's "evolving international personality."[33] By 1989, peacekeeping was considered postwar Canada's major contribution to world politics, with even *Canadian Defence Quarterly*, the official publication of the Canadian Army, dedicating an entire issue to peacekeeping.[34] In 1992, General Manson's evocative vision of the peacekeeping tradition was enshrined in a large monument to peacekeepers in Ottawa entitled *Reconciliation*. At the monument, statues of three UN peacekeepers – two men and one woman – stand with binoculars and radios, calmly observing an imaginary scene. Below, a quotation from Pearson invokes history, reminding viewers of Canada's pioneering role in peacekeeping.[35] When the monument itself was commemorated on the one-dollar coin in 1995, it was evident that peacekeeping had become embedded in the Canadian national psyche.

Scholars on both sides of the political spectrum have recognized peacekeeping's contribution to Canadian national identity. Political scientist and feminist scholar Sandra Whitworth, for example, whose work has analyzed some of the more controversial and gendered behaviour of peacekeeping troops, acknowledged that peacekeeping was a major factor in the construction of a distinctly Canadian identity. Invoking political scientist Benedict Anderson, she stated that the peacekeeping tradition and its symbolism were a crucial part of the "'imagined community' that is the nation."[36] On the other side of the spectrum, political and military historian Jack Granatstein believed peacekeeping was detrimental to the Canadian military because of its encouragement of "do-goodism writ large."[37] Nevertheless, in his bestselling 2004 work, *Who Killed the Canadian Military?*, he too acknowledged the significant role peacekeeping played since 1956 in differentiating Canadian military efforts and identity from that of its southern neighbour – for better or worse.[38] Thus, while academics have interpreted its effects and meaning in different ways, there is a general consensus that peacekeeping contributed to Canadians viewing themselves as peaceful, reticent warriors whose efforts brought stability to embattled parts of the globe.[39] At the end of the twentieth century, the peacekeeping tradition was one of the most prominent threads in the national tapestry.[40] Along with the Mounties, the canoe, and visions of the great white North, peacekeeping was one of Canada's enduring "national dreams," a symbol that expressed some of the fundamental beliefs Canadians held about themselves and their national character.[41]

PEACEKEEPING CHANGES, BUDGET CUTS, AND COVER-UPS

Unfortunately, just as peacekeeping became a national symbol, "peacekeeping" itself morphed into a vague and often euphemistic concept. With the dissolution of the Soviet Union by 1991, a proliferation of local ethnic and nationalist conflicts sprung up across the globe, resulting in an increased need for peacekeeping operations.[42] In 1991 there were only 11,000 UN "Blue Helmets" on eleven peacekeeping operations, but by late 1994 there were 76,000 deployed at seventeen different sites around the world.[43] What had previously been an activity largely "full of subtleties for the governments involved and a bit of romantic adventure for the participating soldiers" became a task of almost metaphysical complexity.[44] UN forces in the early to mid-1990s were expected to intervene in civil wars, patrol dangerous areas, organize elections, engage with and disarm militias, help to rebuild infrastructure, and create and reinforce new borders.[45] In some instances, as in Somalia, UN peacekeepers were given mandates that allowed them to be both heavily armed and legally sanctioned in the use of force against warring parties.[46]

The Pearsonian peacekeeping model that served the world well in the postwar period proved to be antiquated, and "peacekeeping" changed into something often more akin to peace building or peace enforcement.[47] The Canadian 1994 Defence White Paper hinted at such changes when it acknowledged the "changing face of peacekeeping" and noted that the nature of UN missions "now poses far more risk to our personnel."[48] That view was mirrored by UN secretary-general Boutros Boutros-Ghali in his 1992 report *An Agenda for Peace*, and 1995 follow-up report, both produced for the UN Security Council. Boutros-Ghali described a "new breed of intra-state conflicts" that were "often guerrilla wars without clear front lines," and he cautioned that "peacekeeping today can involve constant danger."[49] His assessment of the heightened danger was reflected in casualty figures. Between 1948 and 1990, 400 peacekeepers were killed, most often in accidents. But in just four years between 1991 and 1995, 460 were killed, usually in combat or attacks on UN personnel.[50] As it had done since the UN's creation, Canada dutifully participated in numerous peacekeeping missions throughout the 1990s despite the increased danger and complexity of many operations. In late 1992, Canada had peacekeeping troops under UN authority in Cyprus, the Golan Heights, Cambodia, El Salvador, Kuwait, the Western Sahara, Nicaragua, and the former Yugoslavia.[51] Adding to the challenges they faced, Canadian soldiers participated in these missions under a cloud of socio-economic turmoil at home.

The 1990s was, in many respects, the most difficult decade for the CAF and DND since the Second World War. An increased operational tempo and a series of major scandals coincided with successive rounds of budget cuts throughout the decade, leading one senior figure to retrospectively nickname the 1990s "The Decade of Darkness."[52]

Both organizations struggled to weather the storm as they went from "disaster to calamity."[53] While the decade began with a large CAF presence in Europe and a manageable number of peacekeeping operations, the situation rapidly changed after the fall of the Soviet Union ushered in a new, post-Cold War world.[54] In spite of a rising national debt crisis during the early 1990s, Canadians still felt obligated to do their part. Beginning with the Progressive Conservative cabinet of Prime Minister Brian Mulroney, successive governments committed the CAF to a plethora of peacekeeping operations while concurrently decreasing its resources and personnel levels.[55] The first difficulty related to the Forces Reduction Program (FRP). Begun in 1991, the FRP aimed to decrease the total strength of CAF Regular Force members from approximately 89,000 to 60,000 by decade's end.[56] What this reduction meant for the CAF was essentially that they had to do more with less. Budgetary cutbacks also affected equipment, something made painfully clear during operations in subsequent years.[57]

Although finances were an ongoing concern for senior leaders, inside the walls of National Defence Headquarters in Ottawa, DND and CAF officials also battled numerous scandals that tarnished both organizations' reputations. One source of embarrassment related to sexual harassment and assault in the military. In August 1993 the *Globe and Mail* published an exposé about the harassment of female CAF members, drawing attention to the fact that in the previous year, more harassment claims were filed with the Canadian Human Rights Commission against the CAF than against any other single institution.[58] That statistic was a significant concern for an institution whose membership of 80,000 was, by 1993, 11 per cent women.[59] Though the CAF did not keep statistics on sexual harassment, a DND study released a few months prior to the *Globe* article stated that one in every four female soldiers reported incidents of sexual harassment, with a small number even claiming that they had been raped or subjected to attempted sexual assault.[60] One retired major-general chalked the problem up to men's resentment toward women entering a historically male preserve, but a 1998 *Maclean's* magazine article titled "Rape in the Military" – followed by two more articles that year in which numerous former military women reported "flagrant hostility" and sexual harassment – hinted that the problem went deeper than just male posturing.[61] Under pressure after the June 1998 exposé, Chief of Defence Staff (CDS) Maurice Baril asked women who had been sexually assaulted to come forward, insisting that their cases would be quickly and thoroughly investigated.[62] Despite Baril's admission that a problem existed, a December 1998 *Maclean's* follow-up piece stated that almost all thirty women who came forward to the magazine were disappointed with how their case had been handled. CAF and DND leaders, the article implied, were more concerned with managing their public image than expunging the problem.[63]

THE SOMALIA AFFAIR

Sexual harassment in the military was a recurrent flashpoint throughout the decade, but it was events in Belet Huen, Somalia, on 16 March 1993 that would overshadow the CAF for the remainder of the 1990s. That night, two members of the Canadian Airborne Regiment (CAR) – which was in Somalia as part of Unified Task Force, a UN-sanctioned, US-led peace-enforcement contingent – viciously tortured and murdered a Somali teenager caught hiding in a portable toilet on the Canadian compound.[64] The shock of the crime was matched only by its brutality. For over two hours, Master Corporal Clayton Matchee and Private Kyle Brown blindfolded Shidane Arone, beat him repeatedly, and burned his feet with cigarettes, at several points stopping to take "trophy photos" of themselves with their victim.[65] They were unhindered by numerous witnesses who saw the crime in progress. Another CAR member later found the dying teenager and sounded the alarm, but Arone was declared dead as a result of his injuries when he was taken to a medical unit. Future testimony revealed that Arone had repeatedly screamed "Canada! Canada!" shortly before his death.[66] Military police were not informed until 19 March, at which time Matchee was arrested. Perhaps finally sensing the gravity of his crime, he tried to commit suicide in custody. He was found hanging in his cell a few hours later, alive but in a coma. He was then taken to an Ottawa hospital and subsequently declared unfit for trial on account of severe brain damage.[67] Private Brown was court-martialed, dishonourably discharged, and sentenced to five years in prison, but was released after serving less than two.[68]

Ottawa ordered a full military police investigation within three days of the 16 March crime, but details were withheld.[69] A *Globe and Mail* article published two weeks after Arone's murder, somewhat laconically titled "4 Soldiers Held in Somali's Death," revealed the duration of time the media and public had been kept in the dark.[70] But such secrets could not be kept indefinitely. On 20 April the Canadian Broadcasting Corporation (CBC) was the first to allege a cover-up regarding the Somali teen's death.[71] The parliamentary opposition accused Minister of National Defence (MND) Kim Campbell, an aspirant to the prime minister's office, of failing to bring the matter to light sooner. That criticism was given credence when it took until 27 April for Campbell to announce the creation of a military board of inquiry into the CAR's activities in Somalia.[72] Worse was still to come when military physician Major Barry Armstrong testified that less than two weeks before Arone's murder, on 4 March, two other Somalis were gunned down under suspicious circumstances while attempting to enter the Canadians' Belet Huen compound. According to Armstrong, one of the men, Ahmad Aruush, was killed execution-style with a bullet in the back, before someone "finished him off" with another in the head.[73] The doctor reported being subsequently pressured to leave Somalia and destroy his medical files related to the shooting.[74]

By the end of April a media blitz had ignited, with various outlets reporting that documents related to Somalia had repeatedly been altered or gone missing.[75] Over the following years outrage escalated, and the magnitude of inquiries grew along with it. The flames of public anger were further stoked in November 1994 when a publication ban on the trophy photos taken during Arone's murder was lifted, leading to the pictures' appearance in newspapers across the country.[76] In 1995, a Parliamentary inquiry was created – both to get at the truth and provide much-needed transparency to the public, and to take some heat off the Jean Chrétien Liberal government.[77] The Commission of Inquiry into the Deployment of Canadian Forces to Somalia, which would itself be cut short in January 1997 by MND Doug Young just before it began to investigate Arone's death and alleged cover-up attempts by DND officials, nonetheless brought forth a litany of problems.[78]

The Commission, broadcast nightly on national television, revealed deep structural problems within the CAR and at times questioned CAF/DND leadership as a whole. In a final report over 1,500 pages long, the inquiry spotlighted numerous disciplinary issues within the 2nd Commando Battalion prior to its deployment: "Several witnesses testified that members of the CAR … among other things, misused pyrotechnics, ammunition, and weapons; engaged in antisocial activities ... and abused Red Cross workers in CFB Petawawa."[79] The "most serious and alarming" sign of trouble was the burning of the unit orderly sergeant's car; a crime which led to no charges.[80]

Matters were made worse when two disturbing videos surfaced. The first, aired in early 1994, showed 2nd Commando members in Somalia making several racist comments.[81] A year later, the CBC aired a homemade video of 1st Commando hazing rituals from 1992 that included verbal abuse and extreme degradation, such as soldiers being forced to eat feces.[82] On 19 January 1995, prominent CBC political commentator Rex Murphy's *Point of View* program highlighted not just the photos taken during Arone's murder, but also a video released a day earlier, which showed the lone black member of a unit being tied to a tree and then forced to crawl on all fours with "I love KKK" written on his back.[83] Murphy ended his segment by stating that the Somalia affair, as it became known, cast a "pall of hypocrisy" over Canadians' "much-trumpeted image as peacekeepers."[84]

The Commission provided an equally powerful statement of the Somalia affair's effects when it asserted that "certain events transpired in Somalia that impugned the reputations of various individuals, Canada's military, and the nation itself."[85] By the end of operations in Somalia, Canada was not the only nation whose soldiers were accused of brutally violating proper standards of conduct; but for a country that viewed itself as the archetypal peacekeeper, such conduct was that much harder to bear.[86] The Commission itself also faced a number of challenges. As it tried to investigate strategic and systemic issues, it was constantly stymied by the fact that every witness it called sought legal counsel.[87] The slow, uphill battle those tactics produced led to ballooning costs. By the fall of 1996 the Commission had already cost taxpayers $15 million but was nowhere near completion.[88] With so much media and public scrutiny bearing down, it became an albatross around the government's neck. Prime Minister Chrétien felt that the Commission had descended into a "nasty intra-departmental fight," and when it seemed that the inquiry was "having a negative effect on the morale of the troops and leading nowhere," he decided upon its early termination.[89]

Dubbed "Canada's national shame," the Somalia affair sent ripples across all of Canadian society.[90] Canadians expressed disgust at what they saw as a tarnishing of the country's hard-earned reputation as the foremost peacekeeping nation on earth, and one with a proud military tradition.[91] In the midst of the crisis Prime Minister Brian Mulroney was forced to respond to embarrassing statements, such as those made by Haitian Prime Minister Marc Bazin, that Canadian peacekeepers were "a pack of Nazis."[92] The affair was also the catalyst for several ignominious "firsts." Matchee's crime was the first time that any Canadian soldier had been charged with torture or murder during a UN operation.[93] Although the Commission placed much of the blame at the CAF/DND leadership level, public outcry and media pressure, especially over the images of Arone's torture, provoked a defensive and reactionary posture by DND officials that took aim at the CAF's lower ranks.[94] A subsequent "cover your ass" approach developed in both organizations, with leaders blaming subordinates, who in turn passed the blame further down the chain of command to their subordinates.[95] Identification of the entire CAR with antisocial behaviour and Arone's murder, instead of the smaller group of soldiers responsible for it, led MND David Collenette to decide upon disbanding the whole regiment in March 1995.[96] Given the timing and circumstances, Collenette's actions were seen by some as a "political expedient to take the heat off the Forces as a whole."[97] Louise Frechette, former deputy minister of National Defence, acknowledged as much when she called the regiment's dissolution a "political decision to change the conversation."[98] The CAR's disbanding was the first time that a Canadian regiment was dissolved under disgraceful circumstances.[99]

Public reactions against the Somalia affair were consistently strong from 1993 through 1997. The contradiction between Canadians' usually honourable character as humanitarian peacekeepers, and Arone's torture and murder, tainted the entire CAF in much of the public's mind.[100] Anger took the form of soldiers being spat on in public, and, in some cases, CAR soldiers' children and spouses being harassed.[101] At one point public backlash and media pressure were so strong that a Canadian Forces General Order from the Chief of the Defence Staff to all branches/members of the CAF advised CAF members not to wear their uniforms to and from work, for fear of upsetting the public.[102] As politicians, military leaders, and the public distanced themselves from the Somalia affair, a sense of distrust grew between civilians and soldiers. Canadians simply could not reconcile the prominent displays of racism, brutality, and injustice with the idea of the "peaceable kingdom" that pervaded the national consciousness.

Sergeant James Davis, a CAR veteran who participated in peace-keeping missions in the former Yugoslavia and Rwanda during the 1990s, recalled the fallout from Arone's murder and the hazing videos in his 1997 memoir *The Sharp End*: "Immediately we were all branded as racists. This was news to the blacks, Asians, and Native Canadians serving in the Regiment."[103] Davis admitted that there were "some bad characters" in the CAR during the early 1990s, but remarked that they were just "a couple of double-y-chromosome types" exclusively in the 2nd Commando unit; the unit from which Matchee and Brown stemmed.[104] Regarding hazing rituals, Davis claimed that the only hazing that occurred in his unit, 3rd Commando, involved "new guys running down to the village and buying a case of beer."[105] Davis, along with other former CAR members, lamented the public and politicians' inability to recognize the regiment's predominantly honourable nature and the good deeds it performed on many peace-keeping missions. Particular anger was directed at MND David Collenette: "The minister didn't realize the extent of what he had done to the soldiers, their families and the community … Because he never apologized to the members of the unit that were untainted by scandal, about ninety-nine percent of us, for the pain this [the CAR's disbanding] would cause, he branded all of us as dishonourable murderers and rebels. His failure to separate the bad from the much larger good left us all painted by the same brush."[106] Retired Master Warrant Officer Barry Westholm agreed with the spirit of Davis's assessment, calling the Somalia inquiry and disbanding of the regiment "a real disaster" for CAF morale.[107]

Although politicians, military members, and the public argued over the Somalia affair's root causes, a consensus nonetheless hardened that Shidane Arone's murder was a defining moment for the CAF and Canadian society.[108] Scholars and journalists, also divided on the affair's causes, agreed that Somalia cast a far-reaching shadow, particularly over the CAF. Military historian David Bercuson called Somalia "the deepest crisis of confidence in the history of the Canadian Armed Forces."[109] Carol Off described Somalia as the "worst peacetime crisis in Canadian military history."[110] Sandra Whitworth argued that Somalia forced Canadians into a mode of cultural reflection, similar to how the My Lai Massacre perpetrated by US soldiers during the Vietnam War shocked American sensibilities.[111]

But while the Somalia affair laid bare problems within the CAF and alarmed the Canadian public, it was evident in retrospect that Somalia and its aftershocks concealed as much as they revealed. Specifically, the immense attention Somalia received, combined with the subsequent desire of government and military officials to distance themselves from any potential scandal, caused several other peacekeeping operations to go largely unnoticed.[112] Still mired in a Cold War mindset and unaccustomed to large-scale criticism or scrutiny, CAF and DND leaders "did what they had always done: simply ignore the noise in the expectation that it would go away."[113] In military terminology, they "bunkered." Colonel Jim Calvin recalled his soldiers returning from Croatia and feeling the great weight of the Somalia affair: "When we came home in October of 1993, Somalia was just breaking and the focus was all on what had happened with that particular tour. I think it's fair to say that for the next two years Somalia consumed most of the focus of the public's attention on the military, and all of the other things that had happened, including our tour, were cast into the background."[114] Unfortunately, as the media and public zeroed in on Somalia, Canadian troops experienced the changing nature of peacekeeping across the globe, and in numerous cases returned home traumatized by the danger they faced and atrocities they witnessed. In the divided climate of the time, their difficulties were swept under the rug by CAF/DND leaders who were unwilling to risk any more scandal amidst a historically low civilian approval of the nation's military.

THE NEW FACE OF PEACEKEEPING

Somalia was one of several UN missions Canada contributed to during the 1990s that fell outside of the Pearsonian model of peacekeeping operations. Many of the new UN operations forced peacekeepers to confront an entirely different type of mission than they had trained for or expected. With the Soviet Union's dissolution, a series of ethnic civil wars occurred within the former Socialist Federal Republic of Yugoslavia. As the Yugoslav National Army (JNA) fought to retake territory lost after the secession of its former constituent republics, both military and civilian casualties mounted. In late 1991, UN envoy and former American secretary of state Cyrus Vance proposed to Serb and Croat forces the establishment of a peacekeeping force in Croat territories under Serb control.[115] Both sides accepted, and on 21 February

1992 the UN Security Council authorized the creation of UNPROFOR, a force consisting of 15,000 UN Blue Helmets.[116] The UNPROFOR was deployed to three regions of Croatia, all designated as United Nations Protected Areas (UNPAS). The force's mission included ensuring the withdrawal of JNA troops from all Croat territory, monitoring demili-tarized zones, protecting civilians, and facilitating the return of dis-placed persons.[117] All of these tasks were to be accomplished as a neu-tral party, with the belligerents' consent, and without the use of force.[118] Canada, which initially contributed an infantry battalion of 900 troops and a combat engineering unit in March 1992, rotated thousands of soldiers through the UNPROFOR and subsequent mis-sions, "leaving hardly a Canadian soldier who had not served at least once in the former Yugoslavia."[119]

But throughout the UNPROFOR's existence and subsequent UN/NATO operations, nascent national armies and paramilitary forces fought against neighbouring states, ethnic militias, and local war-lords, with all sides perpetrating ethnic cleansing at various points over the decade.[120] The level of violence that was employed to expel or eradicate perceived enemies was "on a scale not seen since World War II."[121] Canadian peacekeepers, with very little peace in the Balka-ns to keep, found themselves in a morass where traditional, linear mis-sions were no guide. On the surface, the mission resembled previous operations like Cyprus, with peacekeepers wearing blue helmets and riding in painted UN vehicles. But unlike in Cyprus, Canadian peace-keepers delivered humanitarian aid while armed, deployed anti-tank vehicles, and at times used snipers to kill belligerents.[122]

Corporal Gregory Prodaniuk was just twenty-one years old and had only recently completed his training as an infantry soldier when he deployed to Croatia as a member of the 1st Battalion of the Royal Cana-dian Regiment in 1994. Prior to deployment, his unit was given train-ing appropriate for "normal" peacekeeping operations. He summarized his training in the following manner: "Man an OP [observation post]; write a log; come to a riot; search a building for weapons."[123] Neverthe-less, through whispered word of mouth, Prodaniuk was aware of what Canadian soldiers had experienced thus far in the former Yugoslavia, and he sensed that he was entering a mission "irregular to the peace-keeping experience up to that point."[124] He recalled:

When we got over there [to Croatia] it sort of started immediately. We got into theatre and we had to stand in line and exchange equipment with the guys that were coming out. And you noticed the guys that were coming out looked pretty bad, pretty haggard. They definitely didn't look like ... the sort of clean cut Cyprus pictures that you'd seen. You saw guys that hadn't cleaned [themselves] in a few days, had bags under their eyes. Their equipment was all dirty ... At that point we didn't even have our own helmets so we were exchanging helmets. So we were looking for a guy that had the same head size .... to grab a helmet off him. It was a very sort of weird way to be introduced into theatre, and as we're getting off a certain commercial airline we can hear the [artillery] shelling going on in the background.[125]

Prodaniuk's unit spent most of its time isolated across various outposts in a zone of separation between Serbs and Croats. Much of that time was also spent wondering if and when the situation might erupt, while occasionally being shot at, shelled by artillery, and stumbling upon "a lot of gruesome events that had taken place just before we got there."[126] As his tour progressed things started to "ramp up." NATO planes bombed around them. In several instances he was sent with only two or three comrades to inspect Serb or Croat-held buildings for weapons and explosives. Both belligerent forces were unhappy about the UN presence and attempted to intimidate Canadian forces, often in groups numbering fifty or more. Their tactics included not just gruff posturing, but also more serious threats such as "cocking weapons, putting it at your head, that kind of stuff."[127] Prodaniuk characterized the mission as a "really messed up police operation," stating matter-of-factly that "it really wasn't something we trained for." Like numerous comrades, he felt at a loss to grasp the reality of what his peacekeeping duties entailed: "That disconnect between what you *thought* you were going to be doing, and what you ended up doing, was pretty profound."[128]

The biggest testament to how peacekeeping had changed came in September 1993. Members of the 2nd Battalion of the Princess Patricia's Canadian Light Infantry (2PPCLI) were involved in heavy fighting with Croatian forces during what was later termed the Battle of Medak Pocket.[129] That month, Croatian forces attacked Serb-held territory in Sector South, one of the UN's Protected Areas. After five days of battle, a UN-brokered ceasefire led to the imposition of 875 soldiers from 2PPCLI in between the warring parties.[130] Their mandate was to supervise the removal of Croat troops back to their original lines, and likewise to remove Serb troops from a "pocket" that formed during the Croatian offensive.[131] As the Canadian peacekeepers took up positions, local Croat forces refused to let them enter the area, firing on their UN vehicles. A fifteen-hour firefight ensued, during which four Canadians and many more Croats were wounded, and an estimated twenty-seven Croats were killed.[132]

Worse was still to come. After negotiations brought fighting to a close, Canadian peacekeepers moved into the Croats's previously held area and discovered a plethora of gruesome sights. In village upon village Serbian civilians had been murdered, and there were many signs of rape, livestock destruction, and local wells being poisoned. Sergeant-Major Mike Spellen, a member of 2PPCLI's Delta Company assigned to a "sweep team" searching the area, found a wheelbarrow in the middle of a swamp. Thinking it a strange sight, he approached and discovered that it contained the body of an eighty-four-year-old woman who had been shot at least six times.[133] Warrant Officer Matt Stopford recalled seeing a Croatian sergeant throw a "bundle" into a burning house while dancing around with a bloody pair of child's training underwear on his head. Stopford realized after a few moments that the bundle was in fact the dead child to whom the underwear belonged.[134] Echoing Stopford's experience, Master Corporal Jordie Yeo lamented: "The number of times that I saw graves that were only three or four feet long was too many."[135] Traumatic sights were common in the aftermath of the Medak Pocket battle, and were witnessed by many Canadian peacekeepers in the former Yugoslavia throughout the 1990s. In an interview with the author, Mike Spellen stated that there was a pervasive mental and physical exhaustion amongst his comrades, further exacerbated by "being aware that there are atrocities going on around you, [and] seeing some of those atrocities."[136] The UNPROFOR's inability to prevent civilian deaths led Fred Doucette, a Canadian UN military observer in Bosnia in 1995, to argue that the UNPROFOR was as useless as "eunuchs in a whorehouse."[137] The myriad mental and physical challenges that peacekeeping presented took a heavy toll on Canadian soldiers' minds, but recognition of that fact was slow to come because of military leaders' willful blindness and lack of knowledge about war-related mental disorders.

EARLY SIGNS (OF PTSD)

From the beginning of the UNPROFOR and other non-standard peace-keeping missions during the early 1990s, there were rumours inside and outside of military circles that the new peacekeeping significantly impacted its participants. The first publicly visible sign of the aftermath came in September 1993 when a twenty-six-year-old member of 2PPCLI was found dead in full uniform after shooting himself in his apartment.[138] His suicide came shortly after returning from peacekeeping in Croatia. Throughout the 1990s there were widespread stories about suicides and attempted suicides by peacekeepers after their return from the former Yugoslavia, but higher authorities made a concerted effort to downplay the extent of the problem.[139] A soldier who fought at Medak recalled his superiors telling him that he was the only one from his unit with mental health problems.[140] In addition to suicides, there were a number of soldiers who took up heavy drinking, in large part to cope with their experiences or drown out nightmares. Many troops felt that they simply could not relate what happened, or their feelings about it, to comrades or family who were not with them in theatre.[141] It took a number of years before the prevalence of health issues amongst peacekeepers became known to the public – and to soldiers themselves.

Although CAF leaders and medical officers during the early 1990s were aware of the effects of combat stress on soldiers, due to peacekeeping's traditionally lower tempo and ostensibly less stressful character, authorities initially made a strict separation between the stress of "war" and difficulties encountered in "military operations other than war."[142] Peacekeeping operations were not held in the same high regard among military members as war tours, and because they were consequently viewed through the prism of Cold War UN missions, they were deemed largely mundane in character.[143] It was for this reason that the CAF sent a psychiatric resident physician, a psychiatric nurse, and a social worker with the Canadian Naval Task Group during the Gulf War in 1991, but did not send a team during the initial stages of the UNPROFOR mission a year later.[144] A 1991 *Globe and Mail* article written in the midst of the Gulf conflict stated optimistically that, rather than being treated as cowards or malingerers as they were in the past, CAF personnel suffering from combat stress were "treated as victims of a 'combat-related, critical incident, stress event.'"[145] Lieu-

tenant-Colonel James Jamieson, director of Social-Development Services for the surgeon general in Ottawa, affirmed that "the whole philosophy [toward psychological difficulties from war] has changed,"
and that the military no longer considered traumatized soldiers to be
"cowardly or crazy."[146] Captain Judith Pinch, a social worker employed
at Canadian military headquarters in Bahrain, mirrored Jamieson's
hopefulness, painting a brighter picture for soldiers: "They can show
their feelings now ... They don't have to always appear brave and
strong and keep their feelings to themselves. It's not what it used to
be, that's for sure."[147]

But war was regarded as qualitatively different from peacekeeping,
and there were no similar articles describing a new day for traumatized peacekeepers when Canadians were sent to Croatia and Bosnia
in 1992. The idea that Canadian soldiers could become psychologically debilitated because of peacekeeping duties went against decades
of understanding about war trauma and common sense approaches
to military operations. The distinction between the effects of war
and peacekeeping were neatly encapsulated in the terms themselves:
"Combat Stress Reaction," the 1990s' intellectual successor to shell
shock, described the effects that occurred as a result of *combat*, while
peacekeeping, due to its ostensibly peaceful nature, seemed to pre-
clude any instances of trauma or psychological disorders.[148] Thus,
throughout the early to mid-1990s, Canadian military leaders were in
a state of "blissful ignorance" regarding peacekeeping trauma.[149] In
their 2015 book about CAF leadership culture during the 1990s, Bernd
Horn and Bill Bentley described the situation this way: "Due to their
myopic focus and isolation, as well as their anti-intellectual mindset,
the senior leadership of the DND and the CAF had been unable to
anticipate, [or] adapt ... to the myriad of changes that swept over
Canadian society and the globe."[150]

One of the few voices penetrating preconceived notions of war trauma in the early 1990s was that of naval Lieutenant-Commander Greg
Passey.[151] Passey, a psychiatric resident from the University of British
Columbia sent to the Gulf War in 1991, was the first, along with his
supervisor David Crockett, to quantify the psychological impact of
peacekeeping on Canadian soldiers.[152] In 1992–93, Passey, who made
weekly visits to CFB Chilliwack to help medical staff treat CAF psychiatric patients, discovered a number of soldiers who were displaying
signs of PTSD.[153] He had become familiar with trauma symptoms in
civilians a few years earlier while in charge of a hospital in the small

community of Masset, British Columbia. During a 2015 conversation with the author, he recalled a particular case of a two-year-old child dying after being burned in a house fire, and the devastating impact the event had on the child's family.[154] Passey was also an avid reader of military history and from his readings was acquainted with shell shock and battle exhaustion.[155] Lastly, at a trauma studies conference in Amsterdam in June 1992, he discussed the subject with several researchers from America, and heard about a particular study on trauma in Russian veterans from the Soviet-Afghan War. Gradually, Passey became convinced that PTSD could also stem from non-traditional combat and operations resembling war.[156]

Seeing common symptom patterns in Canadian peacekeepers, Passey commissioned a study of Regular Force soldiers and reservists from three peacekeeping regiments: combat engineers in Chilliwack; troops from the Royal Canadian Regiment in Gagetown, New Brunswick; and members of PPCLI in Winnipeg.[157] Study participants filled out confidential questionnaires that measured their stress and depression levels, in order to determine the prevalence of debilitating psychological symptoms among former peacekeepers. The results, published in the *Winnipeg Free Press* and *Globe and Mail* in December 1993, confirmed Passey's suspicions: one Canadian peacekeeper in nine (11 per cent) returned from the former Yugoslavia suffering from combat stress.[158] Amongst the many symptoms soldiers reported, the most prevalent were anxiety or panic attacks, irritability, difficulty falling asleep or staying asleep, diminished interest in work, family, or friends, and "curtailed emotions."[159] A twenty-five-year-old soldier stationed in Winnipeg agreed with the study's conclusion, declaring, "I'm a different person. I have changed for the rest of my life. Over there you're staring at dead kids and starving people and little old ladies who run beside your vehicle so they won't get hit by snipers."[160] Passey ominously predicted that as time passed and new symptoms such as alcoholism and flashbacks manifested, the number of peacekeepers experiencing psychological difficulties might increase.[161]

Passey and Crockett's study was the first to demonstrate something unique about the CAF's historical experience with psychological trauma. They showed that, contrary to contemporary beliefs about combat stress and trauma, peacekeeping missions also exposed soldiers to overwhelmingly traumatic experiences.[162] In a 1994 *Canadian Medical Association Journal* article, Passey further explained the implications of his 1993 study. He maintained that "our people [peacekeepers] are under horrendous stress," and that although "peacekeeping may not be more stressful than battle ... it is certainly more stressful than anyone thought."[163] Unlike war – which often had tangible goals, ways to measure the success or failure of a mission, and clearly defined sides – peacekeeping's success was judged according to more spartan considerations such as "how many people got food or were not killed."[164] Peacekeeping stresses and trauma were often different in kind from combat stresses, but their effect was similar. Passey and Crockett's study was the first powerful piece of evidence that there *was* such a thing as peacekeeping trauma, and also helped confirm that the word "peacekeeping" was in many cases a euphemism for something more menacing.

On the surface, the CAF leadership's response to Passey and Crockett's study, and trauma in general, was one of action. In 1991 the CAF had taken a proactive approach to combat stress during the Gulf War when it sent Passey and the rest of his team to educate personnel about the stresses of war and help them deal with separation from loved ones.[165] A team of specialists was also on hand to provide "Critical Incident Stress Debriefing (CISD)," a process developed in the 1980s, initially targeting emergency response workers to assist them with acute stress and traumatic incidents.[166] Beginning in the 1990s, the CAF implemented CISD, in part due to the efforts of social worker Lieutenant-Colonel Rick McLellan, who likewise saw a need to pay more attention to intense stress' effect on troops.[167] CISD was one of the military's methods for preventing long-term psychological impacts in soldiers exposed to a "critical incident," an event defined as "outside the range of normal experience that is sudden, unusual, and unexpected, disrupts one's sense of control, involves the perception of a threat to life, and may include elements of physical or emotional loss."[168] CISD's purpose was not professional counselling, but rather "to provide a safe opportunity [for soldiers] to deal with reactions to a stressful traumatic event."[169] Ideally taking place within a few days after the event, the goal of Critical Incident Stress (CIS) teams, according to Lieutenant-Colonel Jamieson, was to deal with traumatized troops as quickly as possible and "as close as possible to [the] event."[170] Soldiers were encouraged to express their feelings and emotions, and reassured by the CIS team that their reactions were "experienced by normal people following an abnormal event."[171]

While based on good intentions, CISD and information about critical incidents were inconsistently applied during the early 1990s.

They went up against a closed culture that taught soldiers to spurn outsiders, especially "suits" who did not understand life on the front line. Mike Spellen could not recall any conversations about stress or trauma prior to or during his time in theatre. He said that before Croatia there were "no concerns of that [PTSD] whatsoever," and that he did not even know what "PTSD" meant.[172] Andrew Godin remembered a CIS team arriving from Ottawa during the tail end of his 1992 Croatia tour. They asked Godin and others "a bunch of questions about what we did and saw during the tour," but because the CIS team had no members who were front-line soldiers, "getting answers out of us was like pulling teeth from a chicken."[173] James Davis wrote that he and his comrades instituted an informal and traditional type of CIS therapy: "If someone seemed to be walking too fine a line, the Warrant [Officer] would have a couple of the boys get him drunk and encourage him to let it out."[174] While aware of the existence of CIS teams, Davis maintained that no team visited during his 1992 Croatia tour, and even if they had, "every soldier knows not to talk to these clowns."[175] He cited an instance when a friend admitted to being troubled by his operational experiences, only later to be identified as "an emotionally unstable character."[176] Regardless of its authenticity, such stories ensured that soldiers kept a tight lid on their experiences and sought comrades' ears rather than risk divulging too much to a "suit."

CISD proved incapable of preventing long-term mental health problems for many Canadian peacekeepers returning from the former Yugoslavia. The reasons included a culture of toughness and masculine prowess that inhibited soldiers from speaking out about their psychological difficulties (a type of collective and self-stigmatization which produced outright denial); fears of how reporting a mental illness might affect their military career; a conscious attempt by an old guard among CAF leadership to deny PTSD's existence; and a socio-political milieu that left many soldiers feeling abandoned by both their unit and their country. Living within a culture of denial and suppression, and unable to attach their peacekeeping experiences to any tangible or nationally-supported cause, psychologically injured soldiers suffered in silence. It required several keys events across the 1990s, and a board of inquiry into the seemingly high rate of illness among Balkans peacekeepers, to catalyze a large-scale shift in consciousness concerning the links between peacekeeping and mental trauma.

5

Breaking Down the Wall

I mean my personal sense is that ... psychological trauma in these kinds of situations is one of the toxic exposures that occurs. And it is as valid, if not more valid, than many of the other types of toxic exposures that veterans concern themselves with. But that is – it is more than just an awareness issue. PTSD has baggage with the veterans community.

Testimony of Lieutenant-Colonel Charles Engel,
Croatia Board of Inquiry, November 23, 1999, vol. XXVII, 37.

People were afraid to talk about it [PTSD, stress symptoms], you know. Fear of looking weak or whatever ... Fear of being released from the Forces because, you know, you are either ... a weak sister or [']you have got something wrong with you so we will kick you out['] ... You would hear here and there about things like, you know, guys wondering if they are ever going to have a solid stool again or if they are ever going to sleep the night again without waking up ... or flying into a towering rage at their wife or their family about nothing at all. Guys don't really want to talk about that ... unless they are with their really trusted confidantes. I think a lot of guys kept things inside and guys wouldn't say much ... The system does not reward weakness ... It punishes weakness and ... throws it away.

Testimony of MWO Patrick Lawler,
Croatia Board of Inquiry, October 18, 1999, vol. XIX, 12.

When Corporal Prodaniuk returned from UNPROFOR peacekeeping duties in April 1995, he encountered a "wall of silence" blocking any discussion about what Canadian peacekeepers had witnessed, or actions they had taken against hostile forces.[1] He noticed that military leaders only wanted troops to cite the positive side of peacekeeping:

They wanted us to sort of address what was making the nightly news – show Canadian peacekeepers saving kids, handing out humanitarian aid, something … But they didn't really want to know about us being in actions where we were taking positions or moving belligerents off a hill … sometimes engaging a belligerent force to get them to move, or to do something we wanted them to do. That wasn't something they wanted discussed. And so the command didn't really want to bring it up … So there was this kind of weird repression of what we did and experiences we were involved in … And so when you came home, it was just sort of a 'shut up' culture … So what ended up happening was, you came back and you just moved on with life. You didn't really talk about things.[2]

Prodaniuk initially felt no signs of psychological difficulties, so he channelled his energy into becoming an even better soldier, following the culture that encouraged him to soldier on. Several years went by as he gradually became more "emotionally unstable."[3] He had difficulty sleeping, and was troubled by memories of harrowing incidents that repeatedly played in his mind.[4] Prodaniuk felt that since he had not been in a traditional combat zone, he "shouldn't have any reason to have a problem."[5] Like numerous comrades during the 1990s, Prodaniuk's knowledge of psychological trauma was "razor thin" and consisted of what he saw in Vietnam War films.[6] Thus, he did not make a link between war trauma and his own difficulties.[7] Feeling disaffected, he decided to make a change, and became a materials technician with the Electrical and Mechanical Engineers corps in 1999.

Shortly thereafter, he crashed. He recalled: "I went to a different part of the Army, then, all of a sudden everything sort of unpacked. It was almost as if the social conditions of the battalion were sort of keeping me wired, or keeping me compressed in a way. And once I left, that social support sort of dissolved, and everything became unpacked."[8] Prodaniuk became depressed, and sometimes resorted to alcohol to cope. He found himself "losing perspective all the time," and finally, when his psychological difficulties became almost too much, he decided to get help.[9] He went for numerous rounds of counselling, and in 2000–01 was medically released with PTSD. Reflecting on his gradual deterioration, Prodaniuk affirmed that its primary cause was the "failed processing" of what he experienced in the

Balkans. He declared that above all else, "that in the end is what did me in."[10]

Prodaniuk's poignant recollections and eventual realization of the effects that peacekeeping incidents had on his mind highlight several of the key factors which shaped CAF conceptualizations of trauma during the 1990s. The wall of silence Prodaniuk encountered in his battalion was a microcosm of a much larger wall raised by DND and CAF leaders, designed to prevent scandal and downplay peacekeeping's effects on Canadian soldiers. That silence had profound consequences for many soldiers as they returned to a military that seemed indifferent to their accomplishments and a country that seemed to care little for the sacrifices they had made. For those whose experiences proved debilitating, military leaders' refusal to acknowledge peacekeeping trauma also ensured that numerous soldiers were released from the Forces and denied a pension.

At a social level, this chapter examines the loss and abandonment that numerous peacekeepers felt when they returned home, and how those feelings affected their psychological state in a manner that was all too real, despite being difficult to quantifiably measure. Moreover, Prodaniuk's trouble coming to terms with what ailed him was reflective of a masculine fitness culture that discouraged admitting to injuries and was especially critical of psychological difficulties. Military culture produced a self- and group-policing among its members, causing injured soldiers to deny any problem for fear of being ostracized by comrades or released from the Forces. The situation finally came to a head in July 1999 when the Croatia Board of Inquiry (BOI) was called to determine the cause of a high number of casualties stemming from the UNPROFOR mission. The BOI shone a light on the existence of altered but tenacious ideas about mental disorder reminiscent of discussions from the First and Second World Wars.

UNDER SOMALIA'S SHADOW

CAF and DND leaders had little desire to discuss the possibility of peacekeeping trauma during the 1990s. As recounted in the previous chapter, the shadow of Somalia, and the distrust of the military it created in the Canadian public, loomed large for most of the decade. "If Canadians were thinking of the military at all," their attention was largely focused on the Somalia affair and its aftermath.[11] In his retrospective assessment of the 1990s, Brigadier-General (ret.) G.E. "Joe" Sharpe wrote that "senior Department of National Defence officials were not in the mood to disclose anything about operations that was not absolutely necessary."[12] Their reticence extended not just to operation specifics (e.g., Canadians fighting at Medak), but also to any aftereffects, including peacekeepers' mental difficulties. Thus, for much of the 1990s the problems that soldiers and veterans faced were known to few Canadians outside of the military – and few, for that matter, within it.

Nevertheless, several events throughout the decade slowly put pressure on the CAF and DND to acknowledge that a problem was evidently growing. In addition to Greg Passey's peacekeeping trauma research, other signs of trouble arose in March 1995 when a distraught mother confronted MND David Collenette outside the House of Commons. The woman's son, a member of the Royal 22nd Regiment (the "Van Doos"), committed suicide a year earlier.[13] Although his death was not linked to service in the former Yugoslavia, she confronted Collenette on a day when he was responding to allegations that a "rash" of suicides among Quebec-based soldiers was connected to peacekeeping trauma.[14] While CFB Valcartier spokesperson Jocelyn Laroche admitted that the base had seen nine suicides in the previous two years – the timeline coinciding with the beginning of the UNPROFOR mission – he stated that only three instances involved soldiers who had served in the former Yugoslavia.[15] Nevertheless, the base hospital's chief psychiatrist, Lieutenant-Colonel Louis Berard, said in the same *Toronto Star* article that he had seen over thirty cases of PTSD directly linked to UNPROFOR service, hinting at a much larger problem. Berard, like Lieutenant-Commander Passey, acknowledged that Canadian peacekeepers had been "exposed to extremely traumatic experiences overseas."[16] The article highlighted what became an all-too-familiar refrain later in the decade: peacekeeping veterans were "afraid to seek counselling for fear of hurting their military careers."[17]

A second event in the latter half of the 1990s was the publicity that surrounded Lieutenant-General Roméo Dallaire's personal struggles with PTSD following his ill-fated tenure as Force Commander of the United Nations Assistance Mission for Rwanda (UNAMIR) in 1993–94. Although many Canadians later became acquainted with Dallaire's story because of his bestselling 2003 book *Shake Hands with the Devil*, his battle with PTSD, like those of numerous soldiers, spanned a number of years.[18] Dallaire acknowledged the colossal emotional toll UNAMIR service had on its participants, and took the unprecedented step of requesting mental health assistance for himself, his UN Military Observer officers, and their spouses or partners.[19] In July 1995, Passey, Major Lamontigny (a social worker), and a mental health team spent two days at CFB St Jean conducting CISD and educating officers and their families about stress disorders.[20] Those sessions represented a historic first: they were the first CAF initiatives specifically designed to address PTSD and its effects.[21]

Dallaire's experience with PTSD mirrored many subordinates' struggles during the 1990s.[22] Although he took steps to raise awareness of operational stress and spoke publicly about it after his return from Rwanda, nonetheless, "Camouflage was the order of the day."[23] In a manner akin to Barry Westholm, Greg Prodaniuk, and Andrew Godin, Dallaire became a workaholic. He accepted all tasks sent his way and kept busy to avoid troubling memories.[24] Unfortunately, like Westholm and others, Dallaire's attempts to suppress his inner demons were in vain. Four years after returning from Rwanda, in September 1998, his mind "decided to give up" and he was ordered by CDS Maurice Baril to take a month's sick leave.[25] In an internal e-mail quoted by the *Globe and Mail*, Dallaire cited his "operational experiences" and their effect on his health as the reason for his imposed leave.[26]

Throughout his struggle with PTSD in the 1990s, Dallaire worked with others of a like mind to raise awareness of what was troubling so many peacekeepers. One such ally was Captain Stéphane Grenier, a military officer who served in Rwanda in 1994–95 as UNAMIR spokesperson. Like many other peacekeepers, Grenier returned to Canada "very messed up."[27] In an e-mail to Grenier in 1997, Dallaire espoused the need to produce a video about events in Rwanda and how they affected Canadian UNAMIR participants.[28] Unable to obtain government funding unless he could show that the video had a tangible purpose, Grenier devised the idea of focusing on the "human cost" of peacekeeping missions, thus making it useful as a training video.[29] Dallaire liked the idea and gave him the go-ahead to produce it. Over the next several months Grenier put together something unlike any past CAF video, utilizing candid interviews with UNAMIR peacekeepers about how their Rwanda deployment had affected them. When it came time for Dallaire to be interviewed, he was unsure of what to say about his experiences, and consulted Grenier about different options. Together, they decided it was necessary for both Dallaire and his subordinates to "lay it all down."[30]

In the video, completed in 1998 and titled *Witness the Evil*, Dallaire and other Canadian peacekeepers provided an uncensored report of what they had experienced in Rwanda. Dallaire described his thoughts of suicide after Rwanda and encouraged other sufferers to come forward. But he also candidly acknowledged the barriers for those with mental illness: "Sometimes I wish I had lost a leg, instead of having all those brain cells screwed up. You lose a leg, it's obvious; you've got therapy, you've got all kinds of stuff. You lose your marbles ... very, very difficult to explain; very difficult to gain that support that you need. But those who don't recognize it and go get the help [they need], are going to be a risk to themselves and to us."[31] The image of a high-ranking CAF officer in his UN uniform almost breaking down on camera was unprecedented. The video struck a chord with the public, and excerpts were aired by the CBC on both the radio and *The National* television program in November 1998.[32] Given the wide reach of CBC programming, *Witness the Evil* did much to bring Canadians' attention to peacekeeping trauma and forced the military "to actually pay more attention."[33]

Although Dallaire's rank allowed him the privilege of being spared an ignominious release from the CAF – a fate which befell many rank-and-file soldiers throughout the 1990s – even he encountered resistance to his open advocacy for soldiers suffering from PTSD and other stress-related illnesses. Brigadier-General (then Colonel) Sharpe, future chair of the Croatia Board of Inquiry, recalled that during the 1990s "many senior CAF officers ... felt Roméo was out of line when he started this approach."[34] Sharpe's appraisal was echoed by a high-ranking officer diagnosed with PTSD, who reported that, "When Roméo Dallaire came forward, some senior officers said of him that he's 'always been emotional,' and to them 'emotional' is considered a weakness."[35] Dallaire's openness about mental disorders ran up against a "strong lobby from an old guard" who, like numerous military leaders across the century, dismissed stress disorders as signs of weakness or personal failings.[36] The conflict between traditional and novel approaches to mental trauma in the CAF represented an "ongoing major difference of opinion" between men like Dallaire, and others like Major-General Lewis MacKenzie from the "suck it up buttercup" school of thought, who believed that publicizing the PTSD issue actually *created* more mental health casualties.[37] For much of the 1990s the latter group held the upper hand.

A third crack in the wall of silence came in October 1998 when the House of Commons Standing Committee on National Defence and Veterans' Affairs (SCONDVA) produced a Parliamentary Report, titled "Moving Forward: A Strategic Plan for Quality of Life Improvements in the Canadian Forces."[38] The main catalyst for the committee's investigation was a consistent stream of news reports, many similar to the 1995 *Toronto Star* article, which expressed the anger of injured military personnel and their families at the DND's "apparent indifference to their situation."[39] As one example of that indifference, the report cited instances when medals earned by those killed in action were simply mailed to family members and spouses.[40] The report was based on a year of hearings focused on major issues affecting the daily lives of men and women in the CAF. Its conclusions were less than flattering for military leaders. Among other things, the report provided an unveiled critique of the CAF's handling of psychological casualties, admonishing military leaders that psychologically injured soldiers required "as much care and especially understanding as those injured physically."[41] The committee also contacted serving and former members of the CAF who were injured during service. Firsthand accounts from former peacekeepers confirmed what many injured CAF members felt, namely that the Forces and DND had "lost touch with the realities faced by injured personnel."[42]

Another important step toward reform came with the June 1998 creation of a CAF/DND ombudsman. In the wake of the Somalia affair and sexual harassment scandals, calls for greater transparency and accountability placed pressure on the DND and MND Art Eggleton to take tangible steps to break down the insularity that plagued both organizations.[43] The first ombudsman, André Marin, was a former Crown attorney and director of Ontario's Special Investigations Unit (SIU). Marin's "insistence on openness" and "penchant for news conferences" during his SIU tenure drew displeasure from police leaders and demonstrated that he was unafraid of ignoring political niceties to achieve results.[44] Commenting on Marin's appointment, military historian Jack Granatstein told the *Globe and Mail* that Marin's openness and insistence on accountability was "just what the Canadian military needs right now."[45] Despite Marin's appointment, though, more than a few eyebrows were raised when Eggleton announced that Marin (and future ombudsmen) would report directly to the MND, leaving many wondering whether the position really had the means to conduct "independent" investigations.[46] Achieving true objectivity seemed difficult since reporting to the minister meant that Marin would be investigating an organization headed by his own boss. That approach kept the ombudsman outside the CAF chain of command, but did not allow him or her to be free from DND machinations and politics.

Despite the inherent challenges, Marin quickly moved forward, and true to his pugnacious reputation became a "burr under their [CAF/DND leaders'] saddle" from 1998 to 2005.[47] According to *Ottawa Citizen* reporter David Pugliese, who covered numerous CAF/DND topics throughout the 1990s, although the ombudsman position was created as somewhat of an "escape valve" to deflect criticism, "they [the CAF/DND] got more than they bargained for, because he [Marin] wasn't worried about what the Generals thought. He conducted a pretty high profile campaign. I don't think they expected that."[48] Throughout the length of his seven-year tenure, Marin publicized and investigated numerous systemic issues within the CAF, on several occasions drawing attention to the treatment of soldiers with PTSD.[49] As was also the case during his Ontario SIU directorship, he became a polarizing figure. A federal report commissioned by his successor Yves Coté declared that Marin's staff expressed "overwhelming relief" at his departure.[50] The report moreover stated that 150 staff left during Marin's tenure, a higher than normal turnover rate.[51] Marin's spokesperson countered that he handled 2,000 cases a year, published twenty-six special reports, and was a transformative figure who initiated positive changes for soldiers and their families.[52] A 2005 *Toronto Star* article about Marin's departure agreed, stating that his office was "a welcome arbitrator able to break through the red tape and bureaucratic intransigence that could make life hell" for soldiers.[53]

Beginning in 1992, American – and later British and Canadian – Gulf War veterans began to present a wide array of symptoms, ranging from fatigue to cancer.[54] The symptoms' often inexplicable nature led to investigations into physical exposure to toxins. The main line of inquiry focused on insect repellents and nerve agent antidotes administered to Gulf War participants.[55] Despite the fact that none of the approximately 5,000 Canadians who served in the Gulf War reported serious toxin-related illnesses during the conflict, a great many men and women subsequently complained of fatigue, depression, digestive problems, and a myriad of other problems.[56] Pressure was put on all three governments to act after media reports gave the impression that the issue was transnational and therefore had its roots in the Persian Gulf. Nevertheless, although the commonality of certain symptoms led some to call them "Gulf War Syndrome (GWS)," no single problem was identified as the culprit.[57] GWS, like shell shock and battle exhaustion before it, symbolized and captured the stresses of "a unique war with unique stresses."[58] What produced GWS, a military study affirmed, was the psychological stress of being under constant threat of biological or chemical weapons, rather than the weapons themselves.[59] Colonel Cameron Scott, who reported on the CAF's findings after sending out 6,000 questionnaires to Gulf War veterans, concluded that "the strongest association to adverse health outcomes was [related to] psychological stressors."[60]

In June 1998, Dallaire, then assistant deputy minister (Personnel), agreed with the questionnaire's conclusions and demanded that GWS sufferers be treated in the same manner as physical casualties. It was evident that a small but noticeable shift was occurring within the halls of National Defence Headquarters.[61] The belief that psychological stresses alone could be responsible for causing debilitating symptoms in Gulf War veterans would have been unthinkable at the beginning of the decade, but by the late 1990s it was abundantly clear, at least to a small cadre of military leaders, that traditional ideas of combat stress required revision. Several factors combined to break through traditionalists' attempts to ignore, downplay, or deny the existence of widescale psychological casualties. These included new research into peacekeeping trauma; consistent media reports of soldiers' problems after service; public inquiries into those problems; Dallaire's public battle with PTSD and subsequent advocacy; and the GWS controversy.[62] In July 1999, a military board of inquiry was called which became the culmination of all the previous struggles over the past decade. The Croatia Board of Inquiry (BOI) finally exposed the extent – both numerically and qualitatively – of problems that Canadian peacekeepers faced during and after service. The BOI was a flashpoint that changed the way many military leaders viewed psychological trauma, and highlighted the human cost of peacekeeping for all Canadians to see. It also provided historians with a unique look behind the wall of silence that existed throughout the 1990s. Looking beyond that wall allows us to see the continuation of altered, though still present ideas of proper manliness and soldierly behaviour, the connection made between psychological trauma and personal weakness, and the very real effect that a perceived lack of social support – à la Vietnam – had on Canadian peacekeepers.

THE CROATIA BOARD OF INQUIRY

Two key events occurred in 1998–99 and precipitated the military's calling of the BOI. The first was the case of retired Warrant Officer Matt Stopford, a Medak veteran discharged in October 1998 after becoming partially blind and suffering from a number of symptoms ranging from aching joints to intestinal bleeding.[63] Stopford's case made national news after he, along with two other injured peacekeepers, personally confronted MND Art Eggleton outside the House of Commons about problems that soldiers faced in obtaining a pension for injuries.[64] Stopford's case was particularly mystifying and created a storm of controversy after a 1998 book by journalists Scott Taylor and Brian Nolan mentioned that Canadian peacekeepers at Medak had been forced to use soil "tailings" (materials left after processing ore) that they found around an abandoned mineshaft to make protective sandbags.[65] When it was alleged that the soil contained trace amounts of bauxite and uranium, Taylor and Nolan, as well as Canadian newspapers, implied a link between Stopford's illness and the "red dirt."[66] Connected to this story were reports that Lieutenant (Navy) Eric Smith, a physician who served on a tour in the Medak region and noticed the red soil, wrote a memo in January 1995 warning of possible toxic exposure and had a copy placed in the file of every soldier who served in Croatia and Bosnia from 1992–93.[67] The media revealed that Smith's letter was surreptitiously removed from most soldiers' files, and accusations of a cover-up quickly became national news.[68] The media scrum surrounding the Stopford case, soldiers' ostensible exposure to harmful substances, and an inexplicably high number of peacekeeping casualties proved to be the straws that broke the camel's back. In July 1999, Eggleton ordered a board of inquiry into the matter.[69] Retrospectively, the "red dirt" scare demonstrated the extent to which the media, rank-and-file soldiers, and military leaders still looked to *physical* causes to explain mysterious peacekeeping injuries, despite the piecemeal but nevertheless growing evidence that the cause of many injuries was a more insidious one.

Thus, it was amidst numerous scandals and public scrutiny that the BOI was called to investigate the high number of peacekeeping injuries stemming from UNPROFOR service.[70] The board's initial (and official) mandate was to examine whether from 1993 to 1995 CAF members in an area of Croatia designated Sector South were subjected to "environmental contaminants" in quantities strong enough to pose a health hazard.[71] This very narrow mandate mirrored the desire of most soldiers – and their chain of command – to find a tangible, physical cause for troops' inexplicable health problems. By not responding to early concerns about the "red dirt" and removing Smith's letter from soldiers' files, the military inadvertently encouraged the belief that soldiers' problems were of a physical nature.[72] Throughout the board's existence, its members met and spoke with approximately 2,000 soldiers and their families.[73] From the beginning, Chairman Sharpe was convinced that the only way to gain soldiers' trust was to demonstrate that the board had front-line veterans' confidence. To achieve that trust, Mike Spellen, a retired master warrant officer and Croatia (Medak) veteran, was asked to participate as a board member. Sharpe kept Spellen close at hand throughout the process, especially when speaking at press conferences or with the rank and file.[74]

It was the plethora of face-to-face discussions and initial days of testimony that convinced Sharpe and the other BOI members that "there was a much larger issue" than potential contaminant exposure.[75] When asked to recall the inquiry's initial stages, Spellen focused on how surprised he was to see former comrades arriving to testify with their wives, and in a few cases, their mothers.[76] After testimonies began, it was clear why. Spellen stated: "I had no idea some of these guys were horrifically sick ... and they're showing up with their wives or their mother in a couple of cases, due to the fact that they were so emotionally unstable ... Best of my recollection, there wasn't one testimony from troops where they didn't break down. Everyone broke down, and that's from colonel down [to the lowest rank]."[77] Sharpe noticed a distinct pattern emerging in discussions both on and off the record. Soldiers reported digestive problems, wild mood swings, and great difficulty sleeping, as well as nightmares.[78]

Hence, the board sensed early on that it was only viewing 10 per cent of the iceberg, and decided, with permission from Convening Authority Lieutenant-General Mike Caines, to expand its mandate to include "the much broader issue of how the Canadian Forces and Canada care for military personnel who are injured in the course of their duties."[79] The board was also influenced by military historian Allan English's work on combat stress among Canadian aircrew during the Second World War.[80] Board member Lieutenant-Colonel Brian Sutherland previously took a Royal Military College course offered by English in 1997. At various points in the course English discussed his PhD thesis work on "flying stress."[81] Thus when the board sensed that stress might be a factor in peacekeepers' health problems, Sutherland mentioned English's work to Chairman Sharpe. The latter, who knew English from previous work conducted for the Air Force, telephoned English to discuss the matter.[82] From that conversation Sharpe decided that the BOI could use English's help, and commissioned him in the fall of 1999 to produce a meta-analysis paper on the historical dimensions and interpretations of combat stress and PTSD.[83] English submitted his paper in October 1999, and it constituted one of several crucial factors that encouraged Sharpe and his colleagues to change their direction and mandate. The board's decision to enlarge the scope of its investigation was "not universally accepted and understood within the department [of National Defence]," but it proved to be historic, as the enlarged mandate and subsequent testimonies brought forth themes which had not been thoroughly discussed in Canadian military circles since the First and Second World Wars.[84] From August 1999 until its final report in January 2000, the BOI's proceedings were closely followed by the Canadian media, soldiers, and the public, through both traditional mediums (newspaper articles and discussions during nightly newscasts) and a consistently updated Croatia Board of Inquiry website.[85]

THE FORGOTTEN PAST

Despite the Canadian military's experience with shell shock in the First World War, and battle exhaustion during the Second World War and Korean War, it was clear when BOI testimonies began that the CAF was unprepared for the onslaught of psychological trauma faced in peacekeeping operations throughout the 1990s. Captain Kelly Brett, a physician and one of two senior medical officers who oversaw Canadian medical staff in Croatia in 1993, testified that there was considerable confusion regarding how to handle stress casualties: "We don't know what to really do with them. We have social workers, we have civilian psychologists. We don't really know what to do with it. People try, you know … But I think it was just so foreign … and we just weren't ready to deal with the post-deployment stuff that was going to fall out of these tours."[86] Both military leaders and medical staff were largely unaware of traumatic stress or PTSD, and those who knew about combat stress did not associate such concepts with peacekeeping. That institutional blind spot was best encapsulated in the testimony of Major Dan Drew, 2PPCLI Officer Commanding, Delta Company during the Medak Pocket operation of September 1993. Drew summarized the situation thus:

Stress itself [was] not understood. It was a dead science in the Canadian army. We had not seen combat fatigue probably since Korea. So there was nobody around, no experts to be able to deal with this issue. I don't know – I cannot speak on behalf of everybody else, but for myself I could not accept that we would have some sort of combat fatigue or, you know, some sort of posttraumatic stress syndrome or disorder because in our minds we had not been at war, okay. And yeah, we saw some bodies and we saw destruction and things like this. But probably I did not understand the significance of what this was – the consequences that that would have on all of us later on.[87]

Drew's conceptualization of combat stress and trauma, as with comrades from all ranks, reflected the fact that much of the Canadian military's acquired knowledge about psychological casualties was forgotten after the Korean War.[88] Colonel Ray Wlasichuk, a veteran of two Bosnia tours, maintained, "I above anybody should have known everything I needed to know about post-traumatic stress disorder, and how a human being reacts to the situations we were faced with … but we just didn't have that basic knowledge. It was available in psychiatric journals but it wasn't something that the military focused on."[89] There were, despite Drew's and Wlasichuk's assertions, experts like Passey, up to date with current civilian psychiatric thinking about trauma; but they were few in number. Passey himself testified a week prior that the extent of the CAF's psychiatric team was five psychiatrists for over 60,000 troops, spread across bases all over Canada, with many bases having none.[90] That problem was compounded, Passey said, by the reality that "not all of us [psychiatrists] have got training in this area [stress injuries]."[91] He further expressed incredulity at the general lack of knowledge about PTSD in the CAF, even among the medical staff. He declared: "I am still amazed there is [sic] people on the medical side that don't know anything about this situation, this disorder. And it is like, well, geez if we [physicians] don't know anything about it, what about the front line supervisors."[92] Confirmation of Passey's statement was provided by numerous testimonies to the BOI. When asked about formal mechanisms for dealing with combat stress or PTSD, Lieutenant-Colonel Paul Wynnyk, a "G3" officer responsible for all aspects of training and operations within western Canada, could recall no programs in place during the early 1990s.[93] He chalked the situation up to the fact that the CAF had not "experienced it [PTSD] to the magnitude that we were experiencing it at the time."[94] Beyond revealing a dearth of understanding about psychological trauma, BOI testimonies also demonstrated the persistence of decades-old ideas about mental illness signifying a weakness of character and femininity.

The CAF of the 1990s, consisting of a modest-sized regular force and a smaller reservist element, was far different in character than the large, citizen-soldier armies created in 1914 and 1939. Nonetheless, as in the past, Canadian soldiers in the post-Cold War period looked to military leaders for behavioural cues and adopted CAF cultural attitudes toward topics like proper manliness and soldiering.[95] Far more so than in civilian society, the chain of command ensured that doctrine and attitudes were shaped from the top down. Military culture also gave officers at all levels significant power to resist change and punish thoughts and actions outside the norm.[96] Creating the proverbial "band of brothers" required a starker delineation between acceptable and unacceptable behaviour than that used in civilian society. The term "suit," utilized by CAF members to separate those in the CAF/DND who were part of the organization but not one of "us," provided just one example of how military members defined who was inside and outside of that band.[97] Board testimonies confirmed that despite numerous changes in Canadian society and the military post-

1945, members of all ranks held beliefs about mental illness akin to their forebears several decades prior. Those afflicted with psychological difficulties were urged to suffer in silence, lest they face ostracism for stepping outside of accepted ideals. But as the number of ill and disaffected soldiers increased, the Board of Inquiry gave them a forum through which to finally break their silence and reveal how psychological trauma and CAF cultural attitudes about mental illness had affected their lives. The "shut up" culture had been so effective that – for many soldiers, as with Mike Spellen – it was the first time they saw the true extent of the problem, and how many of their comrades were likewise unduly affected by peacekeeping experiences.

STIGMA

Numerous discussions throughout the Croatia Board revolved around the stigma attached to illness of any sort, and particularly mental illness, in the military. Similar to militaries around the world, the CAF prided itself on members' fitness and ability to deploy at a moment's notice, as well as their resilience under even the most extreme circumstances. That preparedness was how militaries ensured that they were up to the difficult tasks dictated by civilian governments, including operations assigned with little forewarning. The strong sense of self-determination that drove men and women in uniform, and the Forces as a whole, also acted as a shield against anything that deterred operational readiness.[98] That fitness culture had two inadvertent effects on traumatized peacekeepers in the 1990s. The first was that it created in many soldiers' minds a self-imposed stigma regarding their illness, leading them to deny or ignore a health problem until a "crash" occurred.[99] During his testimony, Captain Bob Sparks, chaplain and senior stress coordinator with 2PPCLI in 1993, highlighted the hesitancy soldiers displayed about discussing mental health problems: "The ones that I would see would be ones that the problem had gotten so big that they couldn't hold on to it any more, where the wife was complaining about them waking up in the middle of the night and this kind of thing."[100]

Greg Prodaniuk supported Spark's testimony and underscored the way in which the fitness culture and notions of loyalty to the regiment worked against illness, persuading soldiers to carry on despite mental difficulties: "'Your behaviours are outside the norm. Your efforts are outside the norm. Get back on it. Get back in the run. Get back into the pack' … The shame … that we bring upon ourselves, those stigmas that we put on ourselves, those self-imposed stigmas, were pretty powerful. You were pretty conditioned to do that."[101] Mike Spellen likewise emphasized the immense power of military culture to shape soldiers' mental processes. The voluminous number of testimonies and off-the-record discussions revealed to the board that "most of these guys initially didn't know that there was something going on with them; or they were in denial."[102] The stigma attached to mental illness was sufficiently strong to prevent many from seeking help, even after losing their family and career, ending up on the street, or deciding to commit suicide.[103]

Beyond the stigma soldiers attached to their condition, the fitness culture's second consequence extended to how CAF members perceived their comrades' vulnerability. Board testimonies indicated that many decades after Sir Andrew Macphail described shell shock as a display of femininity, a powerful sense of military masculinity still operated against psychological "weakness" and PTSD. Captain Kelly Brett summarized the situation thus: "The military still has a very macho attitude and certainly in the army it is a male dominated culture and people don't want to come forward. They just don't want to come forward and admit a weakness … And it is [both] the men and officers, it doesn't matter."[104] In other words, weakness was not tolerated. Greg Prodaniuk described the language used in the 1990s against those showing signs of vulnerability as "blunt" and sometimes "brutal" words, implying that a soldier reporting psychological problems was just a "weak piece of shit."[105] And, as stated in the quotation at the start of this chapter, military parlance was infused with gendered terms such as "weak sister" to describe those who displayed physical or psychological vulnerability.[106] Dr Mark Tysiaczny, regional surgeon at Air Command Headquarters in Winnipeg in 1993, described the reticence that soldiers of all ranks displayed about undergoing CISD or discussing mental illness. Tysiaczny faced an "uphill battle" when he attempted to organize CISD sessions with 2PPCLI a month after its return from Croatia.[107] The reason, he said, was that "it [CISD] was seen by some as a sort of … airy-fairy, not very macho thing."[108] Like the figure of John Wayne, real men embraced stoicism when facing adversity, instead of resorting to "feminine" behaviour such as venting their feelings. When queried about whether resistance came from the "combat arms side" or the "medical side," Tysiaczny responded, "It was every side."[109] Mike Spellen further probed the source of resistance, asking Tysiaczny about the participation rate he received from "upper management, senior NCOs and officers."[110] In a sign that military leaders were less than enthusiastic about encouraging the rank and file to express their feelings or problems, Tysiaczny affirmed that, "We [CISD specialists, social workers, etc.] handled more the [lower] ranks than the officers. We had had a couple of officer groups and tended to have only junior officers present."[111]

The stigma attached to psychological vulnerability was present in all ranks and trades. Mike Spellen recalled that the few soldiers who had the courage to come forward about mental difficulties were quickly cast off by their peers.[112] Those diagnosed with a mental disorder found themselves on the outside of the circle, as their friends "all of a sudden wouldn't socialize with them."[113] Higher up, many in the upper chain of command quite simply "thought it [PTSD] was all bullshit."[114] Greg Passey testified that when he started working with the PPCLI, "some senior people" thought PTSD "was all garbage," arguing instead that a high level of discipline and morale made their companies impervious to psychological casualties.[115] Spellen remembered a private meeting with Chairman Sharpe and an anonymous colonel from the Van Doos Regiment.[116] During the discussion, the colonel informed Spellen and Sharpe that he had been diagnosed with PTSD by a civilian physician and he was paying for treatment out of his own pocket, so that he did not have to reveal the condition to his superiors.[117] Passey testified that even amongst the infantry battalions, where there were considerable numbers of soldiers diagnosed with PTSD, "they are not very tolerant of this disorder. It's like you get ostracized, you get marginalized."[118] Master Warrant Officer Ed Larabie, a Reconnaissance Platoon warrant officer in Croatia in 1993, echoed Passey's sentiments: "There are loads of people out there that will not come forward because they are worried about ... the stigma attached to it and having to put up with their peers ... I still sit in the mess [hall] now and they start talking about ... 'Oh, this guy is a loser.' 'He is an idiot.' 'He has lost his marbles.'"[119]

For those unwilling to accept the existence or extent of PTSD within the military, the issue was often perceived as a matter of honour.

PTSD and mental illness were deemed a literal attack on manpower, operational effectiveness, and unit cohesion, but equally important, they were also a metaphorical attack on the Forces' prestige. Sergeant Chris Byrne, a 2PPCLI member who served in Croatia in 1993, explained how notions of honour encouraged hostility against health problems that implied cowardice or weakness: "The people that are the cause of what is wrong with the system are afraid that the honour of the soldiers of the past or regiment itself or the battalion itself is going to be dishonoured in some way."[120] Ed Larabie's testimony before the board likewise demonstrated that penetrating the internalized cultural values about duty to the regiment was a herculean task. He affirmed: "It's a stigma that I don't know you can ever get over ... I guess it is a soldier's honour or whatever but you can't be perceived to be weak."[121] PTSD, like other afflictions, tainted both individual and regimental honour, and, as expressed by many soldiers throughout the centuries, "those that weren't there have no idea what it [soldiers' honour] is about."[122]

CAF members were reluctant to do anything to jeopardize their honour, or that of the military, and quickly closed ranks when approached by those from outside the circle. A soldier's loyalty was – and still is – first and foremost to the battalion, and more specifically to those with whom they shared front-line experiences — colloquially put, their buddies.[123] According to Kelly Brett, when a Critical Incident Stress (CIS) team arrived in Croatia, a colonel forbade them from seeing his soldiers – a move Brett approved of, even as a doctor, because "we understood ... you can't just fly a team in from Canada without any [front-line or other military] experience."[124] Back in Canada, Mark Tysiaczny knew that CISD was most effective at penetrating soldiers' reluctance to speak out when conducted by "a peer counsellor who is from the group," but lamented that "it took some time before that philosophy was accepted."[125] Master Warrant Officer Randy Northrup, 2PPCLI Combat Support company sergeant major in Croatia in 1993, recalled that a few soldiers were willing to speak with CISD counsellors, but "a lot of guys, pure rebuff. 'Didn't bother me at all.'"[126] Northrup indicated that most men in uniform simply did not trust CIS teams, and that treatment success was more likely to come "behind their house having a barbecue with a beer," rather than trying to discuss something perceived as a "manhood problem" in a formal setting.[127]

PENSION AND CAREER CONCERNS

In addition to concerns about social shunning, dishonouring the regiment, or being viewed as lesser men, many soldiers' desires to hide their injuries were further fuelled by career concerns. The military constituted not just soldiers' social world, it encompassed their economic one as well. Those with families, in particular, wore several hats as husband, father, and provider.[128] Similar to their civilian counterparts, Forces members sought job stability and a future retirement life secured by a pension. But unlike civilians, CAF members were subject to the "Universality of Service" principle, mentioned in the introduction. Universality of Service made (and still makes) it the requirement of military members to be "operationally employable" and "operationally deployable," as well as able to perform the functions of their specific occupation or "the more generic type functions of their environment."[129] In short, soldiers had to be physically and mentally fit to serve their country at a moment's notice and able to carry on their trade. Bosnia veteran Fred Doucette laconically summed up the principle: "No deploy, no employ."[130] In a military undergoing significant funding and troop reductions throughout the 1990s, those deemed in violation of the universality principle were at greater risk of being released. Soldiers suffering from psychological injuries were thus between a rock and a hard place as they battled both inner demons and fears over losing their career and calling.

Chairman Sharpe and the Croatia Board members sensed early in the proceedings that not only were many soldiers suffering in silence, but many others were being – and had been – released from the Forces early and denied a pension.[131] Sharpe, later described by Carol Off as a "guardian angel" to injured soldiers and veterans, made no secret of his disgust at what he deemed an archaic and broken system.[132] He did not tread lightly, and placed his career on the line in a number of public criticisms about the way ill soldiers were treated.[133] In a December 1999 *Globe and Mail* article, the Croatia Board's report was quoted as calling the treatment of such soldiers "a disgrace."[134] The report affirmed that the situation "cannot be allowed to continue," and reiterated the board's belief that stress illnesses were neither a fabrication nor a sign of weakness.[135] According to Sharpe, he was so outspoken that the DND assistant deputy minister of Public Affairs sought, unsuccessfully, a court martial against him for bringing disrepute to the military.[136]

As it did with its investigation into the CAF's socio-cultural attitudes, the BOI delved into the organizational factors that shaped how and why psychological injuries were treated as unworthy of monetary restitution by the CAF and Veterans Affairs Canada (VAC). Sharpe and his colleagues discovered that the traditional medical model, largely unchanged for several decades, persisted within both organizations, emphasizing the legitimacy of physical over mental injuries.[137] Since the type of injuries stemming from peacekeeping repeatedly failed to fit that model, many soldiers were treated as malingerers unqualified for a military pension.[138] Mental injuries were not included on VAC's list of covered injuries, and thus were afflictions that soldiers could not prove had been sustained in a "special duty area" (any country or area where Canadian peacekeepers served because of war or a breakdown of law and order).[139] Lastly, the disability insurance program that CAF members paid into, the Service Income Security Insurance Plan (SISIP), had a different definition of "medically unfit" than the CAF. The result was that soldiers could be released from the Forces on medical grounds, but still denied a pension by SISIP with the justification that they were not proven "sufficiently disabled."[140] In short, the organizational deck was stacked against injured troops, and especially those whose injuries were not visible to the naked eye.

Board testimonies also revealed that troops faced a labyrinthine and sluggish process in their fight for restitution. Bernard Butler, acting director of Pension and Operational Services for VAC, testified before the board that prior to 1995 veterans making a pension claim waited an average of eighteen months for a decision in their case.[141] After a series of reforms, Butler happily reported that the turnaround time was down to approximately five to six months.[142] Nevertheless, whatever improvements were made in response times were offset by the organizational factors that made proving a claim, according to retired Colonel George Oehring, "a very, very big uphill battle to fight."[143] Suspicions about VAC's willingness to help psychologically injured veterans were further supported by specialists' anecdotal evidence. Passey related to the board a story of a peacekeeping veteran with PTSD who became an alcoholic after his diagnosis, ostensibly in part because of his illness. Passey indignantly testified, "Veterans Affairs basically said, 'Well, he has got an alcohol problem. We are not paying for that.' And it is like ... The person has got PTSD. He is abusing the alcohol."[144]

One particularly poignant testimony regarding problems with the system came from Master Seaman Wade Kelloway, a preventive medical technician in the Balkans from April to October 1994. Kelloway bluntly told BOI member Lieutenant-Colonel Sutherland early in the proceedings that when dealing with health issues, "I prefer to deal with [the] civilian side of the house, rather than the system."[145] Later in his testimony Kelloway further expounded on his discontent, saying that after experiencing health problems "over in the Medical Unit ... they didn't give two rats about me."[146] But the most scathing comments about the CAF medical system came during the last moments of Kelloway's appearance. When Chairman Sharpe reiterated that "part of our mandate here is to try and make sure that we take care of people properly when they come back," Kelloway quickly interjected: "And they don't sir ... I see it all the time ... I'm a medical person in a medical system and I'm not even taken care – I'm pushed aside."[147] Coming from a member with intimate knowledge of the CAF medical milieu, Kelloway's statement was all the more indicative of systemic problems. Consequently, many in the Forces chose a similar route to Kelloway's and the anonymous Van Doo colonel, seeking treatment away from their posted base. Major Darrell Menard, a doctor who worked in the Directorate of Medical Policy at the National Defence Medical Centre in the 1990s, argued that given the financial implications and his belief that "there is no accommodation left in the system for them [soldiers] if they have a problem that won't allow them to deploy," it was "not hard to understand" why many troops sought help outside of the military.[148]

More than any other testimony, that of Colonel Oehring, the former commander of Sector South in Croatia from September 1993 to August 1994, summed up soldiers' problems with the CAF medical system and VAC's treatment of injured veterans. Late in his testimony Oehring lamented:

We subject each embarking soldier to a medical screening and/or examination as a precondition to deployment, and then when they return in other than the physical or mental shape in which they left we seem not to accept that the cause is attributable to that deployment. This is not only unfair; it is immoral. We seem to be so frightened that one man or one woman will cheat the system that we make it very difficult for any to receive the compensation and/or treatment the country owes them. In this regard, we have made our otherwise excellent medical system the watchdogs and agents of the Pension Board rather than the advocates of the soldiers that they should be.[149]

Oehring's testimony, and the testimonies from soldiers of all ranks, spotlighted certain issues, such as attributability, that remained a problem eighty years after the end of the Great War. For all of the changes during the intervening decades and conflicts, the onus was still on soldiers and veterans to definitively prove their injury was attributable to service; a task made immensely more challenging for those who, like their First and Second World War counterparts, brought home invisible wounds. Fears about individuals cheating the system, which were foremost in pension officials' minds during the post-1918 and 1945 periods, were still present in military leaders' and VAC officials' minds in the 1990s.

CAF doctors were also reluctant to acknowledge psychological illnesses. Sharpe explained in his retrospective book about the Croatia Board proceedings that "doctors in uniform, particularly senior officers, are far more sceptical than civilians when it comes to stress-related injuries."[150] Skepticism mixed with traditional understandings of combat stress, proper soldiering, and manhood to ensure that psychologically injured peacekeepers encountered many of the same difficulties as their forebears when seeking medical treatment or a pension.

A sadly informative case was that of Phil Tobicoe, First Nations member and Croatia veteran with a long family history of military service in the American, British, and Canadian armies.[151] Tobicoe, who developed inexplicable psychosomatic symptoms after Croatia, was turned down for a pension.[152] He spoke for many soldiers when he expressed that he simply wanted to serve his country and be granted a pension for injuries incurred as a result: "I want to do my 20 years [in the military]. I want to do it proudly because I am Missassaugas [sic] of the Credit [River] ... and a First Nations Indian. I am very proud of my service and ... have family [history] in the American army, the British army, the Canadian army and we are very proud. We just want to make sure we are looked after."[153] Tobicoe's response to his predicament reflected the mixture of anger, disappointment, and confusion many soldiers felt towards the military and VAC.

As the Board of Inquiry progressed, it was not just front-line soldiers and officers who expressed anger at how the system was failing men and women in uniform. During the testimony of SISIP president W.D. Roberts, Chairman Sharpe became so angry at the former's "callous and uncaring attitude" and "pride in the fact that he was able to save the insurance company money by denying soldiers' claims" that he was unable to thank Roberts for his appearance before the board; it was the only time during the proceedings when such an event occurred.[154] Sharpe's anger was partially fuelled by Roberts's appearance in a "thousand dollar suit and Italian leather shoes," as well as his apparent mirth when "denigrating the 'unwarranted' requests from near destitute soldiers."[155] Sharpe firmly believed that Roberts was "proud of his ability to find ways to deny [pension] coverage."[156] Mike Spellen described Roberts as akin to a "washed up used car salesman," and stated that he had never seen Sharpe mad in many years, "except for that day."[157] For his part, Spellen stated matter-of-factly that if he was not a board member he "might have" punched Roberts.[158]

SOCIAL SUPPORT

After returning to Canadian soil, most troops were preoccupied with getting back to the basic comforts of life and seeing loved ones. Sergeant Gregory Goudie's thoughts reflected what so many colleagues felt: "We just want to see the wife, you know, get a bottle of bourbon down range."[159] Above all else, they were happy "just to get home."[160] The initial euphoria of being home caused most troops to ignore or suppress thoughts about the tour. Nevertheless, after settling in they discovered that they were relatively invisible, both on and off the base. Given the aforementioned socio-political climate and "shut up" culture pervading the CAF in the 1990s, soldiers returning from peacekeeping tours often found that nobody knew or cared about what they had been through.[161] Despite the fact that senior UN commanders praised the performance of Canadian peacekeepers in the Balkans, and UNPROFOR commander general Jean Cot awarded the PPCLI a special UN citation, most Canadians in and out of uniform knew little about the UNPROFOR mission and its challenges.[162] In fact, it was not until nine years after the Medak Pocket battle, on 1 December 2002, that Governor General Adrienne Clarkson finally presented 2PPCLI members with a special citation, admitting that "your country did not recognize you at the time."[163] BOI testimonies captured the manner in which stigma and CAF culture created socio-economic difficulties for injured soldiers. They revealed the intangible but nonetheless important ways that a lack of military and public support exacerbated psychological injuries as well. Psychological trauma and PTSD had significant medical and financial dimensions. But there were also moral and spiritual dimensions to how peacekeeping experiences were rationalized by troops who were returning to a Canada that looked different to them after they had witnessed the horrors of ethnic cleansing and other traumatic events. Board testimonies and the modest primary literature on 1990s Canadian peacekeeping provide a window into how soldiers dealt with the psychological aftermath of service, and how a perceived lack of support affected the meanings they attached to that service.

One of the biggest obstacles that Canadian peacekeeping veterans faced, especially those suffering from psychological difficulties, was finding a comrade or close friend with whom to make sense of their experiences. Croatia and Bosnia veteran Sergeant Peter Vallée, from the Van Doos, found it difficult to speak about his experiences, especially because most civilians were "so clueless about all of it [that] it's almost laughable."[164] Occasionally people asked Vallée what it was *really* like to participate in peacekeeping operations, but he discovered that few thought of it as anything more than a "flash on the news."[165] Vallée decided the best course of action was to just avoid the subject entirely: "I won't talk about it, *ever*, because immediately you're the outcast. It's not a great icebreaker at parties."[166] Similar to other peacekeeping veterans, Vallée felt a vast gulf between the civilian and military worlds, since for the former group peacekeeping operations were, simply put, "not part of their reality."[167]

Master Warrant Officer Randy Northrup noticed a tell-tale sign that soldiers were attempting to stave off the memories haunting them. Unable to process the immensely troubling evidence of ethnic cleansing and other scenes in the Balkans, many turned to black humour to downplay the effects that such experiences had on their minds.[168] One example of that humour in action during the UNPROFOR mission occurred when Canadian soldiers spray-painted "UN" in UN blue on a group of chickens from a destroyed farm.[169] While their actions symbolically – and sarcastically – expressed how many soldiers felt about the mission's effectiveness at protecting civilians, the joke's darker implication was that the chickens were literally "the only signs of life" in the area.[170] Many troops brought their strategically dark humour home with them. Northrup described to the Croatia Board how soldiers, several years after the events, still used it to shrug off troubling thoughts: "When you talk to individuals that were in the mortar groups and the sweep teams [who investigated and cleaned up after ethnic cleansing] and when you talk about certain [events] ... they go right to black humour. It's immediate defense ... the black humour, for people who are still fighting off the issue ... They try to laugh it away. But you can tell it still bothers them."[171]

Given the social, financial, and career risks associated with venting to the wrong person, most soldiers simply kept quiet about their thoughts except in the presence of someone else who had been there. Naval Lieutenant Michael Brown, a Roman Catholic chaplain to 2PPCLI from April to October 1993, testified about the emotional weight that peacekeeping veterans carried long after their return: "I have had guys over the past six years who have – I guess maybe it is a typical thing. When you get together, you meet in the airport ... or whatever it is and you go off for a beer and they just – it starts to come out. Because they actually found someone who they can tell the story [to] and the person's eyes don't glaze over."[172] As with numerous comrades, Brown felt that he could not speak about his experiences to someone who had not been in theatre, because they did not "get it."[173]

In Brown's estimation, honouring peacekeepers was a moral responsibility and the military and Canada had failed at it. That failure, he angrily testified, carried psychological consequences for veterans: "Have we honoured what they have gone through? No ... We have not honoured their sacrifice. We have not given them what they need ... Part of that process in honouring what they have done is to normalize it for them ... And by doing that [not honouring them] we have added ... to their stress."[174] Colonel Jim Calvin, commanding officer of 2PPCLI during the Medak Pocket battle, likewise believed that the dearth of attention paid to peacekeepers' efforts made an already difficult psychological situation worse. He remembered that "when we came home, there was no recognition of what we had achieved even though if you talked to anybody [other national contingents] in UNPROFOR ... they thought we were all bloody heroes ...

We came back here and it was just you are done ... There was very little assistance and I would have to say a certain amount of an uncaring attitude that was put toward us."[175]

Calvin had encountered first-hand how little the military and DND seemed to want to know about the Medak Pocket, since it was not until April 1998, almost five years after the battle, that a delegation of his soldiers was finally allowed to conduct a presentation about Medak to a Parliamentary committee on defence.[176] Calvin was also ordered a year earlier to break off a promised interview about Medak with *Ottawa Citizen* reporter David Pugliese. That order was later rescinded, but only because Pugliese threatened to change his story to draw attention to Calvin's forced silence.[177] Like Lieutenant Brown, Calvin attributed harmful effects to the CAF/DND's attempts to shield the public from any unpalatable peacekeeping experiences. He inferred that the "uncaring attitude" demonstrated by both departments and lack of recognition "certainly might have exacerbated things."[178] Calvin believed that his soldiers had lived "ten years in that six months [of UN service]," a belief given credence by Sergeant Chris Byrne's affirmation that "what I witnessed during our stay in Medak would haunt me forever."[179]

Lieutenant-Colonel Craig King, 2PPCLI Alpha Company commander in Croatia from July to September 1993, discussed peacekeeping's moral quandaries and the existential questions that soldiers battled with during and after their tour. One of the most troubling questions was whether or not Canadian soldiers had done all they could for civilians who were caught in the crossfire and targeted for ethnic cleansing. Although Canadian troops ostensibly operated as part of a "protection force," some felt they had in fact failed to protect anyone.[180] King testified before the BOI that certain questions, such as "What were we doing? Could we have done more for these people?", plagued soldiers' minds.[181] King told the board that "there is a sort of moral plane that you start to look at these things and start to ask yourself these sorts of questions."[182] For numerous soldiers such as Sergeant Byrne, witnessing the aftermath of ethnic cleansing caused them to question the entire purpose of their mission and sacrifices. He declared: "We were not peacekeepers. We were not soldiers. We were nothing over there. Nobody knew exactly what we were supposed to be doing and what we weren't supposed to be doing ... We weren't to establish peace because there was no peace to begin with."[183] Captain Bob Organ, a CISD trained regimental chaplain to 2PPCLI, emphasized the spiritual and existential dilemmas that disturbed soldiers after returning from the Balkans: "I think you call into question what it means to be human ... if there's a God[,] and if there's a God, what is that God doing? You're confronted with evil and I think you've got to work that through in order to regain an equilibrium and feel that you can re-invest in life."[184] Unfortunately, already-challenging spiritual and moral questions were made all the more difficult to grapple with when peacekeepers returned home and found that their missions were neither widely known nor honoured by the military and civilian society.

RESERVES

Reservists were and are part-time members (soldiers, sailors, and airmen) of the Canadian Forces who are trained to operate with their Regular Force counterparts on operational commitments, such as peacekeeping missions. When the Canadian Forces are committed to multiple operations and greater manpower is required, as was the case throughout the 1990s, reservists often comprise a large portion of the CAF's committed strength. Once a reservist's tour is completed and they return to Canada, they revert to part-time status and go back to their normal job and routine. Essentially, they can be a soldier one day and a welder the next.

Although Regular Force members encountered difficulties finding comrades to trust with their most intimate thoughts and troubles in the 1990s, reservists, who made up a significant number of the Canadian UNPROFOR contingent (and other peacekeeping contingents), were up against even greater challenges if they developed psychological problems or simply needed a colleague's ear. Budget concerns were foremost in military leaders' minds, so upon a reservist's return from peacekeeping duties they were hurriedly rushed through post-deployment medical checks and sent home before their contractual time elapsed.[185] Colonel Calvin said that troops were, for the most part, "scattered to the winds."[186] Chief Warrant Officer D.F. DesBarres, a platoon second in command with 2PPCLI in Croatia in 1993, described the post-deployment situation thus: "A reservist arrived in Winnipeg, walked by somebody who was filling out a medical questionnaire to make sure you had your ten toes and ten fingers and that your head was on the top of your body ... and a day or two later you found yourself in an airport in Halifax, St. John's, Newfoundland, Vancouver and all the way across the country."[187] When the Croatia Board first convened several years later, it quickly became evident that the CAF did not even have a central information source listing which reservists had served in the Balkans.[188] Such embarrassing revelations seemed to indicate that reservists and post-deployment issues were not at the top of the military's priority list, and added to many soldiers' suspicions about "the system."[189]

From evidence provided during the BOI about Regular Force members' psychological difficulties, it stood to reason that reservists must also be facing similar issues. Mike Spellen described how reservists were provided even fewer opportunities to process their tour and seek comrades' support before being sent home. He recalled: "Now we're going home ... before the second plane [with Regular Force members] lands, some of these guys [reservists] are already sent home to Pump Handle Junction, Alberta and Tuna Lake, Newfoundland. And they never got to see each other or socialize with each other ... and that had an effect on guys."[190] Retired Master Warrant Officer Gerald Boyle echoed Spellen's assessment, saying that reservists were "just dispersed," and "some people were on flights that night or the next day and you never seen [sic] them again."[191] Even Regular Force members were not necessarily guaranteed time to readjust and work through their experiences with colleagues before dispersal. Warrant Officer Geoff Crossman, a member of a mortar platoon and sweep team that cleaned up civilian bodies after Croatian ethnic cleansing in 1993, was quickly posted from Calgary to Toronto after his homecoming. His rapid dispersal meant that, like many reservists, he found himself far from his comrades and "with no one to talk to" about the heartbreaking experiences he had endured.[192]

Corporal Anita Kwasnicki, a reservist from Saskatoon who served with 2PPCLI in Croatia in 1993, was in a uniquely challenging social position as the only female infanteer in her battalion. Like her male colleagues, she remained in Winnipeg less than a week after returning, then was sent home to Saskatchewan. Although describing herself as in good health, Kwasnicki stated to the board that she was unable to access any formal (or informal) social or medical support if necessary, since both were only available at CFB Moose Jaw, over two hours' drive from Saskatoon.[193] After joining the Regular Force and moving back to Winnipeg in 1997, Kwasnicki was still unable to discuss her experiences or socialize with her peers, since most were "a whole bunch of 18-year-old guys" she could not relate to.[194] Even after another woman joined the battalion in 1999, Kwasnicki still felt unable to socialize; her colleague was younger and "at a different point in her life."[195] Her testimony demonstrated how geography as well as age and gender affected reservists' ability to discuss peacekeeping tours and seek help if needed. Although Kwasnicki ostensibly escaped her peacekeeping tours without any serious health issues, many of her comrades were not so fortunate.

Captain Kelly Brett, a physician who saw first-hand the effects of trauma on returning soldiers, described how social and medical issues were intimately linked. The problem with immediately disbanding reservists was that "there is some guy in rural Newfoundland who has been exposed to that [traumatic event] and no one around him understands what he was exposed to and he is just not the same guy he used to be and the civilian physician there that is trying to deal with him doesn't have a clue what is wrong with this guy either."[196] Soldiers who had only a few weeks prior witnessed horrific events or been involved in firefights with belligerent forces suddenly found themselves sitting back in their living rooms "with absolutely no support network."[197] As a psychiatrist who had seen the fallout of Canada's peacekeeping efforts, Greg Passey echoed Brett's arguments about reservists' post-tour dispersal. Passey believed that in the future, "the whole issue about the reserves is something that needs to be addressed," because after being sent home without adequate time to be assessed and vent with colleagues, "they didn't have the unit or the normal sort of comradeship that you would expect that would help dissipate some of the PTSD stressors."[198] In most cases, reservists were "sent off to nowhere, wherever that happened to be, often without a job or any employment and often without any sort of medical resources to help them deal with the situation."[199] Master Warrant Officer Larabie echoed Passey's appraisal, lamenting that "we came back, we handed our rifles in and we sent the reservists off on their merry way, never to be seen or heard from again ... and that ... in my mind, is criminal."[200]

ANGER AND DISILLUSIONMENT

Two of the most common feelings that soldiers expressed during the Board of Inquiry were anger and disillusionment. The biggest target of their frustration was, unsurprisingly, the military itself. Throughout the proceedings, numerous soldiers testified that they felt ignored or shunned by their battalion, their regiment, and the Forces as a whole. For Lieutenant and Padre Michael Brown, the issue was one of responsibility. From his experiences as a peer and confidante to soldiers during the Medak aftermath, Brown knew that many took "a lot of rage, disappointment, and loathing" back home.[201] Brown himself also struggled with what he witnessed overseas, and told the board that for months after returning from Croatia his wife said that nighttimes were "like sleeping with a boxer."[202] Brown had nightmares during which he crawled out of bed or rolled under it, and was often totally unaware of his actions the next day when his wife informed him.[203] He, like his peers, was angry that the CAF and DND seemed unwilling to shoulder their share of responsibility for soldiers' health problems stemming from service: "Responsibility is, if I ask you to go do something … I accept the consequence that you may come back not the same as you left. I will own what I am responsible for. So that when you come back, I will hopefully be able to put you back together the way you were before you left. We do not do it."[204] Major Darrell Menard's testimony highlighted the same theme: "When they [soldiers] are destroyed by doing a mission like that, I think the people that sent them there have a responsibility to take care of them."[205]

Kelly Brett expressed anger at how the CAF and politicians seemed willing to send Canadian troops anywhere at any time, usually without considering how many deployments they had already shouldered. Once soldiers signed up, he said, "we somehow feel we have this right to expose them to whatever we feel like we can expose them to."[206] Brett felt it was "simply wrong" to send soldiers on, in some cases, eight or nine tours.[207] The physical and mental weight of multiple tours caused many to collapse under the strain. Brett reported to the board what the results were: "I do their release medicals in Calgary and it is the same story. [Soldiers said] [']I can't take it. I just can't go away again.['] There are huge family problems. There is alcoholism. There is drug abuse. There is all this stuff because guys aren't given a break."[208] Brett's candid assessment reflected his belief that the number of operations and the subsequent treatment that soldiers received were "ruining people's lives."[209] Captain Alain Guevremont, padre and Croatia veteran, agreed with Brett, testifying that the situation was "burning our people, big time."[210] One particularly emotional assessment came from Matt Stopford, himself a medically released soldier whose career was cut short by a litany of inexplicable physical and mental symptoms. Stopford sorrowfully told the board that "when that faith is broken by them [the CAF/DND], it's like somebody's torn your heart out and just tossed it away. That was my life. You guys talk about it as a career. That was my soul, my life. I love what I did. I still would love to do it."[211]

Soldiers also directed their sorrow and frustration at the federal government and Canadian public. Civilian indifference led some CAF members to believe their country had betrayed them. Major Dan Drew lamented that although Canadian troops had represented Canada "in the finest possible fashion" in the Balkans, many civilians did not know about their experiences.[212] Worse still, the Canadian government, more concerned about actual or potential scandals, had "not acknowledged or even cared about their sacrifices."[213] Retired Master Warrant Officer M.B. McCarthy, a regimental sergeant major with 2PPCLI who served in Croatia in 1993, repeated Drew's appraisal. After noting citations that Canadian peacekeepers had received, both from the UN during the UNPROFOR Mission, and much earlier during the Korean War when the regiment received the United States Presidential Unit Citation, McCarthy asked the board: "And what has Canada given us? Absolutely nothing. Whether it is ... [the] Canadian Forces, country, whatever, we have gotten nothing from the country."[214]

Sergeant James Davis likewise vocalized frustration and disillusionment about how Canadian peacekeepers were treated upon their return. He recalled that while they were overseas, soldiers sometimes received supportive letters from schoolchildren – letters that "were like gold" for troops bearing the brunt of Canada's foreign policy decisions.[215] Sadly, such kind gestures inadvertently created a belief among troops that the Canadian public was deeply aware of current peacekeeping missions. After he returned from the former Yugoslavia, Davis noticed a "huge gap" between what he thought people knew and the actual reality.[216] "The Canadian public," he lamented, "just doesn't seem to know what's going on in these places, what's going on with this military."[217] A lack of awareness and societal support caused Davis and other soldiers to question the reasons for their service. Davis expressed his frustration at the public's seeming indifference: "So am I dedicating my life to the Canadian public? At least the government has the decency to abuse you in the open. The Canadian public just doesn't seem to care and that's even harder to take."[218] Instead of worrying about what troops were doing overseas, he argued, Canadians were more concerned with "where we're putting our investments and what's the new plot on *Ally McBeal*."[219] The trouble with being too caught up in day-to-day matters was that "we forget that out there, in the real world, there are real Canadian troops who are doing a damn fine job for Canada. But no one seems to know that."[220]

Andrew Godin further expounded on how Davis and a number of peacekeepers felt about public indifference. He contended that although Canadians were quite willing to honour fallen soldiers, the injured were often forgotten:

> Once a year ... we gather at cenotaphs all across the country to celebrate the fallen ... How many are actually injured? Probably about five times as many, but no thought is given to that. We honour the dead, because they made the ultimate sacrifice, but we don't honour the injured. We don't honour the people that are still alive and functioning. But we feel in our hearts and minds, 'Yeah, I took a moment' ... Well, sorry to say, that's not quite enough.[221]

Sergeant Peter Vallée, a Croatia and Bosnia veteran from the Van Doos Regiment, believed that the problem related to education – a point made evident by the fact that "some Canadians don't know that Canada was even in Korea."[222] He believed the situation could be vastly improved if education was provided about what the military "actually" did.[223] Vallée affirmed that the public, when informed, was "very supportive" and interested, but simply put, "They don't know."[224]

There were ephemeral examples of public interest and support. Master Corporal Phil Tobicoe's Croatia Board testimony revealed the bolstering effect that public displays of support had on returning peacekeepers. He described the welcoming atmosphere that soldiers encountered after landing in Winnipeg: "I loved the greeting that the

Winnipeg people gave us. My God there was – when we arrived in Winnipeg, we felt like something. There were ribbons on trees, signs, a hall greeted us, people. My God I didn't even know some of these families and they greeted us like they knew us. They sort of loved us and shook your hand. It was like the whole city came out for us."[225] Regrettably, the moment was short-lived. When Tobicoe and his comrades arrived in Calgary twenty-four hours later, "there was nothing. There was a six foot table, a box of doughnuts and a coffee urn and there was only maybe one or two families there ... and the CO [commanding officer]."[226]

One of the most stinging criticisms of the public and federal government came from Master Corporal Jordie Yeo, a Balkans veteran physically injured by shrapnel who, like many comrades, was haunted by nightmares after his return.[227] Yeo invoked the United States' Vietnam War experience in his evaluation of Canadian peacekeepers' predicament:

> I can truly understand what soldiers from the United States who were in Vietnam have gone through. They came back and people hated them or just ignored them. That's what happened to a lot of Canadian soldiers. Just about every single guy that's in the Canadian Armed Forces has done some sort of tour of duty in Yugoslavia, Haiti, Rwanda, Somalia and we're doing this because the Canadian people and our politicians believe that it's the right thing. If it's the right thing, then how come when we come back home nobody says, 'Good job'? I would really like somebody to sit down and explain to me why.[228]

Reminding Canadians, "It's your country and your soldiers are your people," Yeo challenged citizens who were unhappy with overseas operations to discuss the matter with politicians.[229] In Yeo's mind, the only worse thing than criticism was indifference. He exhorted Canadians to take action: "Stop sitting on your hands eating your Pringles."[230]

NEW MILLENNIUM, NEW DAWN?

Yeo's invocation of the Vietnam War demonstrated the historical links between traumatized Canadian peacekeeping veterans' experiences, and soldiers' treatment after the First and Second World Wars. What made the Canadian experience unique, though, was that unlike in Britain and the United States, the CAF's first large-scale encounter with PTSD and "combat" stress in the late twentieth century came not from war but from ostensibly innocuous peacekeeping operations. As the Board of Inquiry came to a close and issued its final report in January 2000, it was clear that several traditional notions were under siege. First, while never discounting the possibility of toxic exposure, after scientific tests and expert testimony, the board concluded that the predominant factor in Canadian soldiers' illnesses was the overwhelming psychological stress they endured.[231] The BOI, the CAF, and the Canadian public learned – or more accurately, remembered – that every combatant, or in this case peacekeeper, had a breaking point. Moreover, they learned that soldiers debilitated by traumatic events or plagued with recurring nightmares were not lesser men, but simply exhausted and traumatized by witnessing horrific scenes and living in conditions that, for all intents and purposes, were war zones.[232] The multiple tours that CAF men and women carried on their backs demonstrated that they were far from being cowards, malingerers, or whiners. Nevertheless, as a flood of testimonies made clear, a CAF culture dominated by ideals of heightened masculinity and traditional views of the stoic soldier ensured that those suffering from psychological problems kept it to themselves, for fear of social ostracism, and, equally important, to prevent an early release from the Forces.

Although the Canadian experience was unique in a few key respects, there was one important link between 1990s peacekeepers and soldiers in earlier conflicts. As with the First and Second World Wars, and most prominently the Vietnam War, there was an intangible but nevertheless important connection between the level of medical and social support that troops received upon their return home, and their ability to rationalize and overcome operational experiences. Chairman Sharpe and the Board of Inquiry concluded – unsurprisingly, given the number of testimonies expressing fear, anger, disillusionment, and sorrow – that the low level of public awareness and departmental prevarications "contributed to the problems suffered by returning soldiers."[233] Worse still, a significant number of CAF members, especially reservists, were dispersed almost immediately after their return, leaving them unable to normalize their experiences and seek informal comfort from comrades. As with Corporal Prodaniuk's story at the beginning of this chapter, the "social conditions of the battalion" had a salutary effect on both the social life and mental health of troops.[234] Without that support, some who were already suffering with psychological difficulties collapsed under the strain. There were a number of previous methods for bringing soldiers home, but Master Warrant Officer Ed Larabie, trained in CISD, cited the First and Second World War methods as a potential solution: "Maybe they had the right idea … you put them on a nice slow boat, a chance to [informally] debrief each other on the way home."[235] Whatever the solution, it was evident to the board that the quick disbanding of units after peacekeeping operations contributed, however difficult it was to measure, to an already stressful reintegration.

Canadian UNPROFOR troops, who in the best cases lived under threat of enemy action, and in the worst cases were forced to clean up the aftermath of ethnic cleansing, also returned to find their mission unknown among civilians and unacknowledged by the governments that sent them. Consequently, many men and women in uniform suffered in silence, another point made abundantly clear by the anecdotal evidence provided during the BOI. About 300 soldiers who served in Croatia from 1993 to 1995 reported illness from service, but the board inferred that "many more" were staying in the shadows.[236] Innumerable troops, like Prodaniuk, tried to carry on as usual, only to later succumb to the "failed processing" of their experiences and traumatic memories.[237] Although it was impossible to put a precise figure on the number of psychologically affected soldiers who did not come forward, if Kelly Brett and Greg Passey's testimonies were any indication, that number was likely in the thousands.[238]

As the new millennium approached, the Croatia Board of Inquiry's conclusions cast a light on sweeping changes needed within the CAF. The board's enlarged mandate – from investigating toxic exposure to investigating the overall treatment of injured soldiers – displayed the "frustrations and humiliating treatment experienced by injured soldiers," many of whom served on multiple tours with only twelve months at home between deployments.[239] Chairman Sharpe, critical throughout the inquiry of how the CAF and VAC handled injured soldiers, declared to the Canadian media that "We don't take as good care of our soldiers as our airplanes."[240] Sharpe and Mike Spellen also noted the difficulties that a historically unwavering macho culture caused for injured soldiers, especially the psychologically injured, who were encouraged to stoically bear pain and suffering.[241] At a news conference Sharpe laid out the issue plainly: "The macho image is [still] a major problem for our people."[242] Contrary to what predominant CAF cultural beliefs argued about PTSD and other psychological illnesses, BOI testimonies proved to Sharpe and the board that most soldiers reporting problems were not "whinging and whining" malingerers, but genuinely injured troops who deserved the benefit of any doubts.[243] Unfortunately, the board exposed a recurring theme in Canadian military and medical history: the burden of proof still lay with injured soldiers and veterans to prove that their illness was service-related. Sharpe affirmed that the primary way to tackle that problem was to "focus on the patient, not the illness."[244] In January 2000, it remained to be seen whether or not CAF and DND leaders would heed that advice.

6

Millennium Approaches:
New Reforms and Old Challenges

The soldier is alone in his war with terror and we have to recognize the
first signs of defeat that we may come in time to his rescue.

Moran, *The Anatomy of Courage*, xxi.

The trick is to not let anyone see how much it hurts. To be ostracized
from the group is the secret fear of all combat soldiers. In the end, all you
can truly rely on is the group, and you can't allow others to see you as
weak. If they do, there are thousands of overt and covert means they will
use to shun you, removing your only support structure. So we grit our teeth
against the pain and pretend that it doesn't hurt.

Flavelle, *The Patrol*, 83.

During the early morning of 15 March 2001, thirty-one-year-old Corporal Christian McEachern, a 1PPCLI member, drove his sport utility
vehicle through the doors of garrison headquarters at Canadian
Forces Base Edmonton.[1] He steered the SUV in circles through empty
personnel offices, knocking over desks and causing significant prop-
erty damage.[2] McEachern was discovered sitting behind the wheel,
weeping and incoherent. After his arrest he assaulted a member of the
Military Police.[3] For his actions, the Crown laid five charges against
him, including impaired driving, mischief, and assaulting a peace officer.[4] He was released from the military in July 2001.

McEachern had participated in difficult peacekeeping operations
during the early to mid-1990s, including missions in Croatia and
Uganda. In the former, he was deeply affected after a fellow soldier

died in a land mine explosion.[5] Later, in Uganda, operational restrictions forced him to watch helplessly as a woman was raped outside a military compound.[6] Adding to his trauma, McEachern saw a man beaten to death and was once again forced to stand by as the man's disfigured body was dragged away.[7] By 1997, McEachern struggled heavily with what he had witnessed overseas, and in September 1997 Greg Passey diagnosed him with PTSD.[8] For the next two and a half years he was on sick leave and under Passey's care, until Passey resigned from his twenty-two-year career in the Forces in September 2000, due to what he saw as Ottawa's mishandling of soldiers' mental illness.[9] McEachern's weekly appointments were cut down to one every three months, and this, in combination with a lack of social support, contributed to his unravelling.[10] Just a day before he drove his vehicle into garrison headquarters, McEachern received a medal for his peacekeeping efforts in Africa during a private ceremony.[11] His defence counsel would later point out that the belated medal was bittersweet, since he was on sick leave for two years and felt ostracized from his unit.[12]

McEachern's mother, Paula Richmond, travelled to Ottawa shortly after the incident to plead for help from the Parliamentary Standing Committee on National Defence and Veterans Affairs, but a Liberal committee member prevaricated and refused to hear her grievances, claiming that he was unprepared.[13] Undeterred, Richmond wrote a letter to the *National Post* explaining her son's poor treatment by the military. The same paper subsequently published excerpts of the case, and highlighted McEachern's plight as well as Richmond's claims that the Chrétien government was not doing enough to alleviate a PTSD "crisis" in the Forces.[14] Then, along with her local MP Leon Benoit, Richmond approached the office of CAF/DND ombudsman André Marin. After meeting with Richmond and Corporal McEachern in Edmonton on 4 April 2001, Marin agreed to investigate McEachern's claim that soldiers with PTSD were treated unfairly by the military.[15]

McEachern's story received national attention. His trial, and Marin's 2002 report on the systemic treatment of soldiers with PTSD (which was itself published as a result of McEachern's complaint and numerous similar claims), drew renewed attention to the plight of soldiers psychologically affected by military service. McEachern's case divided military members and, like the Croatia Board of Inquiry, framed discussions throughout the first decade of the new millennium. The trial, extensively covered in the *Globe and Mail* and *National Post*, hinged on whether his actions were deemed voluntary or an involuntary result of his illness. The defence's case pitted Greg Passey's clinical experience and his research on PTSD in Canadian peacekeepers against the testimony of Randy Boddam, the chief of psychiatry and mental health for the CAF.[16] Boddam claimed that McEachern was "distraught, suicidal and intoxicated" during the morning of 15 March 2001, and undertook his destructive actions willingly and voluntarily.[17] In a later 2008 article for *Criminal Law Quarterly*, lawyer Benjamin Kormos examined the case and disapproved of the fact that Boddam testified in the case, despite admitting during cross-examination that he "had not reviewed any of McEachern's personnel or medical files," and so in Kormos's opinion "had a tremendously limited foundation upon which to base any professional opinion."[18] For his part, Passey testified that McEachern was in a "robotic" state of dissociation, a phenomenon he witnessed on several occasions during their weekly appointments.[19] McEachern testified that he could recall little of that night except vague memories of drinking scotch and later seeing a woman looking down at him behind the wheel of his vehicle.[20] Passey also used the trial as a forum to raise awareness of what he judged to be systemic problems within the CAF. He testified that senior officers and DND officials knew that PTSD was an increasing problem throughout the 1990s and early 2000s but they did little to alleviate it, and he cited overwork and frustration at their indifference as the primary reasons for his retirement.[21]

Much of Passey's testimony during McEachern's trial echoed his October 1999 testimony at the Croatia Board of Inquiry. He claimed that CAF and DND leaders in Ottawa kept resources and information centralized in the capital, rather than encouraging an open dialogue and providing adequate services at bases nationwide. He likened the CAF's handling of PTSD to "having a fire brigade in Ottawa and, if you have a forest fire [i.e., suffering soldiers], trying to bring all the trees to Ottawa to put them out."[22] Ultimately, Madame Justice Doreen Sulyma sided with the CAF's take on events, rejecting McEachern's PTSD as a defence for his actions.[23] On 3 February 2003 she ruled that "his actions were voluntary."[24] The Crown sought six to nine months in jail, but Sulyma opted instead for a fourteen-month conditional sentence.[25] McEachern calmly hung his head when the verdict was read.[26] While still in the courtroom his mother sobbed and declared, "It's his whole life they [the CAF] took from him."[27]

Although McEachern was found guilty at the Court of Queen's Bench, a different form of vindication nonetheless came a year earlier in the guise of André Marin's February 2002 Ombudsman's Report. Marin's investigative team, headed by Gareth Jones with advisory assistance from former Croatia Board chairman Joe Sharpe, interviewed approximately 200 soldiers, half of whom had been diagnosed with PTSD.[28] The team discovered a culture that, by and large, even after the events of the past decade and the Croatia Board's January 2000 conclusions, still refused to countenance the existence and prevalence of mental difficulties among Canadian soldiers. Marin's team found "overwhelming evidence that many within the CF are skeptical about whether PTSD is a legitimate illness" and a "distressingly common belief among both peers and leaders that those diagnosed with PTSD were 'fakers,' 'malingerers,' or simply 'poor soldiers.'" That belief persisted despite evidence from medical professionals and caregivers that instances of soldiers exaggerating or faking PTSD symptoms were rare — somewhere around 1 to 3 per cent.[29]

Marin's report contained aspects that were, according to long-time *Toronto Star* columnist Rosie DiManno, "blatantly self-serving and self-congratulating," but his team nevertheless produced a vast array of evidence demonstrating that the CAF was still split between those who deemed PTSD a legitimate illness and an "old guard" who argued otherwise.[30] The report also demonstrated that several past issues, such as stigma, a lack of social support, problems with bureaucracy, and soldiers' career concerns, were still a problem in the new millennium, and that any attitudinal changes would be slow to come. Marin concluded that McEachern's complaints were justified and that the problems in the CAF were systemic in nature. His report concluded: "As is the case for many CF members who suffer from PTSD, he [McEachern] was stigmatized and isolated from his unit, without the support from his peers that could have sustained him."[31] Unbeknownst to McEachern, his case would become another catalyst for change within the CAF. With the case receiving national media coverage, and Marin's report confirming the findings of earlier inquiries, Defence Minister Art Eggleton vowed in February 2002 to eliminate the stigma surrounding PTSD and mental health discussions.[32] With

Canada then engaged in a new war in Afghanistan and the number of
PTSD diagnoses expected to climb, it remained to be seen whether
Eggleton's promise could be realized.

THE CALL TO ARMS

The events of 11 September 2001 were, according to political scientist
Patrick James, "a huge domino, with others toppling over after it."[33]
With Canadian troops already deployed in several peacekeeping missions around the world, the call came for the CAF to participate in a
major, US-led war effort in Afghanistan. Although the military was
tightly stretched, Canadians dutifully sent a battalion of soldiers in
January 2002, preceded a month earlier by elite commandos of Joint
Task Force 2.[34] Ultimately over 40,000 CAF members served in Afghanistan between 2001 and early 2014, when the final army and
police trainers returned to Canada. It was the largest Canadian military operation since the Second World War and the longest war in
Canadian history.[35] In addition to enduring summer temperatures as
high as fifty degrees Celsius, and a constant sense of danger from both
the environment and its populace, Canadian troops also participated
in extensive combat, including Operation Medusa, a 2006 Canadian-
led offensive in Kandahar province that was the nation's largest offensive operation since Korea.[36] Discussing human interactions in
Afghanistan, reservist Ryan Flavelle wrote that "we have an expression
that is supposed to govern our interactions with the locals: 'Be polite,
be courteous, be prepared to kill everyone that you see.'"[37] Flavelle initially thought the expression was "callous," but later understood its
poignancy, telling his readers that "old men detonating 12-year-old
boys from across a field have a way of changing your perspective."[38] In
several respects, the character of the Afghanistan War, a difficult mixture of combat and stabilization efforts, symbolized Canadians'
ambivalence about the nation's appropriate role in the conflict and in
international affairs.

In his 2010 book on Operation Medusa, retired colonel and military historian Bernd Horn argued that the operation "finally put to
rest the peacekeeping myth that it [Canada] had acquired in national
and international psyches since the 1950s and once again overtly
proved itself as a warfighting [sic] nation within the international
defence community."[39] Canadian troops certainly once again proved

the nation's military prowess, but the public's attachment to a peacekeeping identity remained in place, even if tempered by Afghanistan.
Although Canadian civilians broadly supported the Afghanistan War,
as recently as 2012 an EKOS survey reported that 63 per cent of civilians still identified peacekeeping as the CAF's primary role on the
world stage.[40] In their 2013 essay on public opinion and soldier identity, Stéphanie Bélanger and Michelle Moore argued that such surveys
indicated that even after Afghanistan, Canadian civilians still wished
"to be perceived as peacekeepers."[41] Canadians were agreeable about
the use of force in Afghanistan to fight a "war on terror," but an
ingrained sense of peacekeeping as the nation's *raison d'être* in international politics was reflected in intense reactions to every Canadian
fatality.[42] There was particular outrage nationwide in April 2002 when
a US Air Force fighter pilot mistakenly bombed Canadians participating in a live-fire exercise, killing four soldiers from the Princess
Patricia's Canadian Light Infantry.[43] War casualties, whether accidental or not, "signalled activity that many had assumed to be a thing of
the past."[44] The "peaceable kingdom" thesis endured.

The Afghanistan War nonetheless brought home the realization
that the military was participating in something inherently different
from peacekeeping operations – something which by its very nature
involved inflicting and sustaining casualties.[45] Canadians were supportive of the troops, but cautious and watchful of what a shifting role
in international affairs entailed.[46] Unlike previous operations during
the 1990s, *all* aspects of the Afghanistan War were intensely scrutinized by politicians, the media, and the Canadian public.[47] The conflict was in many ways a "national preoccupation" throughout the
first decade of the new millennium, at the centre of debates over
Canada's role in the world after 11 September 2001.[48] As part of that
preoccupation, heated discussions surrounded the effect that Afghanistan service, and CAF operations as a whole, had on not just the bodies, but also the minds of Canadian troops.

RESPONSES TO PTSD AND MENTAL HEALTH

In the late 1990s and early in the new millennium, CAF and DND leaders responded to concerns about PTSD and systemic treatment of
mentally affected soldiers in numerous ways. Given the media coverage the subject received, the CAF, DND, and politicians realized that

tangible actions were necessary to demonstrate that something was being done to combat the problem. The first definitive step came in November 1998 with the announcement of five Operational Trauma and Stress Support Centres (OTSSCs) at CFBs Halifax, Esquimalt, Valcartier, and Edmonton, as well as CAF Headquarters in Ottawa.[49] Implemented in late 1999, each OTSSC consisted of a military psychiatrist, a military mental health nurse, a military social worker, CAF chaplain, and at least one civilian psychologist.[50] OTSSCs provided CAF members suffering from service-related psychological difficulties with diagnostic assessments, individual treatment (psychotherapy and/or pharmacotherapy), group treatment, and family therapy.[51] They also provided outreach programs, helping to educate military and civilian healthcare workers about the unique aspects of psychological problems caused by military service.[52]

Aside from the benefits for CAF members and their families, OTSSCs also helped decrease the CAF's reliance on a "very limited number" of civilian psychologists and psychiatrists with experience treating soldiers.[53] That reliance was, as discussed during the Croatia BOI, a particular problem throughout the mid- to late 1990s, since soldiers were uncomfortable discussing psychological problems with civilian practitioners unfamiliar with the challenges of military life. But while the OTSSCs helped to treat mentally injured soldiers, they also revealed the intricacies of dealing with enduring stigmas. The location of OTSSCs (on- or off-base) became a particularly controversial subject, even amongst those dedicated to aggressively taking on mental illness challenges. In his December 2002 follow-up to the McEachern report, André Marin criticized the CAF's decision to place all OTSSCs on-base, arguing that locating them on-base made psychologically injured soldiers reluctant to come forward.[54] Previously, Marin's February 2002 report had recommended a pilot project involving the establishment of one OTSSC in "more anonymous premises off-base."[55] His rationale was simple. Marin cited an example where an OTSSC was located on the second floor of a base hospital: soldiers colloquially termed the stairway leading up to it the "stairway of shame."[56]

Canadian Forces leaders working to combat stigma saw the OTSSC location issue in a different light. Major Stéphane Grenier, producer of the 1998 video about Rwanda peacekeeping trauma, disagreed with Marin's assessment. He believed that locating OTSSCs off-base was "short sighted" and helped maintain current stigmas.[57] While increasing access to care and potentially encouraging more soldiers to seek treatment in the short term, Grenier nonetheless maintained that off-base OTSSCs would cost significant taxpayer money and imply to CAF members that psychologically injured soldiers needed to be quarantined "like people who have the plague."[58] The CAF unsurprisingly approached the fight against stigma from a strategic perspective, and CAF leaders kept all OTSSCs on-base despite Marin and future ombudsmen's protestations.

Regardless of their intended purpose, OTSSCs and any related initiatives to combat mental health challenges were only effective if injured soldiers actually utilized them – and that required attacking stigma head-on. Thus, the military also took steps to address the inherent challenges of penetrating a culture that shunned discussions of mental "disorder." Grenier, a UN spokesman in Rwanda from 1994–95, was himself deeply affected by his military experiences and subsequently diagnosed with PTSD. After the 1998 Rwanda video was unveiled, Major-General Christian Couture approached Grenier and expressed interest in the subject, asking him to delve into possible solutions and report back.[59] Couture subsequently had Grenier serve under the director of the Casualty Support and Administration so that he could work full-time on his initiatives.[60] Under the director, Lieutenant-Colonel Dave Wrather, a "very empowering boss" with the attitude of "do what's right and later find the policy to support the action," Grenier was given latitude to explore novel ways of approaching stigma.[61] Based on his own treatments, which he deemed somewhat "antiquated" and inconsistently effective, Grenier became "quite obsessed" with examining how the military, as an institution, approached the issue from leadership and clinical perspectives.[62] He explained:

I refused to embrace the notion that I had an illness ... or an ailment called 'post traumatic stress disorder' ... When you're first hit with this whole notion that your brain is sick, that in itself is a huge barrier to recovery; when you learn that you have a 'disorder.' So as a patient, as a human being, as a soldier, I started thinking, 'What the frick is wrong with us?' ... And over the years developed a concept where ... what was needed was to de-medicalize these issues to a certain degree. Not that treatment needs to be de-medicalized, but the way our culture, our organization, our leaders, our employees, our soldiers perceive these conditions, has to be terminology that is accepted *culturally* by our people.[63]

Similar to Roméo Dallaire and Joe Sharpe, Grenier believed that one solution was to convince both the chain of command and rank-and-file soldiers that psychological injuries were as legitimate as physical wounds. For Grenier, this strategy involved relabelling medical words that were anathema to soldiers and military culture. He explained that "it's one thing to blame stigma, but it's another thing to actually strategically address the issue of stigma by rebranding to a certain degree, at one level anyway, many things that happen [e.g., psychological injuries]."[64] From 1998 to 2001 he pondered and researched the problem.[65] During his investigation, he was particularly intrigued by Queen's University professor and retired RCAF air navigator Allan English's 1999 paper for the Croatia Board of Inquiry on historical and contemporary interpretations of combat stress.[66] Encountering the word "injury" while pondering stress's effects on past soldiers gave Grenier the idea for a new term for service-related stress illness: "Operational Stress Injury (OSI)."[67] Utilizing the term "operational stress" was a conscious decision to encompass "wider meanings" than narrow medical diagnoses.[68] It was also demonstrative of how, just as "battle exhaustion" was used in the Second World War to lessen the stigma of diagnostic labels such as "neurosis" or "psychoneurosis," "operational stress injury" was a military solution to a military medical conundrum.[69]

The new OSI term encompassed a wide range of psychological injuries stemming from military service. These included PTSD, but also other anxiety disorders, depression, and various conditions that are less severe but still impediments to daily functioning.[70] Bringing those various maladies under one umbrella, with an emphasis on "injury," was an attempt to reduce the stigma of psychiatric diagnoses and demonstrate that like a broken leg, the psychological and physiological symptoms of PTSD "resulted from injuries to the brain and psyche, caused by exposure to military-related trauma."[71] Grenier and like-minded reformers wished to place unseen psychological injuries on the same plane as visible, physical ones.[72] In his own words, Grenier's intent was "not to transform the way clinicians diagnose PTSD, but it was to allow our [military] culture to understand that if you go to war, or if you go on an operation somewhere, some people might get physically hurt, but those who are mentally hurt are equally as injured as others."[73] He was trying to achieve "a [physical] parallel for mental health whereby people can talk about Bob now from a mental health perspective outside the clinical terminology. They don't have to say 'Bob has post-traumatic stress disorder,' which has a hugely negative connotation in the minds of that [military] culture. They can simply say 'Bob had a real tough tour, Bob had a real tough operation, he's not been the same; he might be injured.'"[74]

Simultaneously Grenier worked to effect change where the rubber met the road. From 1998 to 2001 he developed a support program for psychologically injured soldiers. In March 2001, while posted at Land Force Central Area Headquarters in Toronto, Grenier learned about the McEachern case and asked his commanding officer, Major-General Walter Holmes, for permission to fly to Edmonton and meet with the young corporal.[75] Holmes, supportive of Grenier's work, gave his blessing. Grenier promptly met with McEachern, who was then awaiting trial at the Alberta Hospital, a psychiatric hospital in northeastern Edmonton. Their meeting convinced Grenier that decisive changes were necessary. He recalled:

I go to the Alberta Hospital ... sign him out for the day, to find out that nobody [from the CAF] had visited him. He was there after doing a bit of time in jail ... We spent the whole day together, hit it off, and that's when it came to me, 'Holy fuck, things have to change.' Because, you know, I had always asked myself through my own isolation and struggles ... 'I'm a captain, I'm a major; if it's tough for me imagine what it must be like for the corporal' ... I have the latitude to take walks, to walk away, to go to meetings, to go for coffee, but a corporal doesn't have all that latitude. So that was a huge precipitating moment.[76]

After seeing McEachern, Grenier decided to meet with fellow veterans from the Rwanda mission during a business trip to Ottawa. There he brought a few colleagues to lunch to hear their opinions about his idea for a peer-support-based program for psychologically affected troops. They were enthusiastic about the idea and provided him with further input. Thus, Grenier became what he called a "glue stick" for various ideas stemming from his research, the McEachern case, and ideas from rank-and-file soldiers.[77]

In May 2001, Grenier's efforts came to fruition with the creation of the Operational Stress Injury Social Support program (OSISS).[78] OSISS became operational in March 2002, and combined the timeless belief that soldiers know best the plight of other soldiers with a formal structure under the aegis of the DND and Veterans Affairs Canada. The first major step involved hiring peer support coordinators (PSCs), men or women diagnosed with an OSI but deemed by their psychologist or psychiatrist to be at a sufficient stage of recovery to handle support work.[79] Each PSC was required to attend training provided by a multidisciplinary team of psychiatrists, psychologists, clinical nursing specialists, and social workers at St Anne's Hospital in Montreal.[80] Training activities included learning about peer support, methods of conflict resolution, understanding and respecting boundaries, and ensuring continued self-care.[81] Once hired and trained, PSCs were involved in a consistent dialogue with clinicians and provided continuing education.[82]

As the program expanded nationwide, the tasks of PSCs included providing outreach and one-on-one assistance for OSIs sufferers, organizing peer-based social support groups, mentoring those in recovery, and organizing volunteer programs.[83] For coordinators like peacekeeping veteran Greg Prodaniuk, one of the first PSCs hired when OSISS launched in 2001, support work was more than a vocation: it provided an outlet for helping others who were suffering. Prodaniuk stated: "I think the compassion and care that I got from those around me when I was not doing well is really the thing that I sort of in a way got addicted to. And that's the piece I think that has been a profound change in my life."[84] Prodaniuk's goal, like that of the entire organization, was to help others experience the same profound change. OSISS was highly praised by the ombudsman in his December 2002 follow-up report to the McEachern complaint. Marin noted that his investigators heard "widespread praise for OSISS throughout the CF community and VAC."[85] He argued that OSISS would be a "key contributor to the cultural change required to combat the stigma associated with OSIs and to ensure that CF members who may have an OSI are not too frightened to come forward to get the help they need as soon as possible."[86] Grenier, Couture, and Wrather were all singled out for their efforts, as well as the "commitment and dedication of the OSISS peer co-ordinators."[87] As illustrated by former PSC Fred Doucette in his 2015 book *Better Off Dead*, although at times an emotionally difficult job, peer support work helped some soldiers step back from the abyss, even if it was often a thankless task: "No medals, no good work, job well done, just that overpowering realization that someone is alive because you cared."[88]

Despite the widespread praise OSISS received, resistance to the program and the term "OSI" nonetheless developed from within the civilian and military medical communities. The "most frequent" complaints came from professionals who saw the Operational Stress Injury term as "imprecise and not reflecting the current terminology their professions use to designate those possessing the symptoms of OSI [i.e., using 'OSI' instead of 'PTSD' and so on]."[89] Grenier attributed much of the resistance to "turf wars" and an ingrained belief amongst some senior CAF leaders that when approaching medical issues "the only people that can have a say of any credence are the people ... [with] the doctor's symbol on their door."[90] He noticed particular pushback from colonel and chief CAF psychiatrist Randy Boddam in Ottawa. As the OSISS program took shape, Grenier believed that Boddam felt threatened by the attention given to ideas coming from outside the medical community. He inferred that medical resistance arose from the fact that "now all of a sudden you have this uneducated guy with no PhD, who's at the same table, and his opinion starts to be valued."[91] Joe Sharpe agreed with Grenier's assessment, affirming that "Randy was a serious obstacle to adopting a new approach to dealing with PTSD ... If he hadn't come up with an idea, then the idea must be flawed. He had major conflicts with other psychiatrists – most notably Greg Passey."[92] Sharpe recalled that during one meeting he attended, Passey and Boddam had an especially heated argument that "nearly came to blows."[93]

Grenier was not the only reformer dealing with resistance in Ottawa. At the same time that Grenier was working to get OSISS off the ground, Colonel Christian Barabé, the commander of the 5th Canadian Mechanized Brigade Group at CFB Valcartier from 2000 to 2002, became concerned about the number of soldier suicides occurring there. Barabé paired with the University of Laval chair of Occupational Health and Safety Management, Jean-Pierre Brun, to try and root out the problem.[94] Particularly concerned that there was no holistic effort to understand the psycho-social issues faced by soldiers, Barabé gave Brun and a Laval research team access to the entire brigade group and its troops, with the goal of discovering the most common issues that soldiers encountered. The researchers conducted interviews, spoke with the chain of command, and utilized questionnaires to ascertain what stresses troops were under and how they felt about their workplace environment.[95] The team used the results to produce a study of the prevailing climate on-base.[96]

When the "medical system" in Ottawa got wind of his actions, Barabé was advised to cease further studies.[97] The study's methodology and legitimacy were called into question, much to Barabé's consternation given the academic credentials of the Laval team.[98] Like Grenier, Barabé attributed the resistance of Ottawa research and medical personnel to "turf wars" and a desire to ensure that innovations came from the CAF/DND centre rather than the periphery.[99] Regardless, he continued with various initiatives. Several innovations were produced at CFB Valcartier, including the Deployment Support Group, a mix of Regular Force and reservists whose job was to provide support for families of soldiers overseas and help injured troops back to work.[100] Joe Sharpe later praised Barabé's enterprises as one of the first systematic studies of soldiers' psychological health, and the basic concept of a deployment support group was later utilized for the Joint Personnel Support Unit, discussed below.[101]

While Barabé fought to implement reforms at Valcartier, in Ottawa, Grenier worked to convince clinicians about the benefits of the OSISS approach. During the program's development Grenier noticed that clinicians around Canada could be roughly divided into three categories: a third were extremely supportive, another third were undecided, and the final third were deliberately or passively obstructive.[102] From the latter group Grenier encountered "strong resistance" to the idea that OSISS could provide an adjunct, social method of alleviating OSIs. Opposition usually stemmed from the belief that OSIs were a strictly medical subject under the sole purview of the medical community.[103] Grenier was disappointed by how many practitioners initially dismissed a more holistic, lay approach: "I'm not going to start telling doctors what to do with their patients, but it is perfectly understandable and acceptable to actually influence our [military] leadership in how to deal with these matters. Because ... people who have Operational Stress Injury or PTSD, or whatever you want to call it, don't live in their doctors' offices. They have to contend day in, day out with society, their family, their workplace, [and] their colleagues."[104] While patients might see their doctor once a week if they were lucky, "at the end of the day, all of it comes together on the ground floor ... where others reside."[105]

The OSI term and OSISS were, in Grenier's estimation, a few of the "multiple ingredients" necessary to reshape CAF culture and ensure that psychologically injured soldiers were supported outside of the clinic as well as within it.[106] While he battled for support in Ottawa and elsewhere, Grenier told his first four peer support coordinators to just "focus on supporting" mentally injured troops and he would take care of solidifying the program's expansion.[107] Shortly after the beginning of OSISS in 2002, he noted a shift among previously undecided clinicians: "That clinical group of people who were extremely supportive of what we were doing grew rapidly ... because they saw how effective that human connection was and how it could be used as a strategic lever to actually achieve greater and faster therapeutic gains for their patients."[108] There were, he acknowledged, bumps along the road, and on a few occasions he had to let PSCs go because he "might have chosen the wrong guy."[109] Nevertheless, the program rolled on, and by 2004 OSISS had over 900 registered serving or retired soldiers on the books.[110] At the time of his retirement in 2012, after a decade of the OSI term's percolation in CAF circles, Lieutenant-Colonel Grenier could see positive steps in how the word "injury" was being applied: to mental injuries as well as physical ones.[111] Though there was more work to be done, a mental "injury" was no longer always "that term [PTSD] that says 'that guy has a disorder, what the fuck is wrong with him?'"[112]

NEW WAR, NEW APPROACHES

While metaphorical battles occurred in Canada over how to handle psychological injuries, Canadian troops were engaged in literal battles in Afghanistan. After the lessons of the Croatia Board of Inquiry, and with Canadian media outlets zeroed in on the mission, CAF and DND officials knew that they could not be caught unprepared to handle a rise in the number of troops returning with mental difficulties. Thus, from the beginning of the Afghanistan War, CAF leaders adopted novel approaches to screening troops, conducting post-deployment health checks, and preparing soldiers for reintegration into Canadian society. One decisive break from 1990s peacekeeping deployments involved the introduction of a practice known as third location decompression (TLD). TLD drew on a range of historical, anecdotal, and sociological evidence that soldiers reintegrated more effectively and better processed the events of their tour if provided a rest and recuperation period before returning home.[113] The most compelling argument for TLD came from Lieutenant-Colonel Pat Stogran, a Bosnia veteran and the first commander of Canadian troops in Afghanistan. Stogran knew the subject well since he had personally experienced difficulties reintegrating after his 1990s peacekeeping tours. He proposed a short stopover and rest for troops prior to their return. The DND promptly accepted his advice.[114]

Thus the first Canadian contingent returning from Afghanistan in 2002 spent several days on the Pacific island of Guam before flying home.[115] Ironically, the TLD site was later changed to Cyprus, the island previously described as Club Med by Canadian peacekeepers in the 1980s and 1990s. Third location decompression, as the name implied, aimed to provide troops time to rest and decompress before readjusting to civilian society. The Cyprus stay also included information sessions on family and work reintegration, anger management, mental health, and suicide risk awareness.[116] OSISS peer support coordinators were also present to share their own post-deployment stories and explain the organization's role in aiding psychologically injured soldiers.[117] While Ombudsman André Marin initially believed that TLD was "not a productive or practical approach to addressing reintegration," particularly since it kept soldiers away from their families even longer, in his December 2002 follow-up report he admitted that "so far the majority of CF members and their families view these actions as very positive."[118]

Although TLD provided Canadian troops much-needed R and R and demonstrated the CAF/DND's commitment to new strategies for reintegration and maintaining soldiers' psychological health, after several years of implementation its efficacy was questioned. An August 2009 *Toronto Star* article based on obtained DND documents claimed that "the defence department's preferred method of treating the mental toll of war is taking a personal financial toll on the troops."[119] Some members, the article reported, were finding quick ways to divest themselves of their salaries and danger pay on Cyprus, largely as a result of soldiers' timeless method of blowing off steam: alcohol.[120] Military officials running the TLD program recommended briefings on the responsible use of money during deployment and a two-drink limit for soldiers' first night of decompression, but such rules were almost impossible to enforce.[121]

Master Bombardier Adam Hailey, who twice deployed to Afghanistan in 2007 and 2008 and was subsequently diagnosed with PTSD, stated that alcohol also had an effect on soldiers' attention during TLD mental health briefings: "You're so fucking hung over or still drunk from the night before, you're just really not paying attention. You're just thinking, 'I need some water.'"[122] Given the psycho-social and other factors that contributed to reintegration, it was difficult to assess TLD's long-term impact on the mental wellness of soldiers; but troops, even despite some misadventures, found the experience useful. A 2012 *Military Medicine* article by Drs Bryan Garber and Mark Zamorski of the Canadian Forces Health Services Group Headquarters in Ottawa stated that although it was tough to appraise TLD as a "medical intervention," sociologically speaking, the majority of Forces members supported TLD and found the program to be valuable.[123] Tod Strickland, deputy commander of PPCLI battle group in Afghanistan, agreed with that assessment. Strickland believed that in addition to helping monitor soldiers' immediate post-deployment mental state, TLD also helped troops transition back to "normal standards of behaviour."[124] Behaviours taken for granted in civilian life, such as "leave your boots at the door, stop swearing all the time, wash your hands before you eat" and "just being civil" were relearned prior to returning to Canada.[125] For that reason, Strickland argued, TLD made a "big difference" in soldiers' social and mental readjustment.[126]

On the battlefield itself, the CAF demonstrated that it was also taking a proactive approach to psychological injuries sustained in theatre. While mental health teams were conspicuously missing from numerous peacekeeping operations in the 1990s, CAF leaders made the decision to send a team early in the Afghanistan conflict.[127] A more novel and radical approach was also taken with regards to traumatic stress.[128] To bolster the view that PTSD and other psychological injuries were as legitimate as physical wounds, medical officers and mental health teams ensured that those treated for post-traumatic stress – but not necessarily diagnosed with an OSI – were returned to duty "as soon as possible."[129] Citing the military unit's important role as a mental bulwark, trauma surgeon Major Ron Brisebois told the *Toronto Star* that quickly returning traumatized soldiers to active duty "tends to minimize the amount of post-traumatic stress they have."[130] The reason was simple: "It allows them to remain with their unit, and stay with their comrades and be accepted as one. It's probably the best way for them to vent their feelings."[131] Though this approach went largely unnoticed when first reported in 2002, five years later, in March 2007, chief CAF psychiatrist Randy Boddam, then deployed on a four-month tour in Afghanistan, made headlines when he revealed that the military was sending some soldiers with OSIs to the Afghan theatre.[132]

The military's decision to send soldiers with OSIs once more unto the breach highlighted the thorny issues surrounding psychological injuries. Boddam's view, expressed to the *Globe and Mail*, reflected the CAF leadership's new official attitude toward the problem: "Let's acknowledge it [mental illness], let's bring it out of the shadows and get people in so they get treatment sooner, and be employable and living [sic] their lives the best they can."[133] He clarified the military's stance by insisting that the Forces did not "deploy knowingly anybody who is suffering from a mental illness that would impair their ability to function in this environment."[134] Instead, physicians and psychologists sent only those who were on "maintenance phases of their treatment."[135] Boddam and Dr Mark Zamorski, head of the military's deployment health section in Ottawa, emphasized the vast continuum of mental health states, with Boddam stating that "not all post-traumatic stress disorders are created equal."[136] The problem, as the Canadian media noted, was that physicians seemed unable to predict the *total* effect that an Afghanistan tour would have on soldiers with OSIs, as well as how an OSI would affect their operational performance. Boddam opined that, assuming all else was equal, placing soldiers in an operational setting "may not in any way exacerbate their illness."[137] On the other hand, Zamorski's honest but nonetheless unsettling appraisal reflected the reality that any attempt to treat psychological injuries in the same manner as physical ones required a journey into the unknown: "Is there somebody who's died in Afghanistan because they weren't paying attention because they were mentally ill? It's possible."[138]

The revelation that some soldiers with OSIs – particularly PTSD – were being sent to Afghanistan raised a stir amongst politicians and the public, and led to questions in the House of Commons.[139] Three days after the *Globe and Mail* printed its story, Navy Commodore Margaret Kavanagh, commander of the Canadian Forces Health Services

Group, wrote a letter to the paper reiterating the CAF's confidence in its approach:

> Canada has deployed, and will continue to deploy, individuals who have been successfully treated for mental or physical illnesses or injuries ... To do otherwise would only perpetuate the stigma around these illnesses and injuries, and continue to drive the problem underground. If we want Canadian Forces members to seek treatment for a mental illness or an operational-stress injury, they need to trust they can be given the opportunity to continue with a full and rewarding career, even with such a diagnosis.[140]

While an aggressive stance toward OSIs might be disagreeable to some Canadians' sensibilities, in the battle against stigma, CAF leaders believed the problem must be tackled head-on. Kavanagh argued that rather than shrinking from such an approach, Canadians "should be celebrating the success of those who have overcome such problems and returned to active duty."[141] Kavanagh's letter and the CAF's new approach demonstrated that, in addition to new attitudes, the war against OSIs also required new – and sometimes ethically ambiguous – actions.[142]

TWO STEPS FORWARD, ONE STEP BACK

The new approach to psychological injuries represented broader efforts by the CAF and DND throughout the first decade of the new millennium to implement reforms in the mental health realm. Those reforms in turn took place under the umbrella of the larger Rx2000 project, a major initiative to rebuild the entire CAF medical system, including mental health services, after the Cold War.[143] One of the main goals of the new initiatives, as stated by Brigadier-General Lise Mathieu, director general of Health Services in 2003, was the "gradual reduction of the fear of 'stigmatization' as a result of OSI," though she admitted that "much remains to be done in this area to reach all those afflicted."[144] Mathieu wrote that military health care professionals had "become only too aware of the growing demand on the part of members of the Canadian forces for mental health services, not only for treatment but also for prevention and promotion of psychological fitness."[145]

Although a new official stance on OSIs pointed to an attitudinal shift amongst senior CAF leaders, there were signs that a significant number of soldiers were unwilling to part with traditional beliefs about mental illness. Just one year after the 2002 ombudman's report on systemic treatment of soldiers with OSIs, André Marin released another report about an incident that took place during the "French Grey Cup" at CFB Winnipeg on 22 November 2002. A long held tradition of the PPCLI since the 1950s, the French Grey Cup was the championship game at the end of the regiment's intramural football season.[146] In addition to the game itself, there was a parade for which soldiers from each company designed their own float.[147] As part of the tradition, one male soldier from each company was also made to dress like a woman – a "queen." The winner, judged to be the most "ravishing," was declared "Miss Grey Cup" and carried off the field by other soldiers.[148] Traditions and entertainment involving gender inversion, and allusions to homosexuality, had a long history in the Canadian military. During the Second World War, for example, male soldiers dressed in drag put on elaborate song-and-dance shows for fellow troops, while others staged mock weddings in which one soldier took on the role of bride.[149]

Aside from the obvious gender connotations, which hearkened back to days when the CAF was an all-male institution, the November 2002 parade also featured an especially unique float. One 2PPCLI company constructed a float depicting a train pulling a cage.[150] Inside the cage was a young man dressed "provocatively in women's clothing."[151] At first glance the float appeared to simply portray a caged man in drag, but further details demonstrated that it carried a different message. The ombudsman's investigation revealed that the float had the words "2PPCLI Express" and "Next Stop North Side" written on it.[152] The North Side colloquially referred to the north area of CFB Winnipeg, which housed the 17 Wing of the Air Force. 17 Wing provided health and social services to 2PPCLI members, including soldiers diagnosed with OSIs who had been reassigned for health reasons to employment in the base's northern area.[153] In popular parlance, those diagnosed with OSIs were said to be going "to the North Side on the Crazy Train," the latter term being an allusion to the song "Crazy Train" by Ozzy Osbourne.[154] While some interviewees prevaricated about the meaning, and an internal investigation concluded that the float did not reference mental illness, the ombudsman's findings confirmed that the float was indeed meant to mock perceived malingerers diagnosed with OSIS.[155] For 2PPCLI members the meaning was self-evident. One soldier interviewed by the ombudsman's team stated that "everybody right up to the CO [Commanding Officer] knows what the Crazy Train is."[156]

The ombudsman's investigation concluded that there was "a widespread perception within 2 PPCLI that a significant number of members who have been diagnosed with OSIS are faking or exaggerating their symptoms. The perception is that they are doing this in order to obtain advantages that are not available to other members, such as occupational transfers and/or pensions."[157] Although the float was apparently only intended to deride malingerers, the message affected all members with OSIS in a similar manner. Former Croatia Board member Mike Spellen was an OSISS peer support coordinator at the time of the incident and recalled receiving a phone call on 29 November 2002 about the parade float: "There were two guys that were pulling that float that were suffering from PTSD, unannounced to the idiots that made them pull this float."[158] Moreover, a civilian worker told Spellen that a 2PPCLI member who was experiencing psychological difficulties said he was reluctant to seek treatment because the battalion looked unfavourably upon OSIS, citing the aforementioned parade float as an example of the unit's hostility.[159] Angry at the float's connotations and 2PPCLI leaders' attempts to downplay the incident, Spellen made a complaint with the OSISS program manager, then Major Grenier, and subsequently contacted the ombudsman's office.[160]

Marin and his team, led once again by Gareth Jones, lead investigator of the McEachern complaint, concluded that the float mocked OSI sufferers, that the battalion's internal investigation was "neither thorough nor objective," and that "much work" was left to be done.[161] The Crazy Train incident once again highlighted the problems of attempting to comprehensively penetrate CAF culture and traditional attitudes concerning mental illness. The incident also brought out prominent commentators. Several days after the ombudsman's report was released and scrutinized by Canadian news outlets, retired major-general Lewis MacKenzie weighed in on the controversy in a 10 March 2003 *National Post* article. MacKenzie expressed dismay that "at the very moment this country is trying to decide if we should be putting our military in harm's way ... Canada's military ombudsman, is focused on the design of a company float during a 2PPCLI unit celebration ...

Only in Canada, I hear you say."[162] Himself a retired PPCLI member, MacKenzie believed the French Grey Cup parade was nothing more than a fun and silly tradition.[163] He also pointed out that the float in question was investigated "as a result of a single complaint"; hardly, in his mind, a sign of larger problems.[164] MacKenzie's overall take was that for 2PPCLI members and leadership "there was nothing in Marin's report to accept responsibility for!" He summed up his stance: "Soldier's humour can be pretty black at times, but in this case it was pretty good; an upfront attempt to send a message to those soldiers who use feigned operational stress injuries to excuse their behaviour or seek medical release with compensation."[165] MacKenzie's response to the Crazy Train incident and subsequent investigation reminded soldiers that "regimental tradition is more important than a backhand slap from someone [Marin] who has not walked the walk."[166] In a further nod to traditional views of the ideal soldier, MacKenzie's rebuttal was also, in his own words, a counterattack against Marin and other reformers' "'touchy feely' philosophy."[167]

Although unpalatable to some, MacKenzie's viewpoint spoke to those who valued traditional attitudes and believed that an increased focus on OSIs created further problems in the form of malingering. That belief was a perennial concern for those who viewed psychological injuries in an unfavourable light, and had roots as far back as the First World War. MacKenzie's arguments also addressed concerns that, in a consistently understaffed military, there were nonetheless always men and women looking for the proverbial free ride. As just one example, Master Bombardier Adam Hailey was diagnosed with PTSD but initially hesitated to accept his condition because he believed that some other soldiers were feigning the disorder for personal gain. He recalled: "It's like, OK well if *this* person's got it [PTSD] then I can't have it. How the fuck can I justify it?"[168] Hailey expressed "disgust" at what one particular soldier "got" and how she "played the system so well," stating that "it's people like that that make it difficult for people like me ... or people that are in that situation similar to me."[169] Hailey's view, and MacKenzie's similar take, demonstrated that despite a professionally estimated low percentage of "fakers," there were strong beliefs that a greater acceptance and willingness to discuss OSIs led many individuals to milk the system.[170]

One problem with adopting such a stance, though, was that exactly who was malingering and the true extent of the problem were subjective determinations when made by anyone but professionals.[171] In a discussion with the author, retired brigadier-general Christian Barabé, commander of Land Force Québec/Joint Task Force (East) from 2005 to 2008, said that a small number of individuals "abusing the system because of the openness" about PTSD was to be regarded as a fact of life, but that those cases "should normally be picked up by the [medical] specialist."[172] In Barabé's estimation, some malingerers slipped through the cracks only because military medical specialists were overworked and thus unable to dedicate a proper amount of time to learning each case's specifics.[173] Consequently, a number of rank-and-file soldiers were "aware of those who are abusing the system," and therefore saw those cases as evidence that psychological injuries in general were illegitimate.[174] That knowledge sometimes led to instances of shaming perceived malingerers, demonstrated by the Crazy Train incident. Unfortunately, such actions had the effect, even if unintentionally, of pushing real OSI sufferers further into the shadows.

A NEW OPENNESS

In spite of the Crazy Train incident, by the first decade of the new millennium it was clear that CAF/DND initiatives, the work of reformers, and consistent media interest had led to a more open dialogue about and greater acceptance of soldiers with psychological injuries – at least in theory. A new consciousness about psychological trauma thus emerged in both military and civil society. One noticeable trend was more frequent media investigations dissecting and explaining psychological trauma in Canadian soldiers of all generations, especially veterans of the 1990s and beyond.

Discussions about mental illness among Canadian soldiers and veterans were few and far between in preceding decades, but several documentaries appeared throughout the 2000s. The first was a November 2001 documentary titled *War Wounds & Memory*, directed by Vancouver-based filmmaker Brian McKeown. Aired by the CBC on Remembrance Day 2001, *War Wounds & Memory* examined the plight of Canadian Vietnam War veterans and their struggle to find meaning in their service whilst simultaneously fighting PTSD.[175] McKeown was, in his own words, "pre-disposed" to the subject.[176] His own father, a First World War combat veteran, had a "darkness about him," and as with many veterans of that conflict, "had nightmares until the end, always about the war."[177] McKeown's interest in making a film about traumatized Canadian veterans was thus rooted in his father's experiences; an introduction in the late 1990s to a group of Canadian Vietnam War vets living in Vancouver; and an "insight and fresh understanding of combat trauma that has taken place from the 1990s to the present day."[178]

After 2001 media interest unsurprisingly shifted to the effect of the Afghanistan War on soldiers' minds. In the lead-up to Remembrance Day 2009, the popular CBC program *The Fifth Estate* aired an episode titled "Broken Heroes" about Afghanistan veterans with PTSD.[179] Featuring candid interviews with Roméo Dallaire as well as rank-and-file soldiers, "Broken Heroes" focused on the psychological costs of modern war. Among other topics, the program examined the darker side of avoiding treatment, with one soldier describing his descent from healthy living into cocaine and alcohol addiction.[180] Soldiers also discussed the self- and culturally imposed stigmas attached to psychological "weakness" amongst people who were built up to feel invincible.[181] Chief of the Defence Staff Walter Natynczyk, while citing the great progress made in retaining soldiers with stress injuries, nonetheless highlighted the military's perennial challenge:

> We permeate the culture, that kind of warrior culture, where we want people to be warriors. We want them [warriors], because they have to go into harm's way at sea, at 40,000 feet in the air, or in places like Afghanistan. We need that. We need them to be adventurous. We need them to be strong of heart. But at the same time we need them to be accepting, that we're not all in armour suits; and that when we do have a problem, that they go in for assistance.[182]

Moreover, although there was a louder dialogue about stress injuries and greater efforts made to retain those afflicted, the reality was that, historically, most of those diagnosed with PTSD either left the military or were discharged.[183] When asked by the program's interviewer whether those statistics suggested that it was better for soldiers to "suffer in silence," Natyncyzk countered that the "emphasis here is on recovery."[184] Natyncyzk's response subtly acknowledged that recovery and a continuing career in the military were still often incompatible goals.

War in the Mind, a 2011 documentary produced by TVOntario and narrated by Canadian actor Paul Gross, likewise focused on the dilemmas facing Afghanistan veterans.[185] It, too, featured interviews with prominent figures like Dallaire and mental health adviser to the DND Dr Rakesh Jetly, as well as poignant recollections by traumatized rank-and-file troops. A well-balanced appraisal of both reforms and obstacles, the documentary exposed the reality that despite significant initiatives such as TLD and peer support programs, old prejudices persisted, with Gross reminding viewers that "militaries are still macho cultures, and especially at the lower levels, the 'suck it up' factor still exists."[186] As one example of enduring attitudes, an unidentified veteran told the story of a traumatized comrade whose peers often snuck up behind him and yelled "boo" to provoke a startle response.[187] The storyteller lamented: "They think it's a joke, they think it's funny because they don't understand ... because they didn't experience it themselves."[188] Such examples were, in Dallaire's mind, evidence that it was necessary to continue the battle and slowly "wear down the system."[189]

In addition to a greater number of documentaries and television programs, another outgrowth of the new national consciousness about psychological injuries was the willingness of soldiers to publish autobiographical accounts about their struggle with PTSD. After Dallaire's influential 2003 book *Shake Hands with the Devil*, other Canadian soldiers were encouraged to write about how PTSD had affected their lives. Retired Bosnia veteran Captain Fred Doucette's 2008 book *Empty Casing* not only described his traumatic peacekeeping experiences in Sarajevo, but also provided a vivid description of how he slowly transformed from a "tough soldier" unwilling to admit any weakness, to an OSISS peer support coordinator in 2002.[190] Doucette discussed many of the unique problems inherent in dealing with OSIs, not the least of which was that recovery, when possible, often took many years.[191] Even long after his peacekeeping tours, Doucette wrote, the sight of a pumpkin on Halloween could still conjure up images of a mangled human head.[192] Like Dallaire, Sharpe, Grenier, and other champions for CAF cultural reforms, Doucette emphasized that despite evident progress, there was a long battle ahead: "It will be a long time before the system will consider an OSI an honourable injury, one that is treatable and not a sign of weakness."[193] He concluded his autobiography by reminding readers of the nation's responsibility for soldiers injured during service, declaring that the last things troops wanted was "to be discarded like an empty [shell] casing and left on the battlefield to disappear into the dust."[194]

Retired lieutenant-colonel Chris Linford, a Gulf War, Rwanda, and Afghanistan veteran with over thirty years' experience with the Regular Force and Reserves, likewise wrote about PTSD's effect on him in his 2013 book *Warrior Rising*. Inspired by Dallaire's example, Linford wrote a candid account of how treatment and understanding brought him back from the brink after traumatic experiences, particularly in Rwanda, had led to his mental deterioration.[195] Similar to many soldiers of the 1990s, Linford's peacekeeping and war experiences haunted him for a long time – ten years – before he was diagnosed with PTSD.[196] In that time, he began to feel that he was gradually experiencing "the loss of my soul as a human as well as my identity as Chris Linford."[197] Unlike previous works by soldiers, Linford's book directly addressed how masculine norms and expectations affected his decision to avoid genuinely confronting his thoughts and emotions.

In an especially poignant anecdote, Linford described leaving for the Gulf War and his nervousness about crying in front of his wife: "I think most males of our society would have similar fears given how we were educated as young boys regarding displays of emotion."[198] Carrying the burden of culturally enforced stoicism on his shoulders, Linford described feeling "shame, weakness and failing as an officer and a man" when he finally admitted to himself that he could not handle PTSD alone.[199] But as he received treatment and came to terms with his situation, he noticed the value in accepting vulnerability as an inevitable part of life for anyone: "I had never felt stronger about who I was and how I needed to think about myself in the future."[200] Linford praised the work of OSISS and the Outward Bound Veterans' Program, a program designed to help mentally and physically wounded veterans utilize outdoor activities and teamwork, with assisting in his recovery.[201] He reiterated the argument, made by several reformers throughout the 1990s and 2000s, that treating psychological injuries was not just a medical responsibility but a social one as well. He declared, "Peer support extends to all of Canada! The importance of the 'Community' to the returning Veteran cannot be understated! It can take many forms, from a peer group, to family, to all neighbours and friends, and indeed the whole country."[202] Like Doucette, Linford emphasized that psychological injuries were treatable if CAF members sought help and openly addressed mental difficulties. Both autobiographies were a testament to the power of social support, and a call for the military and Canadian society to cast off the unrealistic expectations placed on civilian men and soldiers. They were also a testament to a new and persistent dialogue about psychological injuries that began in the 1990s and by the mid-2000s brought trauma into the Canadian national consciousness.

THE NEW VETERANS CHARTER AND PENSION PROBLEMS

Discussions about psychological injuries throughout the decade also took place against the backdrop of evolving legislation and programs for Canadian veterans. After the Croatia Board of Inquiry and several aforementioned reports from the 1990s had highlighted the woeful system of care for peacekeeping veterans, slowly but surely the need to amend the Pension Act became clear. One of the biggest game changers was a review of veterans' care needs, conducted by VAC from 1996 to 2000.[203] The review showed that VAC's Canadian Forces client base had grown at an annual rate of 9 per cent a year from March 1990 to March 1999, but its programs and energy were focused almost solely on older veterans of the Second World War and Korea.[204] It was also clear that as the number of younger Canadian veterans grew, greater coordination between the DND and VAC was required. Another obvious anachronism was the fact that VAC did not even consider peacekeepers who served after the Korean War to be "veterans." In July 2000 the VAC Canadian Forces Advisory Council was formed to provide advice on how to address current and future challenges. Chaired by historian Peter Neary, a specialist in the historical evolution of veterans' programs, the council concluded in October 2002 that "despite numerous and ongoing improvements in the existing range of services and benefits available to ... veterans and their families, the time had come to propose comprehensive reform."[205] After investigating the subject from 2000 to 2004, the council's top two recommendations were "a complete and thorough overhaul of the way that Canadian Forces members are compensated for injury," and "the development of a robust program of transition services and benefits."[206]

The Canadian government declared 2005 to be the Year of the Veteran. On 13 May of that year, the House of Commons unanimously passed the Canadian Forces Members and Veterans Re-Establishment and Compensation Act, popularly known as the "New Veterans Charter (NVC)."[207] The NVC was the brainchild of the Liberal government under Prime Minister Paul Martin, but was implemented by the Conservatives under Stephen Harper after the Liberals' 2006 electoral defeat. The idea was first discussed by Harper, Martin, NDP leader Jack Layton, and Bloc Québécois leader Gilles Duceppe during a flight home from the Netherlands in May 2005, after commemorating Canada's efforts to defeat Nazi Germany and liberate Holland.[208] On the surface it appeared that such rare political unanimity was the result of an emotional trip overseas (the *Toronto Star* implied as much), but as the above paragraph makes clear, politicians' consensus was more the result of several years of study which concluded that the system of care for veterans required a serious overhaul. With Canadian casualties in Afghanistan growing as military involvement there increased, a general understanding formed that politicking should take a back seat to updating archaic policies and programs.

Designed as a "living charter" to supersede the Pension Act, an act that had remained largely the same since the first version was passed in 1919, the NVC provided a series of career transition services, rehabilitation services, vocational assistance, and, of course, disability awards for ill or injured Canadian veterans.[209] The NVC's emphasis, as the act's full title suggested, was on helping veterans transition to civilian life, and in that regard, it included a range of services. As one example, for a small fee CAF members and veterans were provided full access to financial advice through SISIP's Financial Services, allowing them to obtain help on topics such as personal money management.[210] In January 2013, the Harper government also modified the NVC's Career Transition Services Program, providing $1,000 for eligible veterans and their spouses to obtain expert help in finding civilian employment.[211] For families in which the veterans themselves could not benefit from vocational rehabilitation services, family members and spouses were also given access to vocational assistance. That assistance took the form of "educational training, career transition services, job search training and help finding a job."[212] Lastly, veterans, spouses, and other surviving family members were granted access to individual and family health benefits through the Public Service Health Care Plan, a large, private plan sponsored by the federal government.[213]

But despite its novel programs and services, upon its implementation in April 2006, the NVC came under intense criticism when it became widely known that its Disability Award replaced a previous lifelong disability pension scheme for ill or injured veterans with a one-time, tax-free payment that as of 2013 was capped at $298,587.97.[214] An investigation by the *Toronto Star* in November 2010 disclosed that the average payout was $38,000.[215] The capped, lump sum payment, which was revealed by columnist Rosie DiManno to be far less than British and Australian soldiers received, became in many peoples' estimation "The core failing of the Charter."[216]

For soldiers released from the CAF due to psychological injuries, the lump sum payment could prove an especially tantalizing way to spend away their troubles. Mike Spellen, who counselled many traumatized young veterans with substance abuse issues while working as an OSISS peer support coordinator, described one fatal flaw of the new approach:

So here you've got a guy that's an addict, self-medicating, PTSD ... and everything else, and he could have a gambling addiction. You're going to give him "X" number of thousands of dollars one-time payment. And those guys will blow that in a weekend ... And now you've got an angry vet ... Because if a guy's twenty [years old] or something like that, at least if you gave him money every month and he's still got his addiction and you're getting him some treatment, hopefully down the road he's ... [going to break the addiction]. But, you know, they do a one-time settlement for these guys and that might be worth five or ten years' of payments, but you've still got the guy with the problem.[217]

DiManno agreed with the spirit of Spellen's assessment, referencing a *Toronto Star* investigation that revealed that some young vets "jumped at the lump sum offer that looks appealing to a person in their mid-20s who has a poor grasp of the long-term future."[218] Numerous men and women, DiManno stated, "youthful, with little financial guidance –

have blown it on stuff rather than arrange investments and structured money management."[219]

Veterans Ombudsman and former Afghanistan commander Colonel Pat Stogran publicly criticized the NVC on several occasions. Appointed ombudsman in 2007, Stogran turned out to be more than Veterans Affairs Canada and the federal government had bargained for. As Canadian participation in the Afghanistan War – the longest war Canada had ever participated in – came to a close, and an increasing number of wounded soldiers returned, there was strong evidence that old departmental attitudes persisted despite the new charter's implementation. After three years on the job and receiving countless veterans' complaints, Stogran said that VAC had an "insurance company culture of denial" that placed financial savings at the top of the organization's priority list.[220] He further added there was "an overwhelming perception within the veterans community that they're being cheated," and after three years he had "seen the evidence" behind their claim.[221]

Stogran's appraisal sounded eerily similar to claims made by many serving soldiers and veterans during the Croatia Board of Inquiry ten years earlier, and it fuelled several media reports that there was "complete onus on the veteran to prove that he or she has been grievously and irreversibly harmed, with no reasonable prospect of returning to service or the civilian labour force."[222] A study reported in the *Globe and Mail* by Alice Aiken and Amy Buitenhuis of Queen's University compared financial benefits under the Pension Act of 1919 and the NVC of 2005. It, too, criticized the latter legislation. Most troubling was the authors' conclusion: "Our study demonstrates that veterans are financially disadvantaged under the New Veterans Charter. In addition, the compensation gap between the charter and the Pension Act widens if a veteran lives longer, has more children, has a higher disability assessment or is released at a lower rank."[223] In Stogran's view, as he stated before a House of Commons committee in October 2010, the NVC was "clearly an attempt to unload the financial liability, the long-term financial burden that the government carries with injured, wounded veterans."[224]

Perhaps unsurprisingly, Stogran's vocal and frank judgements convinced the Harper government to decide against reappointing him to a second term, with Veterans Affairs Minister Jean-Pierre Blackburn saying it was "time for a new ombudsman to offer a new perspective."[225] But during his final months in the position, Stogran made it clear that he would not go quietly into the night. In August 2010 he declared that the veterans ombudsman position was just "window dressing" for an "obstructive and deceptive" bureaucracy, and avowed that one of his final missions was to let Canadians "know how badly so many of you are being treated."[226] Chief of Defence Staff Walter Natyncyzk, Canada's top-ranking soldier, avoided commenting directly on the government's decision not to reappoint Stogran, but nevertheless stated during a news conference in August 2010 that Stogran had "certainly voiced with clarity what the issues are."[227] Stogran continued his battle even after his term ended, and in March 2013 told the CBC that veterans with PTSD were being denied treatment, and in some cases pensions, after their release. He summed up the situation as "different time, different place, but same old story," describing the VAC system as "an empty shell of treatment and services."[228] Stogran vociferously advocated on behalf of soldiers and veterans, and as a popular and experienced leader, his opinions contributed to a reappraisal of the government's "living charter."

In September 2010, the federal government announced new measures to address the needs of the country's severely wounded soldiers. The government earmarked an additional $2 billion dollars for VAC programs, which benefitted an extra 4,000 veterans over the next five years.[229] Also included in the new measures was a lifetime $1,000 monthly stipend for the approximately 500 veterans who were so severely injured that they were not expected to work again in their lives.[230] Recipients of a disability award were also now provided three options: "a lump-sum payment," "an annual installment over the number of years of a Veteran's choosing," or a combination of the two.[231] In all three cases, however, the payment comprised a lump sum paid out until the total amount awarded was reached, rather than a lifelong, monthly pension. Stogran said he was "encouraged" by the government's move, but still worried about the way the VAC system "set the bar as high as any insurance company in Canada in the interests of preserving the public purse … when the legislation actually directs it should be liberally interpreted."[232] He believed the system was still "severely broken" and there was a "black hole of bureaucrats" who had a "deny, deny, deny" method of handling soldiers' claims.[233] Master Corporal Paul Franklin, an Afghanistan veteran who lost both legs during a suicide bombing in 2006 and was the subject of a 2007 book,

said that the measures were a "good start" but that he did not believe
the financial commitment of $1,000 a month for severely injured sol-
diers was "anywhere near enough."[234] He further added his wish that
the lump sum be increased.[235] For his part, Minister of National
Defence Peter MacKay denied that Stogran's grievances were a factor
in the new changes.[236] In March 2011 Parliament passed the Enhanced
New Veterans Charter Act.

OTTAWA REACTS

As soldiers' pension issues and psychological difficulties became persistent news items, the CAF and federal government responded in several ways. One important initiative was the 2007 announcement of
five OSI clinics administered by Veterans Affairs to help CAF members,
veterans, and their families.[237] Located in population centres across
the country, and later with satellite clinics established for rural
regions, OSI clinics provided "assessment, treatment, prevention and
support to serving CAF members, Veterans and RCMP members and
former members."[238] Family members of these groups were also entitled to receive some of the available services.[239] Each clinic had a team
consisting of psychiatrists, psychologists, social workers, and mental
health nurses, with one of the main aims being the mitigation of psychological issues resulting from mental disorder through therapy sessions.[240] The clinical team also liaised with community practitioners
to ensure that follow-up care was provided and no one in need slipped
through the cracks.[241] Along with OTSSCs, OSI clinics supplied another layer of treatment and social support for the numerous men and
women who required help after Afghanistan and earlier deployments.

By December 2008, when almost 5,000 of the CAF's 87,000 Regular
Force troops and reservists were receiving mental health care in one
form or another, the government earmarked even more money for
OSIs.[242] That announcement came on the heels of Mary McFadyen's
December 2008 Ombudsman report which showed that staff short-
ages were a detrimental factor at some bases. One example was CFB
Petawawa, where 5,100 military personnel were served by only one
psychologist and one psychiatrist, requiring many to travel over 160
kilometres to Ottawa for help.[243] That number was in strong contrast
to CFB Valcartier, which had eight psychologists and four psychiatrists
for 4,500 troops.[244] Given that Petawawa was "the home base for many

of the recent deployments to Afghanistan" at that time, it was un-surprising that the ombudsman's investigators discovered that sol-diers were "having difficulty accessing timely mental health care services."[245] McFadyen's report highlighted that strenuous workloads were an issue for many CAF health care specialists, which made attract-ing and retaining clinicians difficult. In the case of OTSSCs, staff short-ages forced outreach to become more "incremental," since there was a "serious shortage of time available for most mental health profession-als," despite "adequate funds."[246] There were evident challenges for the future.

Another important augmentation for existing services was the 2008 creation of the Joint Personnel Support Unit (JPSU).[247] Commanded in Ottawa by the Director Casualty Support Management, the JPSU was the central administrative unit which oversaw Integrated Person-nel Support Centres (IPSCs) dotted across the country, aiming "to pro-vide comprehensive care and integrated support for ill and injured members and their families."[248] Essentially, the JPSU ensured uniform access to care and consistent approaches throughout centres nation-wide.[249] Put another way, the JPSU and the IPSCs it oversaw were intended as a "one-stop service" for soldiers and families, with the JPSU playing a "central [administrative] role in the transition process for CF personnel recovering from serious illness or injury, and either pro-gressing towards a normal work schedule or preparing for a civilian career."[250] Whereas previously injured members had to seek out med-ical, financial, and vocational resources themselves, the JPSU connect-ed members with those services and cut down on efforts to obtain support and care.[251] But although it was a step in the right direction, perspectives still varied on the JPSU's effectiveness. Some felt that re-moving ill and injured members from the "family structure" of their unit and peers during a period of vulnerability was "an abdication of the fundamental leadership principle of caring for one's own."[252] Brigadier-General Christian Barabé believed that having a centralized command system in Ottawa for ill and injured soldiers meant that "you detach the responsible [local] authorities from actually what's happening on the ground."[253] As with other reforms of the new mil-lennium, there was divided opinion on how to construct a compre-hensive system of care.

Moreover, for psychologically injured troops, there were other ob-stacles to overcome. The Universality of Service principle, still intact in the second decade of the twenty-first century, meant that injured personnel, including those diagnosed with OSIs, had a finite amount of time to either return to normal duties or face release.[254] Many such soldiers who had served in Afghanistan or on peacekeeping missions were posted to the JPSU and subsequently released against their will. As the number of those cases grew, there was, as Ombudsman Pierre Daigle stated in 2012, "a sense on the part of some that an organizational promise was made [to retain psychologically injured soldiers] and then reneged upon."[255] Among soldiers, there was a persistent view that going to an IPSC and being posted to the JPSU was a "kiss of death" for one's career. That belief prevented an unknown but likely significant number of soldiers from seeking care.[256] Nonetheless, the ombudsman wrote that the creation and general acceptance of the JPSU/IPSC structure appeared "to be providing improved management of ill and injured."[257] Despite some hiccups, the JPSU promised better and more standardized care for those in need than previously disparate measures.[258]

Master Warrant Officer Barry Westholm, whose story was recounted in the book's introduction, thought that the JPSU was a "stellar idea."[259] In 2009, he quit the Regular Force – a "huge decision" – to sign on as a reservist, which was a requirement to be employed with the JPSU at that time.[260] After numerous interview stages and screening processes he was accepted, becoming the first regional sergeant major for the JPSU in the eastern Ontario region, the most senior position of a non-commissioned officer in the unit.[261] Initially, he felt the staff level was adequate and that overall the unit ran smoothly. What he discovered shortly after work began, however, was that the JPSU was already at an "end state."[262] No provision was made for any staff increases as the number of personnel posted to the unit grew. Thus, after the early "great success," the unit became inundated when existing staff were forced to handle a sharp climb from approximately 100 to 500 soldiers posted to it.[263] In spite of their best efforts, JPSU staff became, in Westholm's words, "overwhelmed."[264] He recalled that "the people that suffered were both the staff and the people posted-in."[265]

As the situation deteriorated, Westholm felt an inner conflict between the need to obey his superiors, and his responsibility to the ill and injured soldiers under the unit's care. The inability of staff to keep up with the heavy workload meant that, in his mind, they were putting ill and injured soldiers "in harm's way."[266] In a testament to the situation's severity, Westholm remembered: "We did lose people to suicide. And although I could never state categorically that the situation in the JPSU contributed to the suicide, I can say that we didn't do enough to prevent them ... because we couldn't get to them all in time."[267] He attempted to carry on, but shortly after the January 2013 death of Master Corporal Charles Matiru, a four-time Afghanistan veteran who committed suicide after suffering from PTSD, Westholm resigned in protest – one of the strongest gestures a military member could make.[268] His very public decision was meant to draw attention to the JPSU's "dire need for assistance."[269] Thus he laid everything on the line and, in his words, "grenaded" all his bridges.[270] He subsequently sent a document to the governor general, prime minister, and numerous military leaders, outlining both the hard work of JPSU staff and their tragic inability to cope with the demands placed on them.[271] Westholm's commanding officer said that his behaviour was "very much a disappointment," and his officer commanding later told him to "just stay home," an order he nonetheless refused to follow.[272] Although his resignation did not make the splash he hoped for, a series of *Ottawa Citizen* articles in 2013, partially responsible for a late-2013 ombudsman's investigation into the JPSU, lent credence to Westholm's claims.[273] A year after his resignation he told *Citizen* reporter Chris Cobb that there was a "spectre of indifference" towards veterans within the federal government.[274]

Ombudsman Pierre Daigle's 2013 preliminary assessment of the state of the JPSU bolstered Westholm's assertions and raised more red flags. Although JPSU commander Colonel Gerry Blais described staff levels as adequate, after soliciting comments from sixteen JPSU staff and 177 clients, Daigle wrote that "60% of interviews referenced insufficient staff numbers relative to JPSU member and client demands."[275] His assessment concluded: "Observations made during this review suggest there may be a requirement to review overall governance of support offered to ill and injured members."[276] Several months later, the *Citizen* once again drew attention to the systemic problems outlined by Daigle, with Chris Cobb writing that the JPSU still remained understaffed.[277] Despite requests for figures on the situation at Petawawa and Ottawa, which were considered "the most overloaded and inefficient units," JPSU staff refused to provide the *Citizen* with the information Cobb wanted.[278] For all of its hard work, the JPSU was, by 2014, "widely criticized by serving soldiers, veterans of JPSU and military mental health specialists."[279]

2014 began as another bad year for the unit, as eight CAF suicides in a little over two months brought more criticism from veterans' advocates.[280] The case of Lieutenant-Colonel Stéphane Beauchemin was another controversial flashpoint. A veteran of Haiti and Bosnia operations in the 1990s, Beauchemin was posted to the JPSU on a return-to-work program when he committed suicide in January 2014. His death implied serious problems within the CAF mental health network.[281] Late in 2014 the situation became more desperate as the Ottawa IPSC, one of the busiest in the country, had two staff members quit, leaving two section commanders to assist more than 225 injured personnel.[282] While the centre attempted to regroup, soldiers with urgent crises, including PTSD, were told to dial 911 or visit Ottawa's Montfort Hospital.[283] IPSC platoon commander Lieutenant (Navy) Adam Winchester said that the centre's tempo had "rapidly increased."[284]

While JPSU staff continued to battle their workload and veterans' groups continued to express dissatisfaction, in 2015 the Department of National Defence "quietly shelved" an internal investigation into the unit, stating that a report would not be completed until sometime in 2017.[285] That decision was a disappointment to Ombudsman Gary Walbourne, who had halted his 2013 probe based on an understanding that the DND would issue its own report by summer 2015.[286] In response, in July 2015 Walbourne resumed his own investigation, stating that given the JPSU's importance for ill and injured troops, a report was necessary "now, rather than later."[287] Others agreed. Retired corporal Chris Dupée, who in 2011 had founded Military Minds, a 130,000-strong online PTSD awareness group, told the *Ottawa Citizen* that the system continued to fail many of its injured, who were "falling through the cracks."[288] In the same article, Westholm commented that the JPSU had great potential but was "horrifically mismanaged at the highest level."[289] Thus, although important initiatives and reforms had been made since the new millennium, fifteen years later there were still many individuals from within and outside the military who believed that the system let many soldiers and veterans down, sometimes with dire consequences. Military leaders and DND officials were cognizant of the need to admit the existence of mental health problems in the CAF and veteran population, but they were still unwilling to admit when they had a tiger by the tail. Instead, they fell back on a tried and tested method: deny the extent of the problem until it blew over. Soldiers and veterans suffered while the PR battle continued.

Enduring Struggles and Enduring Hope

Strong legs protrude out of masses of kit [equipment] as we walk across the field, and I feel as if the shades of Canadian soldiers from battlefields past are walking with us, and are embodied in us. For the first time, I feel part of the long, proud Canadian military tradition that is so often forgotten, misunderstood, or just marginalized.

Flavelle, *The Patrol*, 86.

As the Afghanistan War continued through the 2000s and early 2010s, the number of physically and mentally injured soldiers increased exponentially. Concurrently, the precise number of psychologically injured troops became a disputed issue; as in past conflicts, rates and figures widely varied. A 2007 *Toronto Star* article featuring an interview with Dr Mark Zamorski stated that about 28 per cent out of a total of 2,700 CAF soldiers screened after Afghanistan had symptoms of mental health problems.[1] An April 2009 *Toronto Star* article featuring figures provided by VAC spokesperson Janice Summerby stated that one in five deployed to Afghanistan – 1,053 Canadian soldiers and police officers – later left the CAF and RCMP with PTSD or other psychiatric problems.[2] The article further reported that VAC expected an increase in the total numbers over time.[3] In her 2008 report on OSIs, interim CAF/DND ombudswoman Mary McFadyen avoided using exact figures, but estimated that the number of soldiers and veterans with psychological difficulties was likely in the thousands.[4] Yet another *Toronto Star* article from 2010 said that the number of Afghanistan veterans with PTSD was about 5 per cent – "at least 1250."[5] Figures like those were enough evidence for the conservative and controversial *Globe and Mail* columnist Margaret Wente to agree with

Lewis MacKenzie. She believed that numerous veterans were abusing the system: "When stress is mowing down far more troops than the Taliban, maybe something's out of whack."[6] But in spite of Wente's assessment, a consistent stream of reports suggested that the number of casualties was growing.

While a perennial debate over the extent of psychological casualties continued, the public's attention was drawn to another dark shadow of the Afghanistan War: suicide. Throughout the 2000s, Canadians became increasingly aware of the unsettling frequency of suicide amongst CAF members. In 2009, for example, there were sixteen recorded CAF personnel suicides, the highest annual number since tracking began in 1995.[7] In late 2013, four soldiers committed suicide in just one week.[8] One of them, Master Corporal Sylvain Lelievre from the Van Doos Regiment, had deployed to Bosnia three times before serving in Afghanistan in 2010.[9] The quick succession of suicides in 2013 led the charismatic former chief of the Defence Staff General Rick Hillier – "Uncle Rick" as he was affectionately called by troops – to call for a board of inquiry or Royal Commission.[10] Although suicides were difficult to directly tie to deployments, they nonetheless raised further questions about the CAF's approach to mental illness and the extent to which support mechanisms were failing troubled soldiers.[11] More pressure was placed on the CAF and federal government when DND statistics revealed that between 2002 and 2014, more soldiers had been lost to suicide (160) than combat in Afghanistan (138).[12] Those statistics, which included reservist suicides, a category left out in past tallies, led opposition MPs to accuse the federal government of "lowballing" earlier figures to downplay the issue.[13]

One of the most troubling cases was that of Corporal Stuart Langridge, a "dedicated, loyal and motivated" veteran of Afghanistan and the former Yugoslavia, who committed suicide in his room at CFB Edmonton after struggles with depression, alcohol, and drugs – all potential signs of PTSD.[14] In the aftermath and ensuing investigation, many disturbing details emerged about both Langridge's case and the Canadian Forces National Investigation Service's (CFNIS) handling of the matter. Langridge's stepfather Shaun Fynes accused the CFNIS of withholding Langridge's suicide note for fourteen months. He claimed that the note revealed that Langridge had PTSD and thus was withheld as part of a "very calculated deception to protect the uniform from embarrassment."[15] Mr Fynes later told a Military Police

Complaints Commission (MPCC) inquiry that Langridge was "ping-ponged" between civilian and military medical systems, with the former not wanting to deal with him and the latter not knowing what to do.[16] Both Mr Fynes and his wife Sheila, Langridge's mother, claimed that their son was treated as a drunk and an addict by superior officers.[17] Mr Fynes declared before the commission that Corporal Langridge was essentially "killed by the military."[18] Adding to the controversy, after the MPCC inquiry ended, Ottawa Citizen reporter Chris Cobb revealed that the sixty-two day inquiry and investigation cost more than $3.5 million.[19]

The Langridge case and its aftermath received national media attention and exposed controversies that proved embarrassing for CAF and DND officials. In one particularly strange instance, Cobb's colleague David Pugliese at the Ottawa Citizen claimed that in 2010 he was asked, or rather urged, to discontinue writing about the Langridge case by an officer ostensibly working for the chief of defence staff.[20] Pugliese suggested that CAF and DND leaders were upset because "the Langridge story challenged the military's and government's message that Afghan veterans were being taken care of," and because the story drew national media attention to the implied link between post-traumatic stress and suicide.[21]

In addition to suicide, veteran crime also became a national issue in the 2000s and 2010s. As the McEachern case demonstrated, the DND, VAC, and Canadian criminal justice system were in uncharted waters when handling veterans with PTSD accused of criminal offences. In December 2013, the Globe and Mail reported on the case of John Collins, a British veteran with PTSD who was arrested in Lethbridge, Alberta on several charges, including assault.[22] Collins was held in the Lethbridge Correctional Centre – the same jail where Afghanistan veteran Travis Halmrast, charged with domestic assault, had committed suicide just over a week earlier.[23] For his part, Collins felt that his mental health was not properly taken into account prior to or after his arrest. Ironically, he was arrested by Lethbridge police officers after his wife, Anne, inquired about PTSD services in the community. Fearing that she was being abused, police questioned her and then subsequently arrested Collins at his home.[24] Mrs Collins denied that her husband had done anything wrong.

The appearance of Collins's and Halmrast's cases in national newspapers forced the DND, VAC, and Correctional Service Canada (CSC) to admit that they had no system for tracking – or firm statistics about – veterans in the criminal justice system.[25] The authorities' slow reaction to the problem was demonstrated by a 2010 CSC report which utilized information collected from 2,054 offenders to estimate that there may be "626 offenders who served in the Canadian military" and "633 sentenced or remanded veterans in provincial or territorial corrections."[26] CSC believed that those figures amounted to almost 3 per cent of the offender population.[27] More damning were the report's assertions that "veterans often have treatment needs for psychological injuries such as post traumatic stress disorder" and that "it is possible … the presence of PTSD or unresolved issues surrounding trauma may impact the offender's safe transition to the community."[28] In the three years between when the report was issued and Collins and Halmrast appeared in the news, no uniform system to address those issues had been established. For his part, Veterans Ombudsman Guy Parent stated that the presence of so many veterans in the correctional system was a major reason why the federal government should make it a priority to track soldiers upon release.[29]

The CSC report also noted that officials had examined the prevalence of veterans in American and British prisons. While the proportion of Canadian veterans in prison was roughly equal, Canadian authorities, unlike their American and British counterparts, had done little to remedy the problem. The US was perhaps the most ahead of the game in addressing the issue of veterans and crime. In 2008 the Center for Mental Health Service, part of the US Substance Abuse and Mental Health Services Administration, convened a conference whose purpose was to "decrease the involvement of Veterans with the justice system and to provide them with mental health treatment."[30] Attended by representatives from law enforcement, corrections, the courts, veterans' advocacy organizations, and federal agencies, the conference produced a blueprint for a "Veterans Treatment Court (VTC)."[31] With the goal of avoiding "unnecessary incarceration of veterans who have deployed to war and subsequently developed mental health problems," VTCs allowed veterans with mental health or substance abuse issues to, upon arrest, seek treatment instead of going through a criminal court.[32] A man or woman who opted for a VTC was assessed by mental health professionals and, if deemed eligible, provided with treatment. Participation was voluntary, but their ability to remain in the community hinged on fulfillment of the program's requirements, and their compliance was regularly monitored by a judge. If a participant failed drug tests or disobeyed court orders, they faced community service, fines, or jail time.

The results were encouraging. In Buffalo, New York, after one year of the VTC's implementation there was a 0 per cent recidivism rate among those who had completed the program.[33] Unfortunately, despite coverage of VTCs by national newspapers and the CBC, Canadian officials had not instituted similar programs to prevent veterans from ending up on the wrong side of the law. In December 2015, the case of Master Corporal Collin Fitzgerald showed that the problem was still ongoing. A veteran of Afghanistan and earlier peacekeeping missions, Fitzgerald was one of the first soldiers awarded the Medal of Military Valour (the third highest award for valour in the Canadian Forces), in 2006. Like numerous comrades, he suffered from PTSD and the haunting memory of wartime deeds. After one suicide attempt and several criminal offences, in 2013–14 he spent sixteen months in mental health institutions and under house arrest.[34] By 2015 Fitzgerald decided it was time to get his life back on track. With time he learned to use positive participation in veterans' organizations and public speaking as a way to "turn pain into purpose." In the end it was mainly those outside the military, and his surety, whom he credited with helping him "turn things around."[35] After pulling out of his tailspin, Fitzgerald found a better path, but he knew he still had a long road ahead: "I go to bed at night, and I still see people that I killed in my eyelids … Is that going to go on for the rest of my life? I don't know."[36]

LEGACIES AND DILEMMAS

By the end of Canada's combat operations in Afghanistan in July 2011, over 40,000 service personnel had been deployed there, making the Afghanistan War the largest Canadian military operation since the Second World War.[37] During the war, 158 soldiers died, and 1,859 members were physically wounded.[38] In addition, of the 25,000 to 35,000 military members expected to release from the CAF between 2011 and 2016, at least 2,750 were predicted to suffer from a severe form of PTSD, and a further 5,900 were predicted to suffer from other diagnosed mental health problems.[39] In terms of concrete figures, as of March 2010 VAC psychiatrists had 12,689 total cases, with PTSD numbering 8,758 of those.[40] By 2015, the OSISS network had assisted over 10,000 peers during its fourteen-year existence, indicating both the past and future need for its services.[41] The creation of groups such as Wounded Warriors Canada, a non-governmental organization assisting physically and mentally wounded soldiers through a series of national programs and events, was also a sign that government initiatives were not always enough.[42] Christian Barabé matter-of-factly stated that although Wounded Warriors and similar groups provided excellent and necessary assistance, their very existence demonstrated "that there are deficiencies in the system."[43]

At present, soldiers and veterans with psychological difficulties still face the possibility of ostracism by their colleagues, friends, and superior officers. Even in the second decade of the twenty-first century, problems of the mind are often interpreted by military members as a sign of weakness.[44] Those stigmas, widespread in civilian society as well, are heightened in a military milieu. The John Wayne figure – tough, stoic, brave, and seemingly invincible – still constitutes the manly ideal for much of Canadian and North American society, especially in the military.[45] Despite decades of medical and socio-cultural changes, which saw the dominant image(s) of masculinity bend and mental illness no longer interpreted through overtly gendered medical theories, traditional masculinity still pervades society as a whole.[46] Even the rise of the double-income family and working mother, initially viewed by many as a sign of men's social decline, has not thoroughly damaged the belief that a man's identity is tied to his role as breadwinner and family leader.[47] The military's fitness culture and a heightened need to adhere to masculine norms combine to convince many soldiers that the best approach to any physical or mental problems is to tough it out and soldier on. Former CAF reservist Ryan Flavelle's apt summary of this culture, reproduced at the beginning of the last chapter, demonstrates the perpetual state of attitudes that have only altered slightly over the past one hundred years.

In the Canadian Forces, concerns about remaining with the military, and suffering peer rejection, have led to a perennial stigma and fear surrounding mental illness. Retired lieutenant (Navy) Bruce McKay, a chaplain who served from 1980 until 2013, spoke with hundreds of soldiers about their innermost thoughts and private matters throughout his career. By the late 2000s he saw changes in how troops spoke about mental health problems, with fewer soldiers engaging in outright denial when something was wrong. Nevertheless, he noticed that instead of openly acknowledging problems, many opted for veiled statements such as "I'm just dealing with some stuff at home."[48] McKay also noticed reluctance among soldiers to see military medical staff or social workers, because such information went into their personnel file. The decades-old fear of their problem "getting out" persisted.[49] Troops' worry that private information expressed during their appointments would somehow reach their superiors or colleagues was enough to keep many silent. In an attempt to seek some form of help, soldiers sometimes requested private discussions with McKay. During those conversations they would "talk about 'can't sleep', would talk about nightmares, [and] they would talk about how they've woken up strangling their wife and things like that."[50]

For many dealing with emotional difficulties or psychological stress, social support proved a key factor in their resiliency. Master Corporal Toby Prigione, due to be released from the military in 2014 because of mental and physical health matters, said that family and groups like OSISS were particularly helpful. She stated that, quite simply, "It's always nice just to have someone who's willing to listen."[51] Retired Sergeant Derek Spracklin, a veteran of Bosnia, Kosovo, and Afghanistan tours, likewise believes in the power of support: "You definitely need a good support network."[52] Like Greg Prodaniuk, Spracklin aimed to use his positive experiences with peer support and his "gift of the gab" to help others: "I love sitting down with guys, chatting about coffees, chatting about stories, and trying to help them along ... When you sit down with the groups of guys and girls [in OSISS group discussions] ... it gets people understanding ... everybody has had their own problem ... Out of ten people, nine have gotten through it and you're the one that's waiting to get through it."[53] Spracklin believes that with regard to mental health problems, often there is "more to it" than medical diagnoses.[54]

For retired sergeant Daniel Hrechka, a veteran of two Middle Eastern peacekeeping tours, family and peer support were a critical factor in getting over traumatic events. Since being diagnosed with PTSD in 2010, "it's been family and peer support ... hanging with other guys that are going through ... different stages of their healing process."[55] Hrechka affirmed that "being with like-minded soldiers is a really warming feeling" because "we know we're surrounded by people that get it."[56] He found it difficult to discuss his problems with civilians, particularly because of his injury's invisible character: "You look at me, you don't see anything wrong. That's the constant battle with the civilian population. 'There's nothing wrong with you, Dan, you're fine.'"[57] Myths and misconceptions made support from those that "get it" all the more crucial for normalizing his experiences and path to recovery.[58]

The military must train men and women to be tough, so that they are able to face all manners of physical and mental duress. That axiom was crudely but accurately summarized by one soldier during the Croatia Board of Inquiry: "You have to train them to be dangerous weapons ... You can only put so much of a leash on a pit bull because you know he has still got to be the pit bull if need be."[59] How to train so-called pit bulls and still have them show empathy towards injured comrades is the biggest dilemma the military faces in any attempt to reshape CAF culture. Injuries, especially the mental wounds that are often invisible and subject to numerous discretionary factors, challenge the warrior ethos that the military instills. The ideal warrior of earlier eras has changed in untold ways, and there can be no doubt that soldiers with psychological injuries are, by and large, better off than their counterparts earlier in the twentieth century. Nevertheless, as this book has demonstrated, there are still obstacles ahead. One of the military's biggest challenges will be to convince soldiers to abandon the "cult of the strong, silent individual" who bears all suffering stoically, in favour of a team-oriented approach to health and wellness.[60] When queried about change over time, retired brigadier-general Sharpe stated that in the past fifteen years he has seen "a growing acceptance of the team at the core of the warrior ethos."[61] The challenge, he believes, is "to get that culture to continue to evolve."[62]

By examining trauma in the Canadian military during the post-1991 period, this book has brought together events and themes previously discussed in a disparate manner, and created future opportunities for comparative histories that draw on the experiences of veterans from different eras. This work has begun to fill a gap in the Canadian historical literature on war trauma, much of which has revolved around the historical experience of shell shock during and after the First World War. Recounting the Canadian military experience with trauma after the Cold War, it has also highlighted the persistence of trauma narratives throughout the nation's participation in both wars and peacekeeping operations after 1914, and demonstrated the diverse ways that history can provide signposts for contemporary and future discussions. At the same time, it has examined how individual experiences are shaped by, interact with, and alter prevailing cultural ideas of trauma. Listening to post-Cold War veterans' experiences helps us to understand that while trauma has been an ongoing theme in modern wars and peacekeeping, its expression and conceptualization has been framed by historical contingencies. This speaks to the need to continue exploring those contingencies, as well as the various lenses through which trauma is viewed by physicians, the military, politicians, the public, and of course, the soldiers.

From a historical perspective, Sharpe's aforementioned thoughts on military culture and the many reform initiatives to de-stigmatize mental illness support historian Mark Micale's belief that the early twenty-first century represents a unique cultural and historical moment for discussing topics, such as masculinity and mental illness, that were previously kept hidden from view.[63] Like Paul Jackson's 2004 work on homosexuality in the military during the Second World War, this book is a product of a more open approach to topics that previously were entirely taboo for the military, general public, and historians.[64] One inadvertent effect of Canada's peacekeeping and war operations in the 1990s and 2000s was the reappraisal of decades-old approaches to mental injuries. Traditional approaches, which left numerous troubled veterans to merely reminisce with comrades over a beer at their local Legion, no longer sufficed. In battling psychological injuries, the military, physicians, and the Canadian public were forced to look inward and acknowledge the individual, institutional, and cultural beliefs that kept such topics off the table for so long. Importantly, this introspection also involved addressing predominant views of the ideal man and warrior.

Peacekeeping trauma, and later the Afghanistan War, brought mental health problems out of the shadows, and a dedicated group of CAF reformers contributed to a national dialogue on a previously unseen scale. The lived experiences of those who publicly shared their stories during the Croatia Board of Inquiry, and after Afghanistan, highlighted the political, medical, and cultural factors that shaped trauma discussions throughout the late twentieth and early twenty-first century. Trauma, moreover, helped to force a reevaluation of Canada's role in international affairs. The question, still under debate, is this: If peacekeeping is rarely peaceful, and wars seem no longer winnable in a traditional sense, what role should Canada play on the world stage? The Afghanistan conflict temporarily brought war back as the military's *raison d'être*, but with the mission's recent end in 2014, it remains to be seen how Canadians will reconcile their dual image as peacekeepers and warriors – just as it remains to be seen whether peacekeeping, in whatever form it may take, will once again become the military's primary role in international conflicts. As a member of several major political and military alliances, the image that Canada chooses to project to the world carries significant socio-political and economic consequences, most obviously for the soldiers themselves. Such choices are not easily made, especially in a country that has been an enthusiastic peacekeeper but which remains, in the words of Ian McKay and Jamie Swift, "ever divided and ambivalent about war."[65]

Policy makers in the twenty-first century face an increasingly mobilized and vocal group of post-Cold War veterans. With the rise of the Internet, it is far quicker and easier for veterans within Canada and internationally to connect, discuss issues, and air grievances. When driving by or visiting local Legion branches, younger veterans are often a rarer sight than their elderly counterparts. The former group seems to prefer the relative anonymity and accessibility that the Internet provides to keep up to date with current issues and seek help. Websites such as Military Minds, founded by Canadian corporal Chris Dupee, an Afghanistan veteran who battled PTSD after his return, make it far more difficult for governments to simply ignore a problem until it blows over. Military Minds and similar sites and organizations provide veterans with a chance to share stories and publicize egregious cases of bureaucratic nonchalance or heavy-handedness. The news media, itself facing major changes and downsizing as more Canadians opt for online instead of print news, can now utilize the Internet's ubiquity to place sustained pressure on government officials. While tangibly measuring the Internet's effect on government policy is difficult, it is clear that websites, at the very least, provide a way for veterans to take charge of their military or post-military life with less fear of being "hushed up" or censured. That said, recent reports that physically and mentally wounded CAF members were required to sign a form agreeing not to criticize the military on social media are a sign that authorities and government officials are already practising a form of Internet censorship and damage control.[66] How this battle will play out, and the Internet's long-term effects on government policy, remain to be seen.

This book is in many respects a product of the dialogue and events it has related. The experiences shared by CAF members and veterans, quoted throughout these chapters, represent a unique historical moment when Canadian veterans, for the first time, have been willing to publicly express the consequences of PTSD – or whichever term we choose for psychological injuries resulting from traumatic experiences. The legacy of shell shock, battle exhaustion, PTSD, and more recently OSI support the view held by many historians that psychological trauma and psychiatric language are often shaped by cultural beliefs that are produced and altered within a war, and, in the Canadian case, within peacekeeping contexts. The creation of the OSI term, a military solution to CAF cultural beliefs about "disorders," demonstrates the contingency of language utilized to encapsulate trauma's effects, and psychological illness more broadly.

It is unclear what psychiatrists will choose to call PTSD in the future, and how that term will be altered, but historical evidence suggests that we are far from at an end point when it comes to medical terminology connoting trauma.[67] Despite its status as a non-medical term, the creation of new concepts like OSI suggests a continuing tension between a universal representation of trauma encapsulated in the PTSD concept, and the lived experiences of those exposed to it. It also demonstrates the power of institutions like the military to shape cultural beliefs. Psychiatric terminology, despite numerous attempts, is still unable to capture and keep hold of the myriad ways in which trauma is *socially* refracted by individuals and societies. History suggests that it will be a long time, if ever, before psychiatry is able to accomplish such a formidable task. Equally important, just as shell shock, battle exhaustion, and PTSD stemmed from wartime and peacekeeping encounters with trauma, the creation of the OSI term illuminates the continuing influence of military needs on cultural representations of trauma. The tension between medical authority, sympathy toward psychological injuries, and the CAF's desire to preserve manpower will also likely continue for a long while yet.

Canadians have justifiable reasons to take pride in our nation's military heritage, much of which has been forged by war deeds and peacekeeping operations around the globe. As the title of Jack Granatstein's book on Canada's Army suggests, a large part of our nation's historical experience has been shaped by both "Waging War and Keeping the Peace."[68] This belief was echoed in military historian Tim Cook's assertion that while Canadians deem themselves an "unmilitary people," Canada has nonetheless "also turned readily to war in support of allies, alliances, international obligations, ideals, or humanitarian relief."[69]

Lurking behind the grand narratives are the debilitated veterans; the shell-shocked, battle-exhausted, and mentally injured soldiers from past conflicts whose experiences helped to inform such narratives. They are the men and women whose stories are erased by the powerful whitewashing of history which suppresses the less palatable aspects of our national story. At times our historical record towards injured veterans, particularly those psychologically harmed by military service, has proved wanting. Throughout the past one hundred years, many veterans' road to hell was paved by the ostensibly good intentions of politicians and pension officials. The road was also paved by persistent mental health stigmas and unrealistic expectations of what it meant to be a proper man and soldier. A lamentable ambivalence, or national blind spot, has sometimes characterized the Canadian public's attitude toward traumatized veterans. The scenes of suffering, death, and destruction from conflicts of the past century are symbolized and embodied in the psychologically injured soldier, who stares back at us like a dark mirror we do not wish to gaze into. Thus with each passing conflict Canadians seem to gradually forget about those who have borne the brunt of our foreign policy decisions. This ambivalence has been most evident with regard to the new generation of post-Cold-War-era veterans, those who have participated in peacekeeping missions and conflicts that did not have the easily defined good-versus-evil narratives of the First and Second World Wars. Many Canadians know little to nothing about their deeds. Relatively speaking, their numbers are much smaller than their early to mid-twentieth century counterparts. But, as thinkers across time have held, the true test of a nation's morals and values is how it treats its more vulnerable citizens, regardless of their number.

In our collective desire to form a national identity based on our most treasured values, we in the peaceable kingdom must not forget about those who have witnessed the worst in humanity and committed sanctioned acts of violence on our behalf, for they have in many cases sacrificed their mental health for the nation. In the conflict between how military missions are memorialized and their often grim reality, veterans of all ages represent our closest link to the unfiltered version of the story. They are the nearest that those of us who have never served will get to the "truth" of war – something often buried under a pile of politicking and myth-making.

FINAL THOUGHTS

Since this story opened with an anecdote about Canadian veteran Barry Westholm, it seems fitting to conclude by briefly tracing the subsequent path taken by the reformers and psychologically injured veterans who have been discussed throughout this narrative.

After he left the Joint Personnel Support Unit in 2013, Westholm became an advocate for physically and mentally injured soldiers. He frequently counsels and supports injured soldiers, particularly when it comes to the labyrinthine process involved in seeking compensation. He also acts as the proverbial bee in the bonnet of CAF and DND officials, frequently sending e-mails to politicians and military leaders about an injured soldier's situation, suggesting that remedial action be taken or hastened. Given his long career, his personal struggles with PTSD, and his experiences with the JPSU, Westholm is a fount of knowledge about the treatment of soldiers with injuries, and his thoughts and efforts have been spotlighted numerous times by the *Ottawa Citizen*. He divides his time between advocacy efforts and attempting to convince military and DND leaders to overhaul their system for aiding injured troops transitioning to civilian life, particularly the JPSU.

After his retirement in 2012, Stéphane Grenier began utilizing the lessons he learned from his OSISS experience in the civilian workplace. He founded Mental Health Innovations, an organization dedicated to bringing peer support initiatives and other innovations to the corporate environment, shortly after his retirement from the CAF. Dissatisfied with mere talk, Grenier wants to contribute to a paradigm shift in how mental illness is approached by Canadian civilians, just as he did in the military. He sees many similarities between military and civilian mental health issues, and believes that Canadians as a whole need to address the stigmas that pervade our society: "Both [groups] will have a tendency to isolate, both will resist treatment, both will resist taking medication, regardless of the culture. Both will try to get over this [injury] themselves. Both will be embarrassed at the same level. Both will self-stigmatize."[70] Grenier still firmly believes in the power of social support, stating that "social support will provide hope, and with hope you can open the door to recovery."[71]

Joe Sharpe continues to work in several capacities, including as a patron for Veterans Emergency Transition Services, a non-profit corporation headquartered in Nova Scotia that provides aid to transient and homeless veterans across Canada. Recently, he was "reactivated" as a strategic advisor to the CAF Strategic Response Team investigating sexual misconduct within the Forces – another perennial issue for the military.[72] Given his long and multifarious career with the military, he views the necessary reform of CAF culture not only as a prerequisite for the improved treatment of individual men and women of the Forces, but also "as a matter of operational readiness."[73] He sees the continuing erosion of the "old culture" as one of the main challenges facing the military over the coming decades.[74] After the Croatia Board of Inquiry, Sharpe and Mike Spellen remained friends, and are still in regular contact with one another. When Spellen was asked his opinion about what needs to be done to combat systemic CAF problems, he matter-of-factly replied: "The government's got to stand up. Either that, or next time you want to go to war, send all the politicians over."[75]

For Andrew Godin, life since retirement in 2006 has been "an ongoing battle."[76] After his 1990s peacekeeping deployments he found himself increasingly disconnected from his family, and physicians advised him not to seek employment. Godin found such advice difficult to heed because "every fibre in your body tells you [that] you should be out doing something ... the things that a man or a person is supposed to do."[77] He thus tries to live day to day, and is involved with Wounded Warriors Canada, OSISS, and other veterans' organizations. Like many colleagues, he believes that social support from fellow veterans and Canadian society helps him navigate post-retirement life: "I have that [support] through my military family ... My family family, a little different story. They somewhat understand, but they don't quite get it; which is fine, they weren't supposed to get it. It's not their job to get it. The military family, I'm still close to them. They understand. They know. They were standing there."[78]

As mentioned in the last chapter, Greg Prodaniuk became part of the first cohort of OSISS peer support coordinators in 2001, and

remains in that position at the time of this writing. He believes that
a lopsided focus on the medical dimensions of PTSD has failed to
capture how military operations affect a soldier's beliefs, morals, and
outlook. His appraisal of the mental processes that veterans work
through after war and peacekeeping demonstrates that, like shell
shock before it, PTSD is in many respects a metaphor for the profound
impact that trauma has on a soldier's worldview:

> I think people are [now] looking at these injuries sort of in a soci-
> ety sense, and just wheeling out the psychiatrists to explain what's
> going on is kind of ringing hollow. It's not filling in the parts of
> the story that people really want to engage ... I think the next
> change is we're going to be evolving towards understanding this
> as a process ... in some ways almost looking at it as a grief model
> ... something everyone can relate to. Everyone loses people in
> their lives and it changes their lives, and how do they carry on?
> And I think that's really what happens here. Veterans lose some-
> thing. They lose their youth, they lose their innocence, they lose
> some of their morals, some of their ethics are challenged. They
> lose time, momentum, access to the good life that happens in our
> country. And I think that that's really what we're talking about.[79]

Prodaniuk's story, like several others we have seen, is a testament to
how social support for those dealing with psychological difficulties
can have very positive effects, above and beyond what medical treatment can offer on its own. As this book has shown, social support is
not just an individual, familial, or military concern, but a national
one. In Prodaniuk's final interview for this project, his remarks about
the road to his recovery serve to demonstrate that viewing trauma as
both an injury and a metaphor allows us to trace the difficult historical journeys of both individual Canadians and Canada itself:

> I was prompted, encouraged, and decided to take the high road,
> and because of that I've opened up sort of a richness and under-
> standing in my life, and a quality of life that I may not have
> achieved if I had gone down some other paths. So, when I reflect
> upon the injury, I see it as a definite point of deviation or a course
> change in my life ... I look at it as, [I was a] young guy who went
> on operations and I was impacted. And it moved me a few degrees

at a critical point in a different direction, and I'm grateful that ... I had the wherewithal and the support to gain a perspective on it, and use it in turn to inform my life moving forward. I think it's made me a much better man. It's made me a much better father, better husband. It's made me a better leader. It's made me a more balanced person. It's taught me a lot, about the inner workings of people, and about how people approach impasses in their lives. And it's not so much an understanding as an overarching theory. It's more about the story of life and the things that you do in your youth, and the consequences of it, and where you go. And I think that's how I look at the injury now when I reflect back on it. I look at it as a significant moment in my life, and it's something that has created who I am, who I am now.[80]

Prodaniuk's journey points to a new type of masculinity and leadership, and to the redrawing of what constitutes courage. Although Roméo Dallaire's high-profile battle with psychological difficulties is the one best known to Canadians, this new form of optimistic and courageous leadership goes beyond any one individual. Every soldier and veteran who comes forward about their own trials and tribulations, or who approaches their colleagues' problems with an open mind, encourages greater acceptance of the view that manliness, and what makes the ideal soldier, need not be delineated with such sharp edges. There is room to think that one can be both tough and compassionate, and that requiring help does not make one less of a soldier. While PTSD and related difficulties have brought some soldiers to ruinous decline, new ideas and approaches have provided many others with opportunities not just for medical recovery, but for moral and spiritual recovery as well. This is a new chapter in a story of trauma and recovery that began long ago, and it is one that must continue to be written. If history is any indication, it will be years before Canadians cease to see the psychological fallout of the Afghanistan War, making it an issue that must not fall off the public radar as our memories of the conflict begin to fade.

This book has used oral interviews with veterans to demonstrate the socio-economic and moral and spiritual effects that trauma has had on Canadian military members across a one-hundred-year period. Without claiming that PTSD is simply a successor to shell shock or battle exhaustion, it has nonetheless shown that although terms and symptom patterns have changed, trauma has always had devastating social and moral effects on veterans – something that gets lost when too much emphasis is placed on medical narratives. Moreover, by examining the history of trauma in the Canadian military after the Cold War, this book has waded into largely uncharted territory to show that ideas and representations of trauma have consistently been wrapped up in individual, political, and societal concerns. This narrative has expanded on the earlier historical accounts mentioned throughout, which focused largely on the experience of trauma *during* war, rather than in its wake. Most importantly, this book has built on work by historians who recognize the value of a multifaceted approach which takes into account military, medical, and cultural narratives. Future Canadian scholarship on veterans' trauma, and military history as a whole, will no doubt continue to benefit from the combined use of social and medical histories, and the multidimensional perspective that such an approach provides.

Notes

1 Westholm interview.
2 Ibid.
3 Vehicle technicians in the Canadian Forces are expected to be both technician and soldier, with their role changing based on the tactical situation.
4 A predominantly barren and hilly island, Île de la Gonâve was often a hiding spot for runaway slaves during the French colonial period.
5 Westholm interview.
6 Ibid.
7 Ibid.
8 Ibid.
9 Note about terminology: given that "trauma" can also refer to physical
injury to the body, it is important to note that "trauma" in this book refers
only to psychological/psychiatric trauma.
10 Definition taken from National Defence and the Canadian Armed Forces,
"DAOD 5023-0, Universality of Service," accessed 15 January 2014,
http://www.forces.gc.ca/en/about-policies-standards-defence-admin-orders-
directives-5000/5023-0.page. For a full definition of minimum operational
standards see Canada, National Defence and the Canadian Armed Forces,
"DAOD 5023-1, Minimum Operational Standards Related to Universality of
Service," http://www.forces.gc.ca/en/about-policies-standards-defence-admin-
orders-directives-5000/5023-1.page.
11 Micale and Lerner, "Trauma, Psychiatry, and History: A Conceptual and His-
toriographical Introduction," in *Traumatic Pasts*, 1.

12 Ibid.

13 American Psychiatric Association, *Diagnostic and Statistical Manual of Mental Disorders*, 236–9.

14 Scott, "PTSD in DSM-III: A Case in the Politics of Diagnosis and Disease," passim.

15 Micale and Lerner, "Trauma, Psychiatry, and History," 2.

16 Shephard, *A War of Nerves*, 355, 385. Studies of war trauma in the 1980s dovetailed with an increasing interest in studying civilian traumas such as sexual abuse. The publication of psychiatrist and author Judith Herman's *Trauma and Recovery*, based on experience working with sexual and domestic abuse victims, provides an excellent example of a work that bridges the gap between civilian and war trauma.

17 Micale and Lerner, "Trauma, Psychiatry, and History," 2.

18 The best example of the latter trend was the 1985 creation of the International Society for Traumatic Stress Studies, a collection of researchers from around the world who meet to share research, clinical findings, and strategies, and discuss theoretical knowledge on trauma.

19 Fussell, *The Great War and Modern Memory*; Leese, *Shell Shock*, 182.

20 Fussell, *The Great War and Modern Memory*, xv.

21 Ibid., 38.

22 Ibid., 363. For more on Fussell's personal experiences, readers can also direct themselves to popular American documentarian Ken Burns's multi-episode series *The War*, which includes several candid and moving interviews with Fussell.

23 Ibid., 369.

24 Ibid.

25 Winter, *Sites of Memory, Sites of Mourning*; Vance, *Death So Noble*. Another noteworthy study that examines collective memory is Canadian historian Robert Rutherdale's 2004 monograph *Hometown Horizons*.

26 See Vance, *Death So Noble*, esp. 3, 18, 260–1.

27 Showalter, *The Female Malady*, 2, 167.

28 Ibid., 171.

29 Ibid. Shell shock was, Showalter argued, men's bodily protest against a lack of control imposed on them by politicians, generals, and psychiatrists. See also ibid., 172.

30 Ibid., 190.

31 Drawing inspiration from gender studies, scholars readily responded to Showalter's feminist analysis of psychiatry and began examining the histori-

cal construction of modern masculinity in the West. American cultural historian George Mosse's 1996 work *The Image of Man*, which traced the rise of
modern masculinity, signalled a new, incisive assessment of how masculinity
"touched nearly every aspect of society." Mosse provocatively stated that "all
those who want to change society, as well as those who want to escape their
marginalization, have to take the stereotype of modern masculinity into
account." A concept previously taken for granted, exactly what constituted
masculinity, and how that definition changed at any given time, was increasingly placed under the gaze of historians seeking to unravel its many effects
and meanings. See Mosse, *The Image of Man*, 194, 3, 278, 6; In the Canadian
context, during the 1990s historians likewise analyzed how societal expectations, and particularly gender expectations, have been shaped by medico-
psychological dictates. Mona Gleason's 1999 book *Normalizing the Ideal* provided a thorough critique of how "normalcy" and the "normal" post-1945
Canadian family were constructed through psychological knowledge and its
dissemination. While psychiatry focused on emotional and behavioural
pathology, postwar psychologists proclaimed themselves authorities on what
constituted normal family living. See Gleason, *Normalizing the Ideal*, passim;
the late Mark Moss's *Manliness and Militarism* is another notable work.

32 Micale, *Hysterical Men*. In a testament to Showalter's enduring influence
on the field, Micale's prologue was titled "Hysteria: The Male Malady"; it
was, in his own words, a respectful nod to Showalter's "important book."
See ibid., 288n6.

33 Ibid., 278.

34 Ibid., 6.

35 Ibid., 281.

36 Ibid.

37 Ibid., 282.

38 Ibid., 139.

39 Ibid., 284. In Canada, Christopher Dummitt's *The Manly Modern* represented the rise of masculinity studies. Most pertinent to this book, Dummitt
explored the unintended consequences of the "manly modern" project, especially how such consequences affected Canadian war veterans. His study
highlighted the intricate historical web of medical knowledge, gender
expectations, and pension questions, as well as a recurring pattern in Canadian history: the off-loading of long-term financial liabilities at the expense
of Canadian veterans. See Dummitt, *The Manly Modern*, 2, 4, 29–51, 40.
Recent works such as the 2014 book *Ontario Boys* by Christopher Greig, and

the 2012 collection *Canadian Men and Masculinities* edited by Greig and Wayne Martino, display Canadian scholars' continuing efforts to analyze the effects of masculine norms on both individuals and society.

40 Micale and Lerner, "Trauma, Psychiatry, and History," 6. By the new millennium, historians' interest was self-evident. Demonstrative of the expansive growth in the field of trauma history were Ben Shephard's 2000 book, *A War of Nerves*; Mark Micale and Paul Lerner's 2001 edited collection, *Traumatic Pasts*; and Edgar Jones and Simon Wessely's 2005 work, *Shell Shock to PTSD*, all three of which trace the history of psychological trauma across broad timeframes and places.

41 In the United States, where the PTSD concept originated, this trend happened slightly earlier. For one prominent example that mentions PTSD in connection with earlier battlefield disorders, see Gabriel, *No More Heroes*, 77, 157.

42 Brown, "Shell Shock in the Canadian Expeditionary Force," passim.

43 Copp and McAndrew, *Battle Exhaustion*, 157. Copp's 1992 essay on the development of neuropsychiatry in the Canadian Army during World War Two made no mention of trauma or PTSD at all. See Copp, "The Development of Neuropsychiatry in the Canadian Army (Overseas) 1939–1943," in Naylor, *Canadian Health Care and the State*, 67–84.

44 To the best of my knowledge.

45 Copp, "From Neurasthenia to Post-Traumatic Stress Disorder: Canadian Veterans and the Problem of Persistent Emotional Disabilities," in Neary and Granatstein, *The Veterans Charter and Post-World War II Canada*, 149–59. Allan English's 1996 study of Canadian aircrew, which likewise discussed the role of psychologists and psychiatrists (in this case in aircrew selection, training, etc.), made just one brief mention of PTSD in a footnote. See English, *The Cream of the Crop*, 217.

46 Copp, "From Neurasthenia to Post-Traumatic Stress Disorder," 156.

47 See Young, *The Harmony of Illusions*, passim, esp. 5–6. By the 2000s, in combination with the aforementioned rise of socio-cultural histories, scholars interested in war trauma created more holistic analyses that examined societal mentalities, the medical profession, and traumatized veterans themselves. Leese's 2002 *Shell Shock*, about the "mass trauma" of shell-shocked British soldiers and postwar society, was an excellent example of the "new" historical trauma research. Leese examined the Great War shell shock phenomenon not just during wartime, but also its post-1918 emergence as a metaphor for the war itself. He argued that shell shock was both a medical

phenomenon *and* a symbol of collective trauma. Moreover, that symbolism was not static. Put simply, shell shock "changed its meanings to suit the pre-occupations of British society through the twentieth century." See Leese, *Shell Shock*, 184, xiii, 3. Another noteworthy example was Peter Barham's *Forgotten Lunatics of the Great War.*

48 Young, *The Harmony of Illusions*, 5–6.

49 Ibid.

50 Shorter, *From Paralysis to Fatigue*, ix.

51 Ibid., x.

52 Humphries, "War's Long Shadow," 503–31.

53 Their work reproduced several peacekeeping trauma studies, but did not discuss them in a historical perspective. This was most likely because, as its title suggested, it was concerned primarily with *combat* stress, something from which peacekeeping was traditionally excluded.

54 Some of the sources cited throughout this book discuss historical elements of trauma, but most are within military journals and thus focus on trauma vis-à-vis the military. Others likewise discuss elements of trauma history, but approach the subject from a strictly strategic or medical perspective.

55 To the best of my knowledge, Humphries's 2010 article is the only Canadian academic article of its kind.

56 See above works by Copp, McAndrew, and Brown.

57 Off, *The Ghosts of Medak Pocket.*

58 Whitworth, *Men, Militarism, and UN Peacekeeping*. Whitworth further explored this subject in 2008's "Militarized Masculinity and Post Traumatic Stress Disorder," in Parpart and Zalewski, 109–26.

59 Vance, *Death So Noble*, 8.

60 Allan Young made a particularly strong case in this regard with his discussion of the traumatic memory, a cultural creation of the nineteenth century. The print media is still guilty of using "shell shock" and "PTSD" interchangeably.

61 Leese, *Shell Shock*, 31.

62 Shorter, *From Paralysis to Fatigue*, 271.

63 In philosophical terms, it is a medical project that consistently attempts to defy Johann Wolfgang von Goethe's dictum that "All theory, dear friend, is gray, but the golden tree of life springs ever green."

64 See above cited works, namely Young and Leese, as well as Jones and Wessely.

65 The chapter also draws on correspondence with the former chairman

and brigadier-general Joe Sharpe, as well as others involved in the events covered.

66 Here I must acknowledge Copp and McAndrew's *Battle Exhaustion*. Their interviews with former military psychiatrists in the 1980s were one of the first kernels of thought that led me to wonder if I could conduct similar interviews with soldiers and veterans.

67 Along with this e-mail, I sent a one-page consent form outlining my project's aims.

68 Godin interview.

CHAPTER ONE

1 Binneveld, *From Shell Shock to Combat Stress*, 1.
2 Shephard, *A War of Nerves*, 385.
3 Ibid., passim.
4 English and Dale-McGrath, "Overcoming Systemic Obstacles to Veteran Transition to Civilian Life," in Aiken and Bélanger, *Beyond the Line*, 257.
5 Copp and Humphries, *Combat Stress*, 1; English, "Historical and Contemporary Interpretations of Combat Stress Reaction," in Copp and Humphries, 445.
6 Gabriel, *No More Heroes*, 6.
7 Micale and Lerner, "Trauma, Psychiatry, and History," 11.
8 Ibid.
9 Ibid.
10 Ibid., 10.
11 Copp and Humphries, *Combat Stress*, 6–7.
12 Erichsen, *On Railway and Other Injuries of the Nervous System*, 46–7.
13 Jones and Wessely, *Shell Shock to PTSD*, 14.
14 Micale and Lerner, "Trauma, Psychiatry, and History," 9. Much of the controversy during the nineteenth century revolved around the fact that physicians, many coming from the somatic (physical) school of thinking, could not find significant physical injuries on their patient (or on their brain postmortem), yet the patient still seemed affected by the event. That dilemma, among other things, namely the rise of psychology, led to exploration by some into the psychological realm.
15 Jones and Wessely, *Shell Shock to PTSD*, 14.
16 "Railway Surgeons: Eleventh Meeting of the Association Starts," *The Globe*, 7 July 1898. B.B. Osler was for a time the most famous trial lawyer in Canada.

He died of heart disease a few years after this address, in February 1901. For a brief biography, see his obituary in *The Globe*, 6 February 1901. Erichsen, for his part, rejected any association between railway spine and traumatic hysteria. See Jones and Wessely, *Shell Shock to PTSD*, 14.

17 Jones and Wessely, *Shell Shock to PTSD*, 14.
18 Harrington, "The Railway Accident: Trains, Trauma, and Technological Crises in Nineteenth-Century Britain," in Micale and Lerner, *Traumatic Pasts*, 31–2.
19 Caplan, "Trains and Trauma in the American Gilded Age," in Micale and Lerner, 57–8.
20 Harrington, "The Railway Accident," 55–6.
21 Shephard, *A War of Nerves*, 21.
22 Ibid.
23 Myers, *Shell Shock in France, 1914–1918*, 14.
24 Ibid., 11–12. For an account of Myers's time in France researching and treating shell shock, see ibid.
25 Shephard, *A War of Nerves*, 21. It was the French who first described shell shock in late 1914.
26 Ibid., 28.
27 Binneveld, *From Shell Shock to Combat Stress*, 83.
28 Copp and Humphries, *Combat Stress*, 14.
29 Katherine Kent, "Katherine Kent's Own Column," *The Globe*, 3 October 1918.
30 Shephard, *A War of Nerves*, 25.
31 Ibid. In the rare cases when a soldier's mental state was chronically deteriorated, or he showed obvious signs of being mentally unfit to serve, he was sent to an asylum.
32 Bourke, "Effeminacy, Ethnicity and the End of Trauma," 59.
33 Shephard, *A War of Nerves*, 25.
34 Ibid., 29.
35 Ibid., 26.
36 Manion, *A Surgeon in Arms*, 19.
37 Ibid., 31.
38 Moran, *The Anatomy of Courage*, 184.
39 Russel, "The Management of Psycho-Neuroses in the Canadian Army," in Copp and Humphries, *Combat Stress*, 22. During the war, Myers also agreed with this view, stating that he had seen far too many men who claimed that they were suffering from shell shock with nothing visibly (or otherwise)

wrong with them. See Shephard, *A War of Nerves*, 29. Also, a note about terminology: neuropsychiatry often referred to neurology and psychiatry, since
it dealt with diseases attributable to the mind and nervous system as it was
then understood. This terminology subsequently changed when psychiatry
and neurology split into distinct disciplines with uncommon training,
though neuropsychiatry has again become a growing branch of psychiatry
in the twenty-first century.

40 Copp and Humphries, *Combat Stress*, 11. According to archival material utilized by Shephard, during the first few weeks of the Battle of the Somme
the British alone evacuated "several thousand" due to "nervous disorders."
See Shephard, *A War of Nerves*, 41.

41 Ibid., 31.

42 Ibid.

43 Ibid.

44 Ibid., 32.

45 Estimates vary. The first figure comes from Copp and Humphries's *Combat
Stress*, 8; the latter figure from Humphries's 2010 article "War's Long Shadow," 503.

46 Copp and Humphries, *Combat Stress*, 10. The establishment of "neurological" hospitals for those injuries and genuine physical injuries to the head
was in itself demonstrative of prevailing beliefs about the organic cause of
shell shock and other psychological injuries.

47 Brown, "Shell Shock in the Canadian Expeditionary Force," 310–11. For two
excellent accounts of developments in the somatic and psychological
realms, see Young, *The Harmony of Illusions*, 13–42 (esp. 20–1); Micale, *Hysterical Men*, chapters 3, 4, 5.

48 Manion, *A Surgeon in Arms*, 164.

49 Ibid. It is interesting to note that while Manion seemed to subscribe to a
physical explanation of shell shock (a collapse of the nervous system), his
latter example of seeing a comrade killed, during which time the man did
not necessarily sustain physical injury, implied a purely psychological sap-
ping of the nerves. In that regard, Manion seems to have taken the middle
path rather than subscribing to a strictly physical or mental theory.

50 Brown, "Shell Shock in the Canadian Expeditionary Force," 315.

51 Manion, *A Surgeon in Arms*, 163–4.

52 Quoted in Bourke, "Effeminacy, Ethnicity and the End of Trauma," 62.

53 Manion, *A Surgeon in Arms*, 37.

54 Macphail, *Official History of the Canadian Forces in the Great War 1914–19*, 278.

55 Ibid.

56 Morton, *Fight or Pay*, 151. Physicians in the Great War were also initially influenced by French research into "traumatic hysteria," especially the work of Jean-Martin Charcot. See Micale, *Hysterical Men*, 5–7, 139. For more on hysteria see Micale, "On the 'Disappearance' of Hysteria," passim; Showalter, *The Female Malady*, passim, esp. 133–4.

57 Moran, *The Anatomy of Courage*, 185.

58 Canadian Letters and Images Project. "Nanaimo Daily Free Press Letter: 1916 November 13th." http://www.canadianletters.ca.

59 Letters and Images Project, "Shortreed, Robert Letter: 1917 December 9th." http://www.canadianletters.ca.

60 Moran, *The Anatomy of Courage*, 67.

61 Ibid.

62 Letters and Images Project, "Tripp, George Henry Letter: 1916 October 11th." http://www.canadianletters.ca.

63 Letters and Images Project, "Matier, Alexander Letter: 1918 January 8th." http://www.canadianletters.ca.

64 Ibid.

65 See Humphries, "War's Long Shadow," for an extended analysis of how these discussions evolved during the interwar period.

66 Letters and Images Project, "Andrews, Alfred Herbert John Diary: 1915." http://www.canadianletters.ca.

67 Letters and Images Project, "Richardson, Charles Douglas Letter: 1916 July 14th." http://www.canadianletters.ca.

68 Letters and Images Project, "Bell, William Henry Letter: 1917 March 15th." http://www.canadianletters.ca.

69 At the time of the letter, Leduc was a captain. He ended the war as a major.

70 Letters and Images Project, "Leduc, Thomas James Letter: 1917 July 10th." http://www.canadianletters.ca.

71 Ibid.

72 Copp and Humphries, *Combat Stress*, 14; Macphail, *Official History of the Canadian Forces*, 278.

73 Ibid., 13.

74 Ibid.

75 Shephard, *A War of Nerves*, 32; Winter, "Shell-Shock and the Cultural History of the Great War," 7.

76 Fussell, *The Great War and Modern Memory*, passim.

77 Kardiner, *The Traumatic Neuroses of War*, v. Kardiner was one of the first to

make explicit connections between peace and wartime trauma (traumatic neurosis), stating that the peacetime traumatic neuroses were "the same in structure as those precipitated in war."

78 Brown, "Shell Shock in the Canadian Expeditionary Force," 322.

79 Ibid., 323.

80 Ibid.

81 Canadian Mental Health Association, "History of CMHA," accessed 14 January 2014, http://www.cmha.ca/about-cmha/history-of-cmha /#.VNJ8CS5hwnM.

82 "$20,000 Secured For Institute," *The Globe*, 27 February 1918.

83 Ibid. A testament to the prominence and influence of the CNCMH founders was its board of directors. The early board included: Lord Shaughnessy, president of the CPR; Richard B. Angus, Montreal financier and philanthropist; Dr C.F. Martin, professor of medicine, McGill University; Sir Vincent Meredith, president, Bank of Montreal; and F.W. Molson, president of Molson's Brewery. Each board member pledged $1,000 a year for three years, the not-so-insignificant sum of $13,244.68 per annum in 2014 terms. Lieutenant-Colonel Charles Vincent Massey, future governor general of Canada, was also on the executive committee.

84 Both Owen and McCrae did not survive the war, with the former being killed in action one week before the 1918 Armistice, and the latter dying of pneumonia early that year.

85 Vance, *A Death So Noble*, 305.

86 Bird, *And We Go On*, 93.

87 Ibid.

88 Woolf, *Mrs Dalloway*. The works of British novelist Pat Barker, whose *Regeneration Trilogy* of the 1990s focused on the effects of trauma, were a testament to the enduring nature of the First World War and fascination with its traumatic character amongst both historians and novelists. The first work in the trilogy, *Regeneration*, which portrayed the fictionalized encounter of Sassoon, Owen, and pioneering psychologist W.H.R. Rivers, was quite popular, and was made into a 1997 film of the same name.

89 Morton and Wright, *Winning the Second Battle*, 9. Morton and Wright's account provides an excellent traversal through the labyrinthine and confusing political and legal wrangling of the post-1918 period. It is a testament to their work and the subject's difficulty that no other authors have attempted a grand narrative of this period in Canada since its publication. It is important to note that, as Morton and Wright showed, pensions were

not a new topic in Canada, but rather the *scale* of the problem was unprecedented. For those interested in military history minutiae, it was the Russo-Japanese War which first saw more soldiers killed in battle than by disease.

90 Ibid., 13.

91 Ibid., 18.

92 Neary, *On to Civvy Street*, 21.

93 Ibid., 15.

94 Ibid. This group constituted those who didn't qualify for pensions.

95 Ibid., 17.

96 Morton and Wright, *Winning the Second Battle*, 234.

97 Ibid.

98 These pension values were taken from the table in Morton and Wright, *Winning the Second Battle*, 234, and adjusted for inflation (to 2015 dollars) using the Bank of Canada Inflation Calculator, http://www.bankofcanada.ca/rates/related/inflation-calculator/.

99 McKay and Swift, *Warrior Nation*, 24.

100 Morton and Wright, *Winning the Second Battle*, 234. The number of disability pensioners ranged between 15,335 in 1918 to 80,104 in 1939. These figures did not include dependents, the number of which ranged between 10,488 to 20,015 from 1918 to 1939.

101 Ibid., xi.

102 Morton, *Fight or Pay*, 162.

103 English, *Understanding Military Culture*, 87.

104 Morton and Wright, *Winning the Second Battle*, 56.

105 Ibid., 237. Although Veterans Affairs Canada's latest 2006 Table of Disabilities is vastly more complex and specific than the 1919 Pension Act scale, and does not discriminate between ranks, the basic model of determining a veteran's level of disability is still much the same today. For the latest 2006 table and its earlier, 1995, counterpart, see Canada, Veterans Affairs Canada, "2006 Table of Disabilities."

106 Biggar, "The Pensionability of the Disabled Soldier," 30.

107 This amounts to only $8,061 in 2015 terms; for the full scale of disabilities see Canada, Parliament, *Acts of the Parliament of Canada*, vol. 1, 13th Parliament, 2nd Session, chapter 43, 18–19.

108 Humphries, "War's Long Shadow," 520.

109 Biggar, "The Pensionability of the Disabled Soldier," 29. Biggar listed three ways in which ordinary employment could be reduced: "(1) because by reason of his loss of a normal ability his choice of occupation is restricted; (2)

because he is, by reason of his disease, prohibited from undertaking certain forms of work; (3) because he, by reason of his disease or injury, requires more rest than the normal man."

110 Ibid., 29.

111 Cited in Morton and Wright, *Winning the Second Battle*, 60.

112 Biggar, "The Pensionability of the Disabled Soldier," 30–1.

113 For a list of categories see Morton and Wright, *Winning the Second Battle*, 238.

114 Neary, *On to Civvy Street*, 23.

115 Morton and Wright, *Winning the Second Battle*, 56.

116 Copp and Humphries, *Combat Stress*, 83.

117 Morton and Wright, *Winning the Second Battle*, 56.

118 Ibid., 27. In February 1918 the commission became the Department of Soldiers' Civil Reestablishment, which itself merged in 1928 with the Department of Health, becoming the Department of Pensions and National Health.

119 Ibid. Asylums during this period were viewed by most as a last resort, since the conditions were believed to make an already bad (mental) situation worse. In medical historian Edward Shorter's estimation, "by World War I, asylums had become vast warehouses for the chronically insane and demented." The second chapter of his *History of Psychiatry* provides an excellent overview of the asylum era in the west. See Shorter, *A History of Psychiatry*, 33–68. Historians John Weaver and David Wright pointed out that families' and patriotic associations' attempts to keep soldiers out of asylums spoke to the enduring stigma attached to the mentally ill. See Weaver and Wright, "Shell Shock and the Politics of Asylum Committal in New Zealand, 1916–22," 36.

120 Shorter, *A History of Psychiatry*, 65.

121 Morton and Wright, *Winning the Second Battle*, 96. Cobourg was the only hospital in Canada solely dedicated to caring for traumatized soldiers. It had 425 beds and its mission was to cure shell shock sufferers and return them to civilian life. As noted by Copp and Humphries, the "cure" was more a matter of whether or not a soldier became self-sufficient, rather than any medical recovery. See Copp and Humphries, *Combat Stress*, 95.

122 Copp and Humphries, *Combat Stress*, 83.

123 Healy, *The Creation of Psychopharmacology*, 28–9. The genetic/hereditarian view espoused that a person's constitution and character were largely inherited from previous generations, and if one was afflicted with a mental disor-

der physicians and psychologists most often looked to an individual's family history for the potential source. If a mentally ill relative was found in the family tree, this confirmed the perceived hereditary taint. The insidious and terrifying quality of this view was that many physicians in the late-nineteenth and early twentieth century believed in the concept of "degeneration," a concept which held that inherited mental illness worsened with time, potentially leading to the destruction of a family line and, in theory, an entire population. For a concise overview of degeneration theories see Shorter, *A History of Psychiatry*, 93–9.

124   Copp and Humphries, *Combat Stress*, 83.

125   Morton and Wright, *Winning the Second Battle*, 75. This thinking was most clearly spelled out by Freud in his 1917 *Introductory Lectures on Psycho-Analysis*, where he elucidated the concept of secondary gain. Secondary gain referred to the patient's perceived social advantages gained by their illness; in the case of shell-shocked soldiers the most obvious advantage was a pension, or in wartime the avoidance of duties or combat. Secondary gain comes from external motivations, while primary gain comes from internal motivations, such as in conversion disorder, when a person manifests physical symptoms without any discernible organic causes. The "gain" comes from the removal of anxiety that the symptom produces.

126   This was not a uniquely Canadian stance. In Britain, pension officials were likewise "obsessed" with proving that most mentally ill veterans were malingerers. See Bourke, "Effeminacy, Ethnicity and the End of Trauma," 63.

127   Copp, "From Neurasthenia to Post-Traumatic Stress Disorder," 151.

128   Morton and Wright, *Winning the Second Battle*, 75.

129   Humphries, "War's Long Shadow," 503.

130   Ibid., 530.

131   Ibid.

132   Moss, *Manliness and Militarism*, 15.

133   Ibid., 143. Those fears were based to some degree on an "increasingly visible and vociferous women's movement [that] accentuated self-doubt." See ibid., 110. Worries about societal decline and men's effeminization were also thoroughly covered in a European context by Micale, *Hysterical Men*, passim.

134   Humphries, "War's Long Shadow," 530.

135   Copp and Humphries, *Combat Stress*, 91.

136   Humphries, "War's Long Shadow," 503.

137   Cook, *Warlords*, 151.

138 Morton and Wright, *Winning the Second Battle*, 104.

139 Humphries, "War's Long Shadow," 520.

140 Morton and Wright, *Winning the Second Battle*, 238.

141 Copp and Humphries, *Combat Stress*, 87.

142 Humphries, "War's Long Shadow," 526.

143 Morton and Wright, *Winning the Second Battle*, 133.

144 Humphries, "War's Long Shadow," 522. See also Humphries's excellent summary of contemporary attitudes toward charity and welfare.

145 As Morton and Wright so aptly stated, "History keeps little record of those who did fit in." See ibid., 118.

146 Bird, *And We Go On*, 229.

147 Ibid., 100.

148 Ibid., 223.

149 Ibid., 75.

150 Morton, *Fight or Pay*, 23.

151 Mosse, *The Image of Man*, passim.

152 Ibid., 100. The shell-shocked veteran was also the victim of traditional prejudices about the mentally ill, and sometimes treated as such.

153 Ibid., 61.

154 Vance, *Death So Noble*, 53.

155 Eksteins, *Rites of Spring*, 254.

156 Vance, *Death So Noble*, 53.

157 Ibid.

158 See Shephard, *A War of Nerves*, 67, where he uses archival evidence to refute John Major's stance on physicians and shell shock. See also *The Globe and Mail*, 12 December 2001 and 16 August 2006, for Canadian coverage of this issue. For a recent account of Canadian courts martial in the Great War see Iacobelli, *Death or Deliverance*.

159 Shawn McCarthy, "More Than 80 Years Ago, They Were Shot for Desertion. Today, They'd Be Sent Home with Battle Fatigue. Now, Canada Makes Amends," *The Globe and Mail*, 12 December 2001; Ingrid Peritz, "Britain Set to Pardon WWI Troops," *The Globe and Mail* 16 August 2006.

160 Ibid., 12 December 2001. There are seven Books of Remembrance located in the Memorial Chamber. Each day, a page in the books is turned in commemoration of those who gave their lives in service to the country. The First World War Book of Remembrance was the first book created, and is also the largest, containing more than 66,000 names. There were twenty-five Canadians executed during the war, but only twenty-three names were added to the book, since the other two men were executed for murder.

161 Ibid., 16 August 2006.
162 Randy Boswell, "Top Historian Pans Pardons." Canwest News Service, 17 August 2006, https://www.pressreader.com/canada/leader-post/20060817 /281599530972048.
163 Morton and Wright, *Winning the Second Battle*, 215.
164 Ibid.
165 Ibid.
166 Neary, *On to Civvy Street*, 26.
167 Ibid., 22.
168 Ibid., 22.
169 See Humphries, "War's Long Shadow," and Neary, *On to Civvy Street*, chapters 1 and 2, for an in-depth look at pension-seeking in the Depression years.

CHAPTER TWO

1 Shephard, *A War of Nerves*, 205. Forward psychiatry proved to be quite useful in the Second World War and beyond, but the issue still looming behind any attempt to send soldiers back into combat is whether or not treated soldiers will relapse, or, perhaps even more importantly, whether they will suffer long-term health consequences regardless of early treatment. For more on its history see Jones and Wessely, "'Forward Psychiatry' in the Military," 411–19.
2 In reality, the entire army had to be rebuilt, as Canada entered the war with only 5,000 professional soldiers.
3 Battle exhaustion was also called "battle fatigue."
4 Young, *The Harmony of Illusions*, 92–3.
5 Flavelle, "Help or Harm," 2.
6 Ibid., 4.
7 Ibid.
8 Binneveld, *From Shell Shock to Combat Stress*, 101.
9 Ibid., 96.
10 Flavelle, "Help or Harm," 4.
11 Shephard, *A War of Nerves*, 205.
12 Kardiner, *The Traumatic Neuroses of War*, 6. Kardiner was personally (psycho) analyzed by Freud.
13 Ibid., 69. Kardiner's ideas reflected the gradual rise of Freudian psychology and dynamic psychiatry in mainstream American psychiatric circles. In both America and Canada, shifts in psychology's orientation (in Canada it was somewhat less Freudian) led to the displacement of previous hereditary

views of mental illness, something by the 1930s associated with degeneration and eugenics. For more on developments in psychology and psychiatry
during the late-nineteenth and early to mid-twentieth century see Shorter,
A History of Psychiatry, 145–89.

14 Kardiner, *The Traumatic Neuroses of War*, 233.
15 Kardiner's book later became a focal point for researchers who convinced
the psychiatric mainstream to accept the idea of PTSD.
16 Copp and Humphries, *Combat Stress*, 126.
17 This concept was first employed by the French in 1915, and later developed
by the American psychiatrist Thomas Salmon in 1918. See Jones and Wessely, *Shell Shock to PTSD*, 24–5. The acronym was later created by K.L. Artiss.
See Artiss, "Human Behaviour under Stress," 1011–15.
18 Despite PIE's successes, the question of whether a soldier who is able to
function again in combat will be healthy in the long term is another
matter.
19 Ibid.
20 Shephard, *A War of Nerves*, 195.
21 Ibid., 169.
22 Copp and Humphries, *Combat Stress*, 126. Of course, it is questionable
whether psychiatrists could have made any difference in the Battle of
Dunkirk, given the conditions and its relatively short duration.
23 Ibid., 127. The Sutton was a sub-unit of the eminent Maudsley Hospital in
London that had been evacuated in 1939. It is worth noting that the reason
two civilian physicians were caring for military men was because the British
Army had made no provisions for mentally ill soldiers at home. This was
perhaps more telling of the prevailing attitude and optimism about war
neuroses than anything else. Sargant later became (in)famous for his consul-
tation with those working with the CIA for the MKULTRA mind control program, as well as for his "missionary zeal" for psychosurgery. He consulted
with McGill psychiatrist Ewen Cameron on many occasions. See Shephard,
A War of Nerves, 337; and, for his connections to Cameron, see Thomas, *Journey into Madness*, 189–90. See Marks, *The Search for the "Manchurian Candidate,"* for more on the MKULTRA program.
24 Copp and Humphries, *Combat Stress*, 127.
25 Ibid., 128.
26 Ibid.
27 Ibid., 129.
28 Shephard, *A War of Nerves*, 183.

29 Binneveld, *From Shell Shock to Combat Stress*, 83. Battle exhaustion carried similar connotations to neurasthenia, since both implied an exhaustion of the nervous system and its energy. Neurasthenia was largely reserved for officers of the First World War, since it carried less of a stigma than shell shock, on account of the belief that the man whose nervous system was depleted had fought long and hard before succumbing to breakdown. It is interesting to note that the RAF and RCAF, instead of battle exhaustion, used the term "Lack of Moral Fibre" to classify men who had broken from the strain of too many sorties or could not fly for illegitimate reasons. See English, *The Cream of the Crop*, 81.

30 Copp and Humphries, *Combat Stress*, 145.

31 Ibid., 148-9.

32 There was some evident overlap. For more on these developments in Canada, see Gleason, *Normalizing the Ideal*, 6-8.

33 Shephard, *A War of Nerves*, 188.

34 Copp and Humphries, *Combat Stress*, 131.

35 Shephard, *A War of Nerves*, 187.

36 Copp and Humphries, *Combat Stress*, 131.

37 Ibid., 126.

38 Griffin, *In Search of Sanity*, 101. For its part, the Canadian Mental Health Association, then still termed the Canadian National Committee for Mental Hygiene, sent informal bulletins throughout the war dealing with wartime psychiatry. By the war's end, information was being sent to 250 military psychiatrists, psychologists, and medical officers in Canada and overseas. See ibid. Griffin played a large role in the expansion of the Army's psychiatric branch, especially through the establishment of training courses in psychiatry at McGill and the University of Toronto. Regimental medical officers who had served at least six months in the Army were eligible for the seven-month program. On top of course work, the training included a month in a veterans' hospital and two months at a military establishment. Those "fledgling psychiatrists" provided the manpower for the development of the Canadian Army's psychiatric program between 1943 and the end of the war. See Copp and McAndrew, *Battle Exhaustion*, 34-5.

39 Copp and Humphries, *Combat Stress*, 125.

40 Shephard, *A War of Nerves*, 188; see 187-203 for a detailed description and analysis of the British and American screening systems.

41 Young, *The Harmony of Illusions*, 92-3.

42 Ibid. The myriad ways in which commanders viewed and handled psychi-

atric casualties was, in part, the reason for Young's statement about the story's complexity.

43 Shephard, *A War of Nerves*, 219. The "slapping incident" was dramatically recreated in the 1970 biopic film *Patton*.

44 Shephard, *A War of Nerves*, 219.

45 That relationship involved research and initiatives in the mental hygiene movement, and of course its darker expression – eugenics. For more on Canadian developments see Gleason, *Normalizing the Ideal*, 19–36; McLaren, *Our Own Master Race*, passim; Dyck, *Facing Eugenics*, chapters 1, 2, 3.

46 Copp and Humphries, *Combat Stress*, 132. The Canadian Psychological Association was formed in 1938.

47 English, *The Cream of the Crop*, 64.

48 Chisholm was the first private psychiatric practitioner in Canada (1934), and became the first director-general of the World Health Organization in 1948.

49 Copp and Humphries, *Combat Stress*, 135.

50 Dowbiggin, "Prescription for Survival," in Moran and Wright, *Mental Health and Canadian Society*, 178. Copp and McAndrew likewise assessed Chisholm's approach as "Freudian-influenced psychiatric practice." See Copp and McAndrew, *Battle Exhaustion*, 8.

51 Copp and Humphries, *Combat Stress*, 136.

52 Ibid.

53 Ibid. The rivalry between psychiatrists and psychologists was a reflection of challenges to the former's dominance over the mental health profession resulting from the latter's rise as a distinct and organized discipline in the preceding decades. See Grob, *Mental Illness and American Society*, 264–5.

54 Copp and Humphries, *Combat Stress*, 137. The emphasis on sexual adjustment betrayed Chisholm's Freudian leanings.

55 "Influence of Mothers Held Bane," *The Globe and Mail*, 12 February 1944. Chisholm espoused many opinions considered outlandish or strange by twenty-first century standards. He is famous for arguing that parents needed to get rid of the Santa Claus myth because "we know what myths and magic do to people." In a speech at the New York Psychoanalytic Society and the New York Psychoanalytic Institute in 1946, he affirmed that the fact that "hardly a hotel in New York has a floor numbered 13" implied "enormous and disturbing" things. He seems to have spotted neuroses in many ostensibly benign traditions. See "Hotel Lacks 13th Floor, Fact Bothers Chisholm," *The Globe and Mail*, 26 October 1946.

56 Chisholm's expression of "Momism" reflected a larger trend evident during
    the 1930s, 1940s, and beyond. During that time, psychiatrists, psychologists,
    and other experts blamed the war's social upheaval and a subsequent shift-
    ing of gender roles for the rise of emasculated "girly men." Numerous schol-
    ars have examined anxieties about socio-economic changes and shifting
    gender roles. For two Canadian examples see Gleason, *Normalizing the Ideal*,
    and Greig, *Ontario Boys*.

57 "Dr. Chisholm Clarifies," *The Globe and Mail*, 17 February 1944.

58 Canada, Parliament. House of Commons. *Debates*, 19th Parliament, 5th Ses-
    sion, 1944, vol. 239, no. 1, 14 February 1944, 480.

59 *The Globe and Mail*, 17 February 1944. Given the anonymous nature of the
    article and its deferential tone, it seems possible that Chisholm himself or a
    colleague/friend wrote the piece.

60 Ibid.

61 Ibid.

62 Croft, "Emotional Women and Frail Men," in Carden-Coyne, *Gender and
    Conflict since 1914*, 133.

63 *The Globe and Mail*, 17 February 1944.

64 Jackson, *One of the Boys*, passim, esp. chapters 1, 3.

65 And, as Jackson shows, sometimes even scandal could be overlooked if a
    man's service had been particularly distinguished and he was well-liked by
    his unit. Jackson's work is a reminder that with regard to homosexuality
    and 1940s gender pronouncements, a man's "true" masculinity and accep-
    tance within his unit was ultimately determined by his performance in bat-
    tle. A homosexual man, like the shell-shocked soldier, could prove himself
    to be a "real" man and overcome prejudices about his character if he stayed
    the course and fought well with his comrades.

66 Ibid., passim.

67 Copp and Humphries, *Combat Stress*, 137.

68 Copp and Humphries described the Canadian battle exhaustion experience,
    at least in Normandy, as "fairly typical of the overall Allied experience,"
    though Shephard argued that the Canadians had a particularly tough time.
    Cf. Copp and Humpries, *Combat Stress*, 149; Shephard, *A War of Nerves*,
    254–5.

69 R.A. Farquharson, "Drive to Curb Nerve Shocks of Front Line," *The Globe
    and Mail*, 3 January 1940.

70 This situation reflected the fact that before 1939 the treatment of neuroses,
    at least in academic medicine, was almost exclusively the domain of neurol-

ogists in general hospitals. Thus, neurologists and neurosurgeons were put in one place, and the former given the title neuropsychiatrists. See Copp and McAndrew, *Battle Exhaustion*, 15.

71 Ibid. In fact, the article made two references to the implied financial savings. According to Copp, the contrast between the Army's resistance to psychological testing and its positive response to Russel's proposal was a measure of the status he held in the Canadian medical profession. See Copp, "The Development of Neuropsychiatry in the Canadian Army," 69.

72 Ibid.

73 It is unclear where the author took his statistics from, but it might have been a reference to Granville Canadian Hospital. In his previously cited 1919 article "The Management of Psycho-Neuroses in the Canadian Army," Colin Russel made reference to "upwards of 60% of the patients" in 1917 being returned to the front.

74 Ibid.

75 Russel, "The Nature of the War Neuroses," 554.

76 For a fuller account of Basingstoke see Copp and McAndrew, *Battle Exhaustion*, 16–17.

77 Ibid., 16.

78 Ibid, 16–18.

79 The Canadians had of course been decisively defeated at Dieppe in 1942. A psychological study (discussed in a note below) many decades later hinted that many veterans of the Dieppe raid still carried the psychological scars of battle. Neuropsychiatric figures are taken from Copp and McAndrew, *Battle Exhaustion*, 187.

80 Mowat, *The Regiment; And No Birds Sang*. Mowat was eventually promoted to captain.

81 Mowat, *The Regiment*, 333.

82 Ibid.

83 Ibid., 101.

84 Ibid., 130.

85 Ibid.

86 Mowat, *And No Birds Sang*, 215.

87 Ibid., 216.

88 Ibid., 217.

89 Copp and McAndrew, *Battle Exhaustion*, 9.

90 Copp and Humphries, *Combat Stress*, 139–40. Those labels were a byproduct of the focus on testing and reclassifying soldiers prior to the invasion of

Sicily. According to Copp and Humphries, Army psychiatrists were deeply embarrassed by them after the war.

91 Copp and McAndrew, *Battle Exhaustion*, 149.

92 To put this number in perspective, an infantry division at full strength in the Second World War numbered 18,376 officers and other ranks, of which infantry made up 8,148 and medical staff 945. Although divisions never operated at full strength, especially during the war, one psychiatrist still seems exceedingly low. Divisional numbers taken from Granatstein and Oliver, *The Oxford Companion to Canadian Military History*, 155–7. It should also be noted that Sicily was the first time that a Canadian field formation went into battle with a psychiatrist on strength.

93 Copp and McAndrew, *Battle Exhaustion*, 149–50.

94 Doyle, "The History and Development of Canadian Neuropsychiatric Service in the C.M.F.," in Copp and Humphries, *Combat Stress*, 194.

95 Ibid.

96 As was also implied, this escape was only meant to be temporary.

97 And it, in theory, prevented soldiers from diagnosing themselves, as had occurred with shell shock once the term entered popular parlance.

98 Ibid., 193.

99 Ibid., 196.

100 Ibid., 197.

101 McKerracher, "Psychiatric Problems in the Army," 399.

102 Doyle, "The History and Development of Canadian Neuropsychiatric Service in the C.M.F.," 220.

103 Ibid., 192.

104 Copp and McAndrew, *Battle Exhaustion*, 150.

105 Shephard, *A War of Nerves*, 254.

106 Copp, "From Neurasthenia to Post-Traumatic Stress Disorder," 152.

107 Van Nostrand, "Neuropsychiatry in the Canadian Army (Overseas)," in Copp and Humphries, *Combat Stress*, 297.

108 Ibid., 299.

109 Ibid.

110 Ibid., 300.

111 Copp and McAndrew, *Battle Exhaustion*, 151.

112 Van Nostrand, "Neuropsychiatry in the Canadian Army," 300.

113 Ibid.

114 Ibid.

115 Walter P. Davisson, "Wheat Pit Ghost of Former Self," *The Globe and Mail*, 19

July 1940. Economists have been particularly fond of using psychological trauma and its labels to describe market events. One can see a similar use of this analogy even in the twenty-first century. After the events of 11 September 2001, a *Globe and Mail* article described the US economy as suffering "a devastating bout of post-traumatic stress disorder." See Barrie McKenna, "President Says Report Is Bad News for American," *The Globe and Mail*, 3 November 2001.

116 "89 War Veterans Arrive in First Hospital Train to Bring Casualties Here," *The Globe and Mail*, 4 August 1941.

117 J.A. Kirkwood, "Doctors and Nurses Praised," *The Globe and Mail*, 16 August 1944.

118 Mrs Jimmie Smith, "Boy's Nerves Shattered but Sent Back to Lines," *The Globe and Mail*, 18 November 1944.

119 Ibid.

120 Shephard, *A War of Nerves*, 271–2.

121 Neary, *On to Civvy Street*, 63.

122 Ibid., 66.

123 During the Great War, the federal government attempted to keep responsibility for unemployed veterans at the local level, under the belief that a national relief system would promote idleness and dependence. After the war, the only universal benefit was a gratuity, which was deemed expensive and wasteful. Even King himself viewed the payments as having "encouraged undue periods of idleness." The government wished to avoid a similar mistake by directing funds toward encouraging immediate rehabilitation and employment. See Neary, *On to Civvy Street*, 77 and 82. It is important to note that women were included in postwar plans in recognition of thousands of women's direct and indirect contributions to the war effort during both world wars. In the Second World War, their service was exemplified in women's enlistment in the Women's Auxiliary Air Force, the Canadian Women's Army Corps, and the Women's Royal Canadian Naval Service. It is also important to note that contemporary gender norms and beliefs led to women's pension scale being two-thirds that of men. For more on the subject see Neary, *On to Civvy Street*, 111–16.

124 Ibid., 162. The latter name originated in a July 1944 Finance memorandum. The Department of Veterans Affairs took over from the Department of Pensions and National Health.

125 Ibid., passim. Women's courses still had a very gendered flavour, focusing on traditional women's employment such as hairdressing and dressmaking.

But the encouragement to continued employment was nonetheless ground-breaking in its own right. See ibid., 216; Neary viewed the year's free medical care as a "prelude to medicare."

126 Ibid., 284.

127 Ibid., 86.

128 Ironically, one of the expected results of IQ tests, personality profiling, and personnel selection systems in general was a decrease in postwar pensions through the screening out of neurotic and "unfit" men. See Copp, "From Neurasthenia to Post-Traumatic Stress Disorder," 151.

129 Copp and Humphries, *Combat Stress*, 350.

130 Although it is difficult to tangibly measure the postwar result, Copp highlighted that "dozens" of Canadian Army physicians were introduced to psychiatry through a short course run at Basingstoke. Copp argued that the Canadian neuropsychiatric hospitals and program were "a crucial episode in the development of the profession of psychiatry in Canada." See Copp, "The Development of Neuropsychiatry in the Canadian Army," 81.

131 The use of hypnosis seems to have been a source of embarrassment for military authorities, probably on account of its association with pseudoscience and the occult, as well as hypnosis often being a plot device in Hollywood horror films of the 1930s and 1940s. When writing of the history of Canadian neuropsychiatry during the war, A.M. Doyle noted how several war correspondents published newspaper articles about the use of hypnosis. He wrote that "some higher authorities were upset about this," but it is unclear whom he was referring to. See Doyle, "The History and Development of Canadian Neuropsychiatric Service in the C.M.F.," 195. For one such example of those articles see Relman Morin, "Shell Shock: Condition Curable, Say Experts," *The Globe and Mail*, 24 August 1943. Jones and Wessely noted that one British physician in the First World War eschewed hypnotism because it "conveyed a sense of occult power in the doctor." See Jones and Wessely, *Shell Shock to PTSD*, 27.

132 Dancey and Sarwer-Foner, "The problem of the Secondary Gain Patient in Medical Practice," 1108. Concisely stated, psychodynamic understandings of mental illness "saw illness vertically rather than cross-sectionally: trying to understand the patient's problems of a given moment in the context of his or her lifetime history." See Shorter, *A History of Psychiatry*, 99. According to Copp and McAndrew, Canadian psychiatrists showed little passion for Freudian theory, though it seems to have coloured much of their thought and practice nonetheless.

133 Dancey and Sarwer-Foner were director of psychiatry and consultant in psychiatry, respectively.

134 Ibid., 1110.

135 Kardiner, *The Traumatic Neuroses of War*, 70. The connection between compensation and continued illness was a thorny issue even prior to Freud's conceptualizations of it in the 1910s, having been debated in the nineteenth century, particularly with the rise of litigation related to industrial and railway accidents. Erichsen wrote in 1866 that physicians were fast becoming the go-to experts in such litigation because "actions for damages for injuries alleged to have been sustained in railway collisions" had become "a very important part of medico-legal inquiry." He lamented that "no little discrepancy of opinion has arisen as to the ultimate result of the case, the permanence of the symptoms, and the curability or not of the patient." See Erichsen, *On Railway Injuries*, 44.

136 Copp and Humphries, *Combat Stress*, 344.

137 This article was highlighted in "Combat Fatigue Carrying Over into Civil Life, Survey Shows," *The Globe and Mail*, 7 August 1947.

138 Billings, Chalke, and Shortt, "Battle Exhaustion – A Follow-Up Study," 153. Most of the men included in the study had taken part in the invasion of Normandy on D-Day or joined the fight soon after.

139 Ibid., 154.

140 Ibid.

141 Ibid.

142 Wasylenki, "The Paradigm Shift from Institution to Community," in Rae-Grant, *Psychiatry in Canada*, 51.

143 Neary, *On to Civvy Street*, passim.

144 Copp, "From Neurasthenia to Post-Traumatic Stress Disorder," 154.

145 It should be noted at this stage that the Canadian Pension Commission also took the approach that neuroses had their roots in childhood. Dancey outlined the details of the original post 1946 treatment plan for veterans: "At the expiration of this period [one year after service] he may receive treatment for his pensionable condition or for certain acute illnesses provided only that he has had meritorious service and provided he is relatively indigent." He went on to write, "This would mean that the thrifty veteran with a neurosis could not obtain treatment" ("Treatment in the Absence of Pensioning for Psychoneurotic Symptoms," in Copp and Humphries, *Combat Stress*, 344). It is clear that the DVA was recognizing "psychiatric disabilities" immediately after the war though. The DVA listed 641 men as having "psy-

chiatric disabilities" in 1947, though it is unclear who fell under this category. See Neary, *On to Civvy Street*, 235.

146 Dancey, "Treatment in the Absence of Pensioning," 345. This program included both hospital and outpatient treatment.

147 Healy, *The Creation of Psychopharmacology*, 28–9.

148 Dancey, "Treatment in the Absence of Pensioning," 345.

149 Ibid.

150 Ibid.

151 Ibid. One cannot help but notice the psychodynamic understanding inherent in this view. Since the illness was deemed to stem from unconscious factors and earlier life events, physicians saw a patient's lack of symptoms as progress in working through their internal conflicts and an increase in their "ability" to remain symptom free. Such a view seems to have sometimes confused remission, spontaneous or otherwise, with patients' willpower and "ability" to make their minds healthy.

152 Ibid., 346. Dancey did not elaborate on what the diversions consisted of, though one can infer based on contemporary mental hospital care that they were akin to recreation and other stress-free activities. It is not hard to notice a hint of nineteenth-century "moral" therapy in that approach. For a description of group psychotherapy conducted at Queen Mary Veterans Hospital see "Group Psychotherapy: DVA Psychiatrists Subject their Patients to Discussion of Own Ailments," *The Globe and Mail*, 14 January 1952.

153 Cook, *Warlords*, 214, 308; quotations about "psychotics" and therapies are taken from the *Globe* article below.

154 "Horizon for Veterans Broadened by Research of Medicos Aiding VAD," *The Globe and Mail*, 23 March 1946. St Anne's was a DVA administered hospital.

155 Westminster was likewise a DVA hospital.

156 Lex Schrag, "Neurosis Therapy for Afflicted Vets Given at Hospital," *The Globe and Mail*, 17 March 1947.

157 There were evident gender assumptions and stereotypes inherent in that comment.

158 Ibid.

159 Nancy White, "Sunnybrook 1945," *The Toronto Star*, 7 November 2009. This was of course true of all mental illnesses during that time, and is arguably still the case.

160 Dancey, "Treatment in the Absence of Pensions," 345.

161 Ibid., 347.

162 Copp and Humphries, *Combat Stress*, 351. One man, J.N.B. Crawford, direc-

tor of Treatment Services, Hong Kong veteran, and a former prisoner of war, felt so strongly about this stance that he even argued that he too needed to avoid gratifying his own "dependency needs" with a pension, fearing it would cause him to lose his desire to work and avoid stressful situations.

163 Ibid. Dancey's belief that a lack of publicity was a key reason why few veterans went that route is somewhat questionable, particularly given veterans' mass participation in the Royal Canadian Legion, where rumours about such a route would have flown freely. Stigma seems like an equally likely candidate.

164 Dancey, "The Interaction of the Welfare State and the Disabled," 275.

165 Ibid., 276.

166 Ibid.

167 Dummitt, *The Manly Modern*, 45–6.

168 Humphries, "War's Long Shadow," 503.

169 Dummitt, *The Manly Modern*, 44.

170 "Horizon for Veterans Broadened by Research of Medicos Aiding VAD," *The Globe and Mail*, 23 March 1946.

171 Ibid.

172 Kenneth Cragg, "Pensions Aggravate Neurotics," *The Globe and Mail*, 31 January 1948.

173 Dummitt, *The Manly Modern*, 45.

174 Ibid.

175 Ibid., 46.

176 Ibid., 50.

177 Copp and Humphries, *Combat Stress*, 349.

178 Copp and McAndrew, *Battle Exhaustion*, 155.

179 Copp and Humphries, *Combat Stress*, 349.

180 Copp and McAndrew, *Battle Exhaustion*, 157.

181 Copp and Humphries, *Combat Stress*, 349. Most cases were initially sent to Japan, since there was little provision and no organized program for dealing with them.

182 Jones, "Army Psychiatry in the Korean War: The Experience of 1 Commonwealth Division," 257; Watson, *Far Eastern Tour*, 104.

183 Watson, *Far Eastern Tour*, 104.

184 Ibid.

185 Ibid., 107. The Canadians were not the only army that went to Korea unprepared. The Americans also prepared hastily and early in the war saw entire groups of men running for their lives. See Shephard, *A War of Nerves*, 341.

186 Jones, "Army Psychiatry in the Korean War," 258. Jones argued that F.C.R. Chalke's appointment as an expert in personnel selection was an "attempt to stem the flow of evacuees." This was a result of the fact that Canadian troops were hastily assembled and recruited, as the Canadian military was relatively small and poorly prepared after five years of demobilization. Many soldiers were lost to chronic medical conditions or psychiatric problems within the first six months, before the situation levelled off. In a few particularly egregious cases, a seventy-two-year-old man was signed up, as well as a man with an artificial leg. See ibid., 257; Binneveld, *From Shell Shock to Combat Stress*, 129–30; Copp and McAndrew, *Battle Exhaustion*, 158.

187 Watson, *Far Eastern Tour*, 105.

188 Haycock and Hennessy, "The Road from Innocence: Canada and the Cold War," in Bernd Horn, *The Canadian Way of War*, 245.

189 Tyhurst et al., *More for the Mind*, 2.

190 Shorter, *A History of Psychiatry*, 65.

191 Brown, "Shell Shock in the Canadian Expeditionary Force," 324. The term "Therapeutic State" was coined in 1963 by the "antipsychiatrist" author of *The Myth of Mental Illness*, Thomas Szasz.

192 Copp, "The Development of Neuropsychiatry in the Canadian Army," 67.

193 Houts, "Fifty Years of Psychiatric Nomenclature," 940.

194 Rae-Grant, "Introduction," in Rae-Grant, *Psychiatry in Canada*, ix–x.

195 Greenland and Hoffman, "Psychiatry in Canada from 1951 to 2001," in Rae-Grant, *Psychiatry in Canada*, 1.

196 Ibid.

197 Among McNeel's many interesting forays was a 1966 tour of medical facilities in the Soviet Union.

198 Occasionally APA meetings were held in Canada. There was a Section of Psychiatry in the Canadian Medical Association since 1945, but it had limited influence. More rarely, Canadians went across the Atlantic to Britain to discuss ideas.

199 Pankratz, "The History of the Canadian Psychiatric Association," in Rae-Grant, *Psychiatry in Canada*, 29. Many Canadian provinces had (and still have) their own provincial organizations, but their affiliation was loose and lobbying power limited.

200 Ibid. The CPA started off as a relatively modest operation and was almost entirely run by volunteers for its first ten years, until a head office was created in Ottawa, in 1961. See ibid., 44.

201 Tyhurst et al., *More for the Mind*, 5–6.

202 Ibid., 6.

203 Even in 1963, the authors of *More for the Mind* noted that one of the misconceptions still commonly held by Canadians was that "psychiatrists are
different from 'real' doctors in some undiscoverable way – they are not fully
qualified as physicians or not to be trusted." See ibid., 9–10.

204 Greenland and Hoffman, "Psychiatry in Canada," 3.

205 Tyhurst et al., *More for the Mind*, 12.

206 Canadian Mental Health Association, "History of CMHA," accessed
27 January 2014, http://www.cmha.ca/about-cmha/history-of-cmha/#
.VNJ8CS5hwnM.

207 Tyhurst et al., *More for the Mind*, 3.

208 Ibid.

209 Shorter, *A History of Psychiatry*, 298.

210 Ibid. As Shorter pointed out, before the 1950s, psychiatric classifications
reflected the fact that most psychiatrists worked in mental hospitals. Since
many of the hospitals were filled with those suffering from dementia and
other chronic (and major) forms of mental illness, the naming systems
reflected what psychiatrists saw and treated on a daily basis.

211 Ibid.

212 Shephard, *A War of Nerves*, 363.

213 Van Nostrand, "Neuropsychiatry in the Canadian Army," 297.

214 Shorter, *A History of Psychiatry*, 298.

215 Ibid. *DSM-I* was also influenced in part by the work of Abram Kardiner.

216 Houts, "Fifty Years of Psychiatric Nomenclature," 937. William also founded,
along with his father Charles and brother Karl, the famous Menninger
Clinic in Topeka, Kansas, in 1919. William and Karl were, according to
Shephard, two of the "intellectual leaders" of American psychiatry. See Shephard, *A War of Nerves*, 203.

217 Houts, "Fifty Years of Psychiatric Nomenclature," 941. American psychoanalyst and historian Mitchell Wilson described this mixture of thought as
"the theory of personality and intrapsychic conflict developed by Freud
and the more pragmatic and environmentally oriented mental hygiene
movement influenced by Meyerian psychobiology." See Wilson, "DSM-III
and the Transformation of American Psychiatry," 400; it was Meyer who
suggested using the term "mental hygiene." For more on Meyer's influence
on American psychiatry see Lamb, *Pathologist of the Mind*, passim.

218 The "biopsychosocial" approach.

219 Office of the Surgeon General, Army Service Forces, "Nomenclature of Psychiatric Disorders and Reactions," 289.

220 Ibid.

221 For example, while Medical 203 said that combat exhaustion occurred in "more or less 'normal' persons," *DSM-I* similarly stated that Gross Stress Reaction occurred in "previously more or less 'normal' persons." Even a superficial comparison between the two documents demonstrates the undeniable borrowing of the latter from the former.

222 Wilson, "The Historical Evolution of PTSD Diagnostic Criteria," 688. That link was no doubt also due to the "traumatic neurosis" concept, which likewise characterized individual responses in civilian trauma in the same vein as those seen in war.

223 Wilson, "DSM-III and the Transformation of American Psychiatry," 400.

224 Grob, "Origins of DSM-I," 429.

225 Paris, *The Fall of an Icon*, 3. In Canada, with its feet in both European and American traditions, the spread of psychoanalysis was more intermittent than in the United States. With many British and European-trained psychiatrists in Canada, who adhered to a more biological approach, formal psychoanalysis was "relatively invisible" outside of large cities like Toronto and Montreal. In western Canada, for example, most psychiatrists during the postwar period still practised in large mental hospitals and according to Paris, "only a few" had an intense interest in psychotherapy. See Paris, "Canadian Psychiatry Across 5 Decades," 35.

226 Ban interview. In his *History of Psychoanalysis in Canada*, Alan Parkin saw this situation differently, stating that the establishment of the Canadian Psychoanalytic Society at McGill in 1955 was not "a sign of [Ewen] Cameron's sympathy," but a "matter of expedience to stem the loss of the residents from his post-graduate program in psychiatry to centres of Canada where training in psychoanalysis could be found." See Parkin, 84.

227 Shorter, *A History of Psychiatry*, 145.

228 A telling statistic about the number of psychiatrists who had moved from hospitals to private practice was this: By 1956, only about 17 per cent of the roughly 10,000 members of the American Psychiatric Association (which included many Canadians) were employed in hospitals. This stood in stark contrast to 1940, when more than two-thirds of its members were employed in hospitals. See Grob, "Origins of DSM-I," 428.

229 Shorter, *A History of Psychiatry*, 146. Though Shorter's interpretation might seem harsh, even a more sympathetic account of the psychoanalytic movement stated that the expansion of psychiatrists into psychoanalytic territory was, from an economic point of view, "an imperialistic extension of psycho-

analytic practice." See Hale Jr., *The Rise and Crisis of Psychoanalysis in the United States*, 274–5.

230 Paris, "Canadian Psychiatry Across 5 Decades," 35. By extension it was believed that psychoanalysis could explain societal motivations as well.

231 Parkin, *A History of Psychoanalysis in Canada*, 66–7.

232 "Home and School Clubs Survey Urgent Problems," *The Globe and Mail*, 22 January 1947.

233 Greig, *Ontario Boys*, 18.

234 "Homelife Causes Maladjustments, Psychiatrist Says," *The Globe and Mail*, 9 May 1946.

235 Greig, *Ontario Boys*, 18.

236 Ibid., 121.

237 Ibid., 122.

238 Grob, "Origins of DSM-I," 427.

239 Ibid.

240 Ibid.

241 Parkin, *A History of Psychoanalysis in Canada*, 71.

242 Social psychiatry here means "psychiatry engaged in socio-economic issues and health policy." GAP was comprised of an abundance of prominent American psychiatrists, many of whom had served during the Second World War. This included the Menninger brothers, William and Karl, and Roy Grinker, among others. For more on GAP see Grob, "Psychiatry and Social Activism," 477–501. For a comprehensive overview of the many CMHA activities throughout the 1950s to 1980s, see Griffin, *In Search of Sanity*.

243 Tyhurst et al., *More for the Mind*, 38. This became known colloquially as the "McNeel Ideal."

244 Griffin, *In Search of Sanity*, 169.

245 Tyhurst et al., *More for the Mind*, 3; the Medical Care Act was implemented in 1968.

246 Shorter, *A History of Psychiatry*, 247.

247 For a more comprehensive history of chlorpromazine see Shorter, *A History of Psychiatry*, 246–55 and Healy, *The Creation of Psychopharmacology*, passim. McGill University had the first division of psychopharmacology in the world.

248 Paris, "Canadian Psychiatry Across 5 Decades," 35.

249 Ibid.

250 Shorter, *A History of Psychiatry*, 239.

251 Ibid., 154.

252 Paris, *The Fall of an Icon*, 3.

253 Shorter, *A History of Psychiatry*, 299.

254 Ibid., 300.

255 Wilson, "The Historical Evolution of PTSD Diagnostic Criteria," 690.

256 Ibid. The other two examples were: "Resentment with depressive tone associated with an unwanted pregnancy and manifested by hostile complaints and suicidal gestures"; and "a Ganser syndrome associated with death sentence and manifested by incorrect but approximate answers to questions."

257 Ibid.

258 Scott, "PTSD in DSM-III," 297.

259 Wilson, "The Historical Evolution of PTSD Diagnostic Criteria," 691.

260 For example, Archibald, Long, Miller, and Tuddenham, "Gross Stress Reaction in Combat – A 15-Year Follow-Up," 317–22; Archibald and Tuddenham, "Persistent Stress Reaction after Combat: A 20-Year Follow-Up," 475–81.

261 Scott, "PTSD in DSM-III," 297.

262 Ibid. As Shephard argued, by the end of the Second World War, the Americans had become convinced that every man had his breaking point. See Shephard, *A War of Nerves*, 326.

263 Ibid., 341.

264 Bourne, *Men, Stress, and Vietnam*. Among other factors listed for the low rate of psychiatric breakdown were: one-year tours of duty; short battles; few artillery barrages; and high morale. The twelve-month rotation of soldiers turned out, in some ways, to be a hindrance rather than a help. See Shephard, *A War of Nerves*, 348–9.

265 Scott, "PTSD in DSM-III," 296.

266 Quoted in Shephard, *A War of Nerves*, 340.

267 Scott, "PTSD in DSM-III," 298. Scott pointed out that, in a testament to clinicians and military psychiatrists simply adhering to whatever practice works best "in the field," some psychiatrists still felt that GSR was useful and valid, and stuck to applying the concept in their work even after its removal from *DSM-II*.

268 Ibid.

269 Shephard, *A War of Nerves*, 355.

CHAPTER THREE

1 Shephard, *A War of Nerves*, 358.
2 Ibid., 357. Shephard wrote that this event took place in Chicago, in a liquor store, but Johnson was actually killed in Detroit, robbing a grocery/variety store.
3 Jon Nordheimer, "How a Medal of Honor Winner Ended Up Dead in a Holdup," *The Globe and Mail*, 27 May 1971.
4 Ibid.
5 Ibid.
6 Ibid.
7 Jon Nordheimer, "Black Medal of Honor Winner May Have Been Trapped by Ghetto Mentality, Lawyer Says," *The Globe and Mail*, 28 May 1971.
8 Jon Nordheimer, "Pressures that Pushed a Medal of Honor Winner Toward Crime," *The Globe and Mail*, 29 May 1971.
9 Ibid.
10 Ibid.
11 For more on postwar Detroit and racial relations see Sugrue, *The Origins of the Urban Crisis*.
12 Shephard, *A War of Nerves*, 372.
13 Ibid., 357.
14 Scott, "PTSD in DSM-III," 300.
15 This was the title of his twenty-seventh chapter in *A War of Nerves*.
16 Shatan lived in Canada from the 1920s, obtaining his medical degree from McGill University. He moved to New York City in 1949.
17 *The New York Times*, 6 May 1972.
18 Lifton, *Witness to an Extreme Century*, 184–5; *Death in Life: Survivors of Hiroshima*. Lifton's 2011 memoir is a captivating account of his work throughout the second half of the twentieth century.
19 Ibid., 185. Lifton was opposed to the Vietnam War even before it began. He became convinced of his position after a 1954 discussion with a group of Frenchmen in a Saigon café, shortly after the battle of Dien Bien Phu. See ibid., 167.
20 Chaim Shatan, "Post-Vietnam Syndrome," *The New York Times*, 6 May 1972.
21 Lifton, *Witness to an Extreme Century*, 130.
22 *The New York Times*, 6 May 1972; Scott, "PTSD in DSM-III," 300. Essentially, Shatan believed that the symptoms listed in his article stemmed from an "unconsummated grief" that soldiers were unable to exorcise on the battle-

field. The apathy which developed as a result manifested itself in the symptoms presented at the rap sessions.

23 Lifton, *Witness to an Extreme Century*, 187.
24 Ibid.
25 Ibid., 189.
26 Binneveld, *From Shell Shock to Combat Stress*, 41.
27 Shephard, *A War of Nerves*, 359.
28 Scott, "PTSD in DSM-III," 299.
29 Shephard, *A War of Nerves*, 360.
30 Ibid. Copp and Humphries argued that part of Lifton and Shatan's quest to get a Vietnam syndrome recognized was based on a desire to use the disorder's recognition as a further way to undermine the legitimacy of the war itself. Lifton's 2011 memoir confirmed that view. See Copp and Humphries, *Combat Stress*, 415–16, and Lifton, *Witness to an Extreme Century*, 184–91.
31 Shephard, *A War of Nerves*, 360.
32 Ibid., 362.
33 Scott, "PTSD in DSM-III," 301.
34 Ibid., 302.
35 Lifton, *Witness to an Extreme Century*, 185.
36 Ibid., 303.
37 Shorter, *A History of Psychiatry*, 301.
38 This event received coverage in Canadian news circles. See "Homosexuality Not a Mental Disease, U.S. Psychiatrists Say," *The Globe and Mail*, 17 December 1973.
39 Scott, "PTSD in DSM-III," 304. Those events were extensively covered by Ronald Bayer in *Homosexuality and American Psychiatry*.
40 Shorter, *A History of Psychiatry*, 304.
41 Scott, "PTSD in DSM-III," 304.
42 Ibid.
43 Ibid., 305.
44 Ibid.
45 Ibid.
46 Horowitz, *Stress Response Syndromes*, 26.
47 Ibid.
48 Ibid., 28.
49 He also cited and was influenced by Holocaust survivor literature.
50 Ibid., 23–4.
51 Shephard, *A War of Nerves*, 367.

52 Horowitz, *Stress Response Syndromes*, 41.

53 Shephard, *A War of Nerves*, 367.

54 Scott, "PTSD in DSM-III," 307.

55 Ibid., 308.

56 Ibid.

57 Wilson, "The Historical Evolution of PTSD Diagnostic Criteria," 692.

58 Ibid.

59 Copp and Humphries, *Combat Stress*, 352.

60 Ibid., 353.

61 Edward Shorter termed this the "second biological psychiatry," to differentiate it from the "first," which occurred roughly from the nineteenth to the early twentieth century. See Shorter, *A History of Psychiatry*, 69–112.

62 Ibid., 300.

63 Ibid. Of course, saying that psychodynamic-leaning psychiatrists were uninterested in diagnostics and classification must be considered a slight generalization, since Horowitz, Shatan, and other psychoanalysts who fought to ensure the creation of a "stress syndrome" were very interested in developing, at least in the case of PTSD, a model and framework that could be, and was, used as the template for PTSD diagnostic criteria. Nevertheless, it is evident that during the time of psychoanalytic/psychodynamic prominence, diagnostics were not at the top of their priority list.

64 Feighner et al., "Diagnostic Criteria for Use in Psychiatric Research," 57–63; see also Kendler, Munoz, and Murphy, "The Development of the Feighner Criteria," 134–42.

65 Wilson, "DSM-III and the Transformation of American Psychiatry," 404.

66 Shorter, *A History of Psychiatry*, 300–1.

67 Spitzer, Endicott, and Robins, "Research Diagnostic Criteria: Rationale and Reliability," 773.

68 What Spitzer called "shared symptomatology."

69 Shorter, *A History of Psychiatry*, 301.

70 Klerman, "The Significance of DSM-III in American Psychiatry," in Spitzer, Williams, and Skodol, *International Perspectives on DSM-III*, 3.

71 Ibid.

72 Ibid.

73 The story of *DSM-III*'s creation, told in numerous accounts, reads like the story of a coup d'état, with, in Shorter's words, a group of "Young Turks," APA medical director Melvin Sabshin among them, ensuring that Spitzer was appointed as head of the *DSM-III* task force, since he was known by

then as someone determined to make significant changes in psychiatry's orientation. See Shorter, *A History of Psychiatry*, 301.

74 Wilson, "DSM-III and the Transformation of American Psychiatry," 400; Spitzer and Williams, "International Perspectives: Summary and Conclusion," in Spitzer, Williams, and Skodol, *International Perspectives on DSM-III*, 352.

75 Shorter, *A History of Psychiatry*, 301.

76 Healy, *The Creation of Psychopharmacology*, 302.

77 Shorter, *A History of Psychiatry*, 302.

78 Ibid.

79 Ibid.

80 Ibid., 297.

81 Wilson, "DSM-III and the Transformation of American Psychiatry," 403.

82 Hale, *The Rise and Crisis of Psychoanalysis*, 300.

83 Psychopathology here means "deviations from normal behaviour or manifest symptoms."

84 Gurland et al., "Cross-National Study of Diagnosis of Mental Disorders," 24.

85 Rosenhan, "On Being Sane in Insane Places," 250–8.

86 Ibid., 256.

87 Ibid.

88 Shorter, *A History of Psychiatry*, 274. As Shorter noted, much of this movement stemmed from the spirit of the 1960s and its emphasis on hostility to authority, which the medical profession, and especially psychiatry with its emphasis on controlling deviant behaviour and thoughts, seemed to represent. There are any number of works that could be cited here, but several of the most prominent are: Szasz, *The Myth of Mental Illness*; Scheff, *Being Mentally Ill*; Laing, *The Politics of Experience*; Foucault, *Madness and Civilization*; and Goffman, *Asylums*.

89 Spitzer, "More on Pseudoscience in Science and the Case of Psychiatric Diagnosis," 469.

90 Mayes and Horwitz, "DSM-III and the Revolution in the Classification of Mental Illness," 263–4.

91 Shorter, *A History of Psychiatry*, 302.

92 Wilson, "DSM-III and the Transformation of American Psychiatry," 408.

93 Healy, *The Creation of Psychopharmacology*, 305.

94 Mayes and Horwitz, "DSM-III and the Revolution," 263.

95 Shephard, *A War of Nerves*, 385.

96 Summerfield, "A Critique of Seven Assumptions," 1450.

97 Arial, *I Volunteered*, 9. As Fred Gaffen highlighted, despite Canada not being officially involved, Canadian businesses participated obliquely in the Vietnam War through billions of dollars of war materiel supplied to American firms. See Gaffen, *Unknown Warriors*, 9 and 36. Participant figures are taken from Gaffen, 36.

98 Gaffen, *Unknown Warriors*, 9.

99 Ibid.

100 Doug Clark, "The Loneliness and Pain of Canadian Veterans of the Vietnam War," *The Globe and Mail*, 9 July 1984.

101 Gaffen, *Unknown Warriors*, 14.

102 Ibid., 13.

103 Ibid.

104 Those signs went largely unnoticed by all except for specialists and a few interested researchers.

105 *Globe and Mail*, 9 July 1984; Clark's figure was taken from an estimate that 80 per cent of US veterans returned home and adjusted without major difficulties.

106 Ibid.

107 Ibid.

108 McKay and Swift, *Warrior Nation*, 160.

109 Brian McAndrew, "Viet Nam Vets in Canada Still Feel Isolated. While Americans Faced Rejection, Canadians Returned Home to a Void," *The Toronto Star*, 6 July 1986.

110 Ibid.

111 Ibid.

112 Ibid.

113 Christopher Wren, "Vietnam War Also Haunts Canadians Who Volunteered," *New York Times*, 24 January 1985.

114 Ibid. Canadians were entitled to most benefits through the United States Veterans Administration, except for a few, such as housing loans. The problem for most was that free medical care for war-related problems had to be sought at a Veterans Administration hospital or other approved American facility. This meant in practice that some men had to travel extremely long distances into the United States for care.

115 Ibid.

116 Ibid.

117 Ibid.

118 Ibid.

119 Ibid.

120 Ibid.

121 Paris, e-mail message to author, 14 April 2015.

122 Woods, "Canadian Physicians in World War II," 1103.

123 Sullivan, "War Ended Decades Ago, but PoWs' Problems Continue," 837.

124 This number marginally rises to three when including a 1980 case report
     that utilized the concept of traumatic neurosis. The author, George
     MacLean, a child psychiatrist and assistant professor of psychiatry at McGill,
     displayed his psychodynamic (Freudian) leanings when he described the
     case of a three-year-old boy attacked by a leopard. He stated that the boy's
     "well-endowed ego was overwhelmed" due to "coexisting feelings of fear,
     anger and guilt resulting from the age appropriate oedipal strivings." See
     MacLean, "Addendum to a Case of Traumatic Neurosis," 506.

125 Kuch, "Post-Traumatic Stress Disorder after Car Accidents," 426–7.

126 Varadaraj, "Management of Post Traumatic Stress Disorder and Ethnicity,"
     75.

127 Ibid.

128 To the best of my knowledge, as of 2015 Stretch's studies are still the only
     ones of their kind.

129 Stretch, "Effects of Service in Vietnam on Canadian Forces Military Person-
     nel," 571–85; Stretch, "Post-Traumatic Stress Disorder and the Canadian Viet-
     nam Veteran," 239–54; Stretch, "Psychosocial Readjustment of Canadian
     Vietnam Veterans," 188–9. The first article focused on Canadian military
     personnel serving in a peacekeeping role while the second focused on com-
     bat soldiers.

130 Stretch, "Psychosocial Readjustment of Canadian Vietnam Veterans," 188–9.

131 Stretch, "Effects of Service in Vietnam," 583.

132 Ibid., 584.

133 Binneveld, *From Shell Shock to Combat Stress*, 83.

134 Jones and Wessely, *Shell Shock to PTSD*, 131.

135 Copp and Humphries, *Combat Stress*, 419; Trimble, *Post-Traumatic Neurosis*,
     153.

136 Trimble, e-mail message to author, 22 April 2015.

137 Ibid.

138 Trimble, *Post-Traumatic Neurosis*, 3; Jones and Wessely, "A Paradigm Shift in
     the Conceptualization of Psychological Trauma," 173.

139 Copp and Humphries, *Combat Stress*, 419.

140 Shephard, *A War of Nerves*, 378.

141 Ibid., 378.

142 Jones and Wessely, *Shell Shock to* PTSD, 136.

143 Shephard, *A War of Nerves*, 378.

144 Ibid., 378–9; Jones and Wessely, *Shell Shock to* PTSD, 166.

145 Shephard, *A War of Nerves*, 378.

146 Ibid., 379.

147 Ibid.

148 Ibid., 381.

149 Ibid.

150 McGeorge, Hughes, and Wessely, "The MOD PTSD Decision: A Psychiatric Perspective," in Copp and Humphries, *Combat Stress*, 489.

151 Alun Rees, "Suicide of Falklands Veterans," *The Mail on Sunday* (London), 13 January 2002. The South Atlantic Medal Association, which represented and aided Falklands veterans, believed that 264 veterans had committed suicide, as opposed to 255 who died during the war.

152 McGeorge, Hughes, and Wessely, "The MOD PTSD Decision," 493.

153 Ibid., 492.

154 This support was, if not financial, at least social.

CHAPTER FOUR

1 Godin interview.

2 UN forces were first deployed to Cyprus in 1964 to quell and prevent intercommunal violence between Turkish and Greek Cypriots on the island. As part of United Nations Security Council Resolution 186, UN peacekeeping forces were established to create and maintain a buffer zone between the two sides. As of 2015 the mission is still ongoing, and is one of the longest running UN peacekeeping efforts, despite being largely unknown. See United Nations, "Resolutions Adopted by the United Nations Security Council in 1964."

3 This does not mean, of course, that the mission was one of complete relaxation. Godin recalled a few "unnerving incidents," which included having to quell a large Greek Cypriot women's demonstration with no weapon while being subjected to spitting, shoving, and yelling. In one particular instance, over 3,000 women were involved in a march into Turkish held territory that led to numerous injuries and arrests. See Nick Williams Jr, "Greek Cypriot Women, Turkish Police Scuffle: 3,000 Cross Border, Protest Island's Division; 9 hurt, 50 Reported Arrested," *Los Angeles Times*, 20 March 1989, for

coverage of an incident Godin was personally involved in quelling. Fred Doucette likewise highlighted some of the harrowing moments he encountered in Cyprus during the 1970s, including the bombing of the Nicosia law courts. See Doucette, *Empty Casing*, 17.

4 Godin, e-mail message to author, 5 May 2015. Godin's appraisal is backed up by numerous other accounts from Canadians who participated in the Cyprus mission. See, for example, Warrant Officer Matt Stopford's comments about Cyprus: "I'm tempted to say that Cyprus was like a holiday. Now and then somebody got shot or there was a riot, but it wasn't a big deal and you did your job. It was like a picnic." Doucette wrote that in Cyprus he "saw drunkenness on a level" that would shock both civilians and soldiers. See Wood, "Matt Stopford: Warrant Officer" in *The Chance of War*, 124; Doucette, *Empty Casing*, 16.

5 Testimony of CWO M.B. McCarthy, *Croatia Board of Inquiry – Potential Exposure of Canadian Forces Personnel to Contaminated Environment*, 25 November 1999, vol. IX, 28; hereafter referred to as *Croatia Board of Inquiry*.

6 Godin interview.

7 Ibid.

8 Ibid.

9 Ibid.

10 Ibid; Carol Off, *The Ghosts of Medak Pocket*, 2.

11 Godin interview.

12 Ibid.

13 Ibid.

14 Ibid.

15 Ibid.

16 Sarah Hampson, "'I'm Getting Some Hawk Wings,'" *The Globe and Mail*, 4 December 2004.

17 English, "From Combat Stress to Operational Stress," 11.

18 The British invaded largely because the Suez Canal was at that time considered the "swing-door of the British Empire," due to its crucial role in the shipment of oil, and also as a strategic throughway for British ships in case of war. See Kyle, *Suez*, 7–21.

19 Kyle summed up the situation by stating that, after Suez, Britain became convinced there would be "no more solo flights" in foreign policy. See Kyle, *Suez*, 583.

20 Cooper, *The Lion's Last Roar*, 282.

21 Coulon, *Soldiers of Diplomacy*, 25. The UNEF's goal was to oversee the with-

drawal of British, French, and Israeli troops, as well as to monitor the Israeli-Egyptian border. Peacekeeping was not invented during the Suez Crisis. What *was* created was the belief that Canadians were natural born peacekeepers. See Granatstein, *Canada's Army*, 342–4.

22 Ibid.; James, *Canada and Conflict*, 10.

23 For an example of criticism "from below" see William Kinmond, "Suez Efforts Saved Commonwealth Ties, Says Liberal Leader," *The Globe and Mail*, 4 March 1958, which described a talk by Pearson in Flin Flon, Manitoba, when he was asked to justify his decisions during the Suez Crisis.

24 "Pearson Saved World at Suez, Nobel View," *The Globe and Mail*, 11 December 1957.

25 Pearson, "Nobel Lecture: The Four Faces of Peace."

26 Neither the government nor the military were initially enthusiastic about peacekeeping, since it was seen as a distraction from "the big show" in Germany, where Canadian troops were stationed as part of NATO forces in case of a superpower conflict between the United States and the Soviet Union. See English, *Understanding Military Culture*, 89.

27 Lewis MacKenzie, "Foreword," in Horn, *The Canadian Way of War*, 7.

28 Coulon, *Soldiers of Diplomacy*, x.

29 Horn, "Introduction," in Horn, *The Canadian Way of War*, 11. Clarkson used this term on a few occasions, such as during a memorial ceremony for four Canadian soldiers killed by American airstrikes in a friendly fire incident in Afghanistan, in 2002. See Governor General, "Her Excellency the Right Honourable Adrienne Clarkson Speech on the Occasion of a Memorial Ceremony for the Fallen Soldiers of 3 PPCLI." The phrase originated in America as the title of an 1833–34 painting, "The Peaceable Kingdom," by Quaker painter Edward Hicks. It was later used in the 1960s by Northrop Frye in reference to Canadian literary endeavours. Thereafter it became popularized after its use in the title of a 1970 book by Canadian author, historian, and Toronto city councillor William Kilbourn. See Kilbourn, "The Peaceable Kingdom Still," in Graubard, ed., *In Search of Canada*, 27–8.

30 English, *Understanding Military Culture*, 89; MacKenzie, "Foreword," 7.

31 Manson made this statement during a speech to the Empire Club in Toronto. Quoted in Whitworth, *Men, Militarism, and UN Peacekeeping*, 85.

32 Department of National Defence, *1994 Defence White Paper*, 24. This argument has been made by several authors. See, for example, Granatstein, *Who Killed the Canadian Military?*, 30; Last, "Almost a Legacy: Canada's Contribution to Peacekeeping," in Horn, ed., *Forging a Nation*, 382.

33 *1994 Defence White Paper*, 24.

34 Last, "Almost a Legacy," 382. The publication is now titled the *Canadian Army Journal*.

35 Pearson's quotation reads: "We need action not only to end the fighting but to make the peace ... My own government would be glad to recommend Canadian participation in such a United Nations force, a truly international peace and police force."

36 Whitworth, *Men, Militarism, and UN Peacekeeping*, 34; Anderson, *Imagined Communities*, passim.

37 Granatstein, *Who Killed the Canadian Military?*, 23.

38 Ibid.

39 Horn, "Introduction," in *Forging a Nation*, 11.

40 Ibid.

41 Francis, *National Dreams*, 10.

42 Coulon, *Soldiers of Diplomacy*, ix. Some of these conflicts began because of the Soviet Union's collapse, others were unrelated.

43 Ibid.

44 Ibid., ix–x.

45 Ibid.

46 Ibid., 8.

47 James, *Canada and Conflict*, 10; Windsor, Charters, and Wilson point out that there were many examples of non-Pearsonian peacekeeping operations prior to 1991. They state, rightly so, that the UNEF model was "the exception, not the rule." What perhaps changed was that amidst the uncertainties of a post-Cold War world, peacekeeping operations were followed with greater scrutiny and interest by the Canadian media, the UN, and Western society. More research is needed on this subject. For Windsor, Charters, and Wilson's take, see Windsor, Charters, and Wilson, *Kandahar Tour*, 12.

48 *1994 Defence White Paper*, 3.

49 Boutros-Ghali, *An Agenda for Peace 1995*, 8. Boutros-Ghali further elaborated on this point using statistics. In 1988, of the five UN operations in existence, only one was related to an intra-state conflict. By 1995, thirteen out of twenty-one operations were to mediate intra-state conflicts. See ibid., 7–8.

50 Coulon, *Soldiers of Diplomacy*, x.

51 Bercuson, *Significant Incident*, 220–1.

52 The term, coined in 2003 by Lieutenant-General (ret.) Al DeQuetteville, former chief of the Air Staff, originally referred to a successive wave of budget cuts that occurred across the board throughout the 1990s, and their impact

on how senior CAF/DND leadership viewed the future of operational capabilities. There was a very real sense of frustration and uncertainty amongst senior leadership regarding the ability to conduct long-term planning, as well as concerns about whether or not the CAF would be equal to the tasks requested of it, particularly given the increased operational tempo that occurred early in the decade. While the term originally referred to budgets cuts and a sense of uncertainty, it later took on a metaphorical meaning describing the many difficulties that the CAF faced throughout the decade. See English, "From Combat Stress to Operational Stress," passim. Part of this historical background was provided to the author by Brigadier-General (ret.) Joe Sharpe via email correspondence (e-mail message to author, 7 November 2014). More background is also taken from Sharpe and English, "The Decade of Darkness."

53 Sharpe and English, "The Decade of Darkness," 1.

54 Ibid., 3.

55 Coulon, *Soldiers of Diplomacy*, 26; Granatstein, *Who Killed the Canadian Military?*, 127–59. Granatstein laid the blame for the many scandals of the 1990s largely on the Mulroney government, who "agreed to commitment after commitment while failing to ensure that the forces had the necessary manpower, the funds, the equipment, and the training to do the jobs they were being asked to undertake." See ibid., 159.

56 *1994 Defence White Paper*, 8.

57 See Corporal Gregory Prodaniuk's anecdote about exchanging helmets with outgoing peacekeepers earlier in the chapter.

58 Ann Fuller, "Sex and the Military: Battling Harassment," *The Globe and Mail*, 7 August 1993.

59 Ibid.

60 Ibid. In 1989, a Canadian Human Rights Tribunal criticized the CAF for its slow rate of gender integration, and ordered that all women be allowed to fill all military roles within the next ten years. See Granatstein, *Who Killed the Canadian Military?*, 139–48.

61 Ibid.; O'Hara, "Rape in the Military," *Maclean's*, 25 May 1998; O'Hara, "Speaking Out on Sexual Assault in the Military," *Maclean's*, 1 June 1998. The May 1998 article as well as the aforementioned 1993 *Globe* article also tangentially mentioned some of the women having been diagnosed with PTSD, in all cases by civilian doctors. This issue was also covered in the *Toronto Star*. See Allan Thompson, "Woman Soldier Tells of Rape," *The Toronto Star*, 11 June 1998.

62 O'Hara, "Of Rape and Justice," *Maclean's*, 14 December 1998.

63 O'Hara, "Speaking Out."

64 Bercuson, *Significant Incident*, 8. Operation Deliverance, as it was known, was sanctioned by the UN Security Council under Chapter VII of the UN Charter, which authorized the dispatch of peace-enforcement troops rather than peacekeeping troops. In Somalia, their job was to impose peace on warring factions so that relief efforts and supplies could be brought into the country, which had experienced months of famine. See ibid., 2–3.

65 The horrific details of this event and its surrounding circumstances have been reconstructed by several authors. See, Bercuson, *Significant Incident*, passim; Coulon, *Soldiers of Diplomacy*, 88–100; Winslow, "The Parliamentary Inquiry into the Canadian Peace Mission in Somalia." Reports differ on Brown's actual participation in the physical torture, but at the very least he was a willing accomplice. Winslow served as an academic researcher for the Somalia Inquiry.

66 Coulon, *Soldiers of Diplomacy*, 94.

67 Ibid., 94–5.

68 Ibid., 97; Whitworth, *Men, Militarism and UN Peacekeeping*, 96.

69 Horn and Bentley, *Forced to Change*, 48.

70 Geoffrey York, "4 Soldiers Held in Somali's Death," *The Globe and Mail*, 2 April 1993. In fact, were it not for Jim Day, a reporter for the *Pembroke Observer*, being present at the compound when the incident occurred, it seems likely that the event would not have come to light until even later. See Winslow, "The Parliamentary Inquiry," 6.

71 Horn and Bentley, *Forced to Change*, 48.

72 Coulon, *Soldiers of Diplomacy*, 95.

73 Ibid.; Whitworth, *Men, Militarism, and UN Peacekeeping*, 91; McKay and Swift, *Warrior Nation*, 199–200.

74 Whitworth, *Men, Militarism and UN Peacekeeping*, 91; McKay and Swift, 200.

75 Winslow, "The Parliamentary Inquiry," 6. Moreover, documents requested by journalists had been altered, in some cases illegally. For more on this see Horn and Bentley, *Forced to Change*, 48–9.

76 "Soldier Not Guilty in Death of Somali," *The Globe and Mail*, 8 November 1994.

77 Winslow, "The Parliamentary Inquiry," 11.

78 The Commission's final report was tabled, in five volumes, and published in July 1997. See Commission of Inquiry into the Deployment of Canadian Forces to Somalia, *Dishonoured Legacy*. It was revealed during the inquiry

that there was ample evidence of disciplinary problems within the CAR prior to its deployment to Somalia. As recounted by Bercuson, this included, among other things, the burning of an officer's car, an illegal discharging of fireworks, and the presence of several skinheads within the Second Commando. Some CAR members adopted the Confederate flag as a symbol of their values, and one commanding officer even performed a training jump with the flag attached to his leg. See Bercuson, *Significant Incident*, 211–14. The extent of racism and anti-social behaviour within the CAR will never be fully known, but there is a scholarly consensus that a "cancer" had grown inside at least part of it. The Liberal government truncated the inquiry because it claimed that "Canadians already knew all the important facts and … the whole process was keeping open a wound for an unnecessarily long period of time." See Winslow, "The Parliamentary Inquiry," 15. See Horn and Bentley, *Forced to Change*, 51, for Chrétien's statement on why the inquiry was terminated.

79 *Dishonoured Legacy*, vol. 3, 681.
80 Ibid.
81 Horn and Bentley, *Forced to Change*, 48.
82 Bercuson, *Significant Incident*, 216, 241. For a brief but excellent analysis of the role of masculine posturing in the affair, see Jackson, *One of the Boys*, 225–6.
83 "Rex Murphy on the Somalia Affair: 'Bloody and Contemptuous Images,'" *The National*, CBC, 19 January 1995, http://www.cbc.ca/archives/entry/rex-murphy-on-the-somalia-affair-bloody-and-contemptuous-images. Videos that contained the damning evidence were first obtained by Scott Taylor, editor of *Esprit de Corps* magazine. Ironically, his plan was to show the Canadian public the adverse conditions the paratroops had been exposed to and the humanitarian work they performed. The media's airing of the segments which contained racist remarks ended up taking the lion's share of attention. This was perhaps unsurprising, given that in one video, a CAR member was taped during the Somalia operation saying that they "ain't killed enough niggers yet." See Davis, *The Sharp End*, 260; Whitworth, *Men, Militarism and UN Peacekeeping*, 93.
84 "Rex Murphy on the Somalia Affair."
85 *Dishonoured Legacy*, vol. 1, xxx.
86 The Italians, Belgians, and Americans, among others, also had similar incidents occur under their watch. See Coulon, *Soldiers of Diplomacy*, 98–9.
87 Horn and Bentley, *Forced to Change*, 51.

88 Ibid.

89 Quoted in ibid. According to Horn and Bentley, Chrétien's assessment was verified by Doug Young.

90 Winslow, "The Parliamentary Inquiry," 7.

91 Coulon, *Soldiers of Diplomacy*, 89. This was not the first time that Canadian soldiers had been charged with homicide, as there had been three prior homicide trials in Germany involving Canadians. But the nature of the crime, its brutality, and the circumstances – Canadians soldiers sent to provide humanitarian aid and defence for the Somali populace murdering a teenager ostensibly under their guardianship – made the situation uniquely explosive. See *The Globe and Mail*, 2 April 1993.

92 Geoffrey York, "Soldiers Charged in Death of Somali," *The Globe and Mail*, 20 May 1993.

93 Ibid.

94 Winslow, "The Parliamentary Inquiry," 21.

95 Off, *The Ghosts of Medak Pocket*, 233–4; Bercuson, *Significant Incident*, vi.

96 Collenette himself later resigned in October 1996, with some commentators feeling that although his resignation was unrelated to the inquiry, it was a convenient way to "let go of a very hot potato." Winslow, "The Parliamentary Inquiry," 12.

97 James, *The Sharp End*, 264.

98 Quoted in Horn and Bentley, *Forced to Change*, 50.

99 Bercuson, *Significant Incident*, 130.

100 Winslow, "The Parliamentary Inquiry," 6.

101 Ibid., 7. This claim, mentioned by Winslow, is supported by anecdotal evidence in James Davis's *The Sharp End*: "In the schools, children whose fathers were in the Regiment were teased and taunted. They had to go home and ask their fathers if they really did those things ... The wives, who loved the regiment as much as their men, were even more deeply hurt ... The wives were now isolated and unable to fight back against the pain and disgrace forced on their husbands." See Davis, *The Sharp End*, 263.

102 Westholm interview; James, *Canada and Conflict*, 59–60.

103 Davis, *The Sharp End*, 260.

104 Ibid. The inquiry and scholarly works on the Somalia affair concluded that although there were leadership and disciplinary problems within the CAR, the incidents which caused public outrage were indeed limited to the 2nd Commando, though given the role of the 1st Commando in the hazing rituals as well, that seems doubtful.

105 Ibid.

106 Ibid., 263.

107 Westholm interview.

108 Bercuson, Granatstein, and others on the "right" blamed budget cuts and a move away from traditional military preparedness, values, and operations, while those on the "left," such as Sandra Whitworth, saw Somalia more as the outcome of a "crisis of legitimacy" and "crisis of masculinity" that occurred when militaries, driven by hyper-masculine goals and attitudes, were forced to adopt a more "feminine" role as peacekeepers. Cf. Bercuson, *Significant Incident*, 238–9; Granatstein, *Who Killed the Canadian Military?*, 148; Whitworth, *Men, Militarism and UN Peacekeeping*, passim, esp. 16.

109 Bercuson, *Significant Incident*, 13.

110 Carol Off, *The Ghosts of Medak Pocket*, 96.

111 Whitworth, *Men, Militarism and UN Peacekeeping*, 108.

112 Whitworth and others have noted how Arone's murder, and other prominent events such as the 1993 dragging of American soldiers' bodies through the streets of Mogadishu after a failed attempt to kill faction leader Mohamed Farrah Aidid, led to a "Somalia syndrome." Traditionally enthusiastic troop-contributing countries such as the United States and Canada were far more reluctant to participate in the "new" UN operations in the wake of such events. See Whitworth, *Men, Militarism and UN Peacekeeping*, 41.

113 Horn and Bentley, *Forced to Change*, 24.

114 Wood, "Jim Calvin: Colonel," in *The Chance of War*, 116.

115 Coulon, *Soldiers of Diplomacy*, 113.

116 Ibid.

117 Ibid.; United Nations, Department of Public Information, "Former Yugoslavia – UNPROFOR."

118 Coulon, *Soldiers of Diplomacy*, 114.

119 Off, *Ghost of the Medak Pocket*, 63. Nearly 9,000 CAF members served in the Balkans between 1991 and 1995 alone.

120 Granatstein and Oliver, *The Oxford Companion to Canadian Military History*, 259–60.

121 Ibid., 260.

122 Maloney, "In the Service of Forward Security," in Horn, *The Canadian Way of War*, 314–15.

123 Prodaniuk interview.

124 Ibid.

125 Ibid.

126 Ibid.

127 Ibid.

128 Ibid.

129 Off, *The Ghosts of Medak Pocket*, passim; Granatstein and Oliver, *The Oxford Companion*, 257–8; Canada, National Defence and the Canadian Armed Forces, "The Battle of Medak Pocket." The story of Medak, and the Yugoslav Wars, were well covered in Off's 2004 book.

130 Ibid. That contingent also included some French troops.

131 Granatstein and Oliver, *The Oxford Companion*, 258.

132 Ibid. The casualty figures are estimated because the Croatian government subsequently denied that anyone died, or that the battle even took place.

133 Off, *The Ghosts of Medak Pocket*, 215.

134 Wood, "Matt Stopford: Warrant Officer" in *The Chance of War*, 135. For Stopford and others, the worst part of seeing such atrocities was that they were forced to watch without being able to intervene.

135 Wood, "Jordie Yeo: Master Corporal," in *The Chance of War*, 222.

136 Spellen interview.

137 Doucette, *Empty Casing*, 86.

138 "Canadian Troops Suffering Combat Stress," *The Globe and Mail*, 6 December 1993.

139 Off, *The Ghosts of Medak Pocket*, 256–7.

140 Ibid., 257.

141 Ibid., 256.

142 English, "From Combat Stress to Operational Stress," 11.

143 Ibid. In the US context, peacekeeping operations were judged even at the highest command levels as something emasculating in character, with the chairman of the Joint Chiefs of Staff declaring that "real men don't do moot-wah [military operations other than war]."

144 Birenbaum, "Peacekeeping Stress Prompts New Approaches," 1485.

145 Rod Mickleburgh "New Treatment for 'Shell Shock,'" *The Globe and Mail*, 16 February 1991. The combat-stress-intervention team was a new concept for the military, and due to the fact that Canada had not been at war in a long time (since Korea), the Gulf War was the first chance to test its effectiveness.

146 Ibid.

147 Ibid.

148 English, "From Combat Stress to Operational Stress," 11.

149 Ibid.

150 Horn and Bentley, *Forced to Change*, 37.

151 The Royal Canadian Navy at that time was still called Maritime Command. In the civilian realm it is worth mentioning that psychologist Dr A. Lynne Beal examined PTSD symptoms in prisoners of war and combat veterans of the Dieppe Raid. Like Passey's work, studies such as Beal's were few and far between in Canada during the 1990s. See Beal, "Post-Traumatic Stress Disorder in Prisoners of War and Combat Veterans of the Dieppe Raid," 177–84; Spears, "Psychologic [sic] Scars Remain 50 Years after Dieppe Raid," 1324–6.

152 Birenbaum, "Peacekeeping Stress Prompts New Approaches," 1485. Passey was also a former general duties medical officer. Passey and Crockett's study was the first of its kind in the world.

153 CFB Chilliwack officially closed in 1997.

154 Passey interview.

155 Ibid. Passey stated that one of the books which had an impact on his conceptualizations of trauma was Copp and McAndrew's 1990 book *Battle Exhaustion*.

156 Ibid.

157 Birenbaum, "Peacekeeping Stress Prompts New Approaches," 1485.

158 *The Globe and Mail*, 6 December 1993.

159 Birenbaum, "Peacekeeping Stress Prompts New Approaches," 1485.

160 *The Globe and Mail*, 6 December 1993.

161 Ibid.

162 Off, *The Ghosts of Medak Pocket*, 245.

163 Birenbaum, "Peacekeeping Stress Prompts New Approaches," 1485.

164 Ibid., 1486.

165 *The Globe and Mail*, 16 February 1991.

166 Developed by Dr Jeffrey Mitchell in the early 1980s, the approach was first laid out in a 1983 article. See Mitchell, "When Disaster Strikes," 36–9. CISD seems to have been first utilized by the CAF in 1993 after a C-130 Hercules transport plane crashed at CFB Wainwright (Alberta) on 22 July 1993. See Testimony of Captain John Organ, *Croatia Board of Inquiry*, 24 September 1999, vol. XIII, 6. For media coverage of the crash see Miro Cernetig, "Hercules Crash Kills Five at Alberta Air Base," *The Globe and Mail*, 23 July 1993.

167 Passey interview.

168 This definition was taken in large part from the *DSM-III*, which defined a traumatic event as one "outside the range of usual human experience" and one that likewise involved a threat to the person, such as war, torture, rape, or natural disaster. See American Psychiatric Association, *Diagnostic and Statistical Manual of Mental Disorders*, third edition, 236–9. For an example of

information about CIS the CAF provided its troops, see Canada, Department of National Defence, Directorate of Medical Policy, *Preparing for Critical Incident Stress*. Greg Passey stated during an interview that McLellan was one of the key persons behind the push to introduce CISD and pay more attention to stress among troops.

169 Department of National Defence, *Preparing for Critical Incident Stress*, 9. By the end of the 1990s, CISD was heavily utilized in civilian situations as well, such as during the aftermath of the Swissair Flight 111 crash at Peggy's Cove in Nova Scotia, on 2 September 1998. Over 7,000 people, ranging from pathologists who examined body fragments to children who saw the tragedy unfold, received a form of CIS counselling from military and civilian CISD teams. See Kevin Cox, "Emotional Aftereffects of Swissair Targeted," *The Globe and Mail*, 21 October 1998.

170 Birenbaum, "Peacekeeping Stress Prompts New Approaches," 1484.

171 Department of National Defence, *Preparing for Critical Incident Stress*, 10.

172 Spellen interview.

173 Godin, e-mail message to author, May 27, 2015.

174 Davis, *The Sharp End*, 112.

175 Ibid.

176 Ibid.

CHAPTER FIVE

1 Brock and Passey, "The Canadian Military and Veteran Experience," in Scurfield and Platoni, *War Trauma and Its Wake*, 91.

2 Prodaniuk interview.

3 Ibid.

4 Ibid.

5 Ibid.

6 Ibid.

7 Ibid.

8 Ibid.

9 Ibid.

10 Ibid.

11 Sharpe, *Croatia Board of Inquiry: Leadership (and Other) Lessons Learned*, 3.

12 Ibid., 4.

13 The "Van Doos" are so termed because of the anglicized pronunciation of the regiment's French name, "vingt-deux" (twenty-two). The Royal 22nd Regiment was originally the 22nd Battalion during the First World War,

the only combatant battalion in the CEF whose official language was French. It was later given the "Royal" title in 1921, in honour of its war service, a year after it was reactivated as a regiment.

14 "Dead Soldier's Mom Confronts Collenette," *The Toronto Star*, 31 March 1995. For another article that examined the issue of suicides in the Van Doos see André Picard, "After Johnny Comes Marching Home," *The Globe and Mail*, 8 April 1995.

15 Ibid. A 1996 independent study by a team at Toronto's Clarke Institute of Psychiatry into suicides in the military found "few direct links" between peacekeeping duties and any of the sixty-six suicides in the CAF from 1990 to 1995. Nevertheless the study highlighted the "macho military culture" that prevented many from coming forward. The CAF responded by implementing (at least in theory) a plan whereby peacekeepers were given at least a year at home between deployments. See Jeff Sallot, "Military Maps Action on Suicide Report," *The Globe and Mail*, 8 November 1996.

16 *Toronto Star*, 31 March 1995.

17 Ibid.

18 Dallaire, *Shake Hands with the Devil*.

19 Ibid., xii.

20 Brock and Passey, "The Canadian Military and Veteran Experience," 92. Passey and Lamontigny were deployed to Rwanda in 1994, along with a mental health team, to appraise the mental health impact of UNAMIR service on Canadian participants.

21 Ibid.

22 Although it cannot be doubted that Dallaire's rank helped him avoid many of the problems his subordinates faced, what this book suggests is that his slow, gradual decline and mental processing of his situation, as well as his attempts to stave off the inevitable crash, were similar in kind to those lower in rank.

23 Dallaire, *Shake Hands with the Devil*, xi.

24 Ibid., xii.

25 Ibid; Dallaire's "final straw" came when he testified before the International Criminal Tribunal for Rwanda in 1998: "The memories, the smells and the sense of evil returned with a vengeance."

26 Ibid.

27 Grenier interview. Grenier was later diagnosed with PTSD.

28 Ibid.

29 Ibid.

30 Ibid.

31 Canada, Department of National Defence. *Witness the Evil – A Canadian Forces Video.*

32 "Canada's Veterans: Veterans and Post-Traumatic Stress," *The National,* CBC, 25 November 25 1998, http://www.cbc.ca/player/Digital+Archives/War+and+Conflict/Veterans/ID/1842315607/; "Witness the Evil," *As It Happens,* CBC, 26 November 1998, http://www.cbc.ca/archives/entry/blue-berets-shell-shock.

33 Grenier interview.

34 Sharpe, e-mail message to author, 14 October 2014.

35 Quoted in Ombudsman, National Defence and Canadian Forces, *Report to the Minister of National Defence, Special Report: Systemic Treatment of CF Members with PTSD,* 65.

36 Off, *The Ghosts of Medak Pocket,* 245.

37 Sharpe, e-mail message to author, 14 October 2014. One cannot help but notice the similarity of the latter's view to that expressed by historic military figures such as American general George Patton. It also resembles the "contagion" theory espoused by some military leaders in the First World War.

38 Canada, Parliament, *Moving Forward.* The CAF had undertaken its own internal investigation in 1997, led by chief social worker Lieutenant-Colonel McLellan, in response to bad press. His report, the *Care of Injured Personnel and their Families Review,* aimed to determine the extent to which the CAF/DND were succeeding or failing in their care of injured personnel and families. Made public in 1998, the review concluded, among other things, that the problems experienced by those physically or psychologically wounded as a result of service were symptomatic of a larger, systemic problem with how the CAF and VAC handled injured personnel. The review's acerbic tone reflected McLellan's anger toward what was evidently an antiquated system; and one which left many Regular Force soldiers and reservists without proper care. See Canada, Department of National Defence, Injured Personnel and Family Review Team, *Care of Injured Personnel and their Families Review.* For an example of McLellan's public outspokenness about the issue see Jeff Sallot, "Forces Can't Keep Track of Casualties, MPs Told," *The Globe and Mail,* 1 May 1998. An even less publicized report was also prepared earlier in 1997 that focused on CAF members released on medical grounds. See Canada, Department of National Defence, *A Study of the Treatment of Members Released on Medical Grounds.*

39 Parliament of Canada, *Moving Forward.*

40 Ibid.

41 Ibid.

42 Ibid. The SCONDVA's report proved to be a "turning point" in overall Canadian military quality of life, as its broad scope and recommendations set forth a number of tangible goals that were required to improve a moribund system. For more on quality of life initiatives and their connection to civilian practices see Cowen, *Military Workfare*, passim, esp. 220–2.

43 Taylor and Nolan, *Tested Mettle*, 247.

44 Kim Honey, "Director's Exit Rocks Ontario SIU," *The Globe and Mail*, 8 June 1998.

45 Ibid.

46 Taylor and Nolan, *Tested Mettle*, 246–7; Erin Anderssen, "Forces Sex-Complaint Hotline Gets 40 Allegations to Probe," *The Globe and Mail*, 10 June 1998.

47 Bruce Campion-Smith, "For André Marin, Success Measured in Complaints," *The Toronto Star*, 29 March 2005.

48 Pugliese interview.

49 Discussed in the subsequent chapter.

50 David Brusher and Moira Welsh, "André Marin Left Dysfunction and Discontent as Military Ombudsman," *The Toronto Star*, 2 June 2010.

51 Ibid.

52 Ibid.

53 Ibid., 29 March 2005.

54 Jones and Wessely, *Shell Shock to PTSD*, 167.

55 "Gulf War Syndrome," *The Globe and Mail*, 17 May 1996. Jones and Wessely linked the fear of physical toxins to "powerful cultural themes" in the civilian context brought into a military milieu. The general fear of radiation, pesticides, etc., that began in the post-1945 era became even more heightened in the 1980s and beyond. Events such as the Bhopal disaster, Chernobyl, and other mass exposures to human-made weapons and chemicals made death by toxic materials seem like a legitimate fear. The Vietnam War and Agent Orange also played a key role in raising fears among soldiers of chemicals. See Jones and Wessely, *Shell Shock to PTSD*, 198–9.

56 Allan Thompson, "Study Links Gulf War Ills to Stress," *The Toronto Star*, 30 June 1998.

57 Jones and Wessely, *Shell Shock to PTSD*, 167.

58 Allan Thompson, "Study Links Gulf War Ills to Stress," *Toronto Star*, 30 June 1998.

59 Canada's lone clinic for assessing those suffering with GWS from 1992 to 1998 was the Chronic Fatigue Syndrome Clinic, later renamed the Gulf War Veterans Clinic. It was established and run by Colonel Ken Scott. For more information on Canadian research and treatment of GWS, see the testimony of Major Timothy Cook, *Croatia Board of Inquiry*, 19 November 1999, vol. XXVI, passim.

60 Ibid. This number included those who stayed in theatre after the initial conflict was over, thus the discrepancy in the numbers – 4,500 initial participants plus those who served after in Kuwait or elsewhere. A 2005 Statistics Canada report on Persian Gulf veterans' health concluded that "Canadian Gulf War veterans (both retired and currently serving) did report symptoms and common illnesses at significantly higher rates than other veterans of the same era," but were not at increased risk of developing cancer or dying, further pointing to the possibility of psychological causes. See Statistics Canada, *The Canadian Persian Gulf Cohort Study*, 47.

61 Ibid.

62 This of course is not an exhaustive list, but some of the key events/factors.

63 Sharpe, *Croatia Board of Inquiry*, 8. Stopford became a "poster boy" for soldiers suffering ill effects from deployment. Sharpe and board member Mike Spellen later convinced Stopford to testify at the BOI, because Sharpe was convinced that if "we could get him to come and talk to the board then we would be able to get most of the soldiers to open up" (e-mail message to author, 8 October 2014).

64 Graham Fraser, "Eggleton Fails to Placate Peacekeepers," *The Globe and Mail*, 5 November 1998. One of Stopford's comrades, Tom Martineau, who was paralyzed from the waist down after being hit by a sniper bullet in Bosnia in 1994, had his wheelchair taken away by Veterans Affairs due to bureaucratic considerations. On another occasion, doctors would not authorize his release because his parents' house did not have a wheelchair ramp, something which VAC initially refused to pay for. Even after Stopford's case made national news his disability was still initially placed at only 25 per cent, entitling him to $432 a month. See Graham Fraser, "Ill Ex-Soldier Offered Pension of 25 Per Cent," *The Globe and Mail*, 17 August 1999.

65 Taylor and Nolan, *Tested Mettle*, 233–4.

66 Ibid.; also referred to as the "red soil." See also *The Globe and Mail*, 5 November 1998, for an example of how Taylor and Nolan's book was utilized to make a link between contaminants in Croatia and Stopford's (and other soldiers') health issues.

67 Off, *The Ghosts of Medak Pocket*, 245. Stopford learned about the memo because someone slipped a copy under his door. See Daniel Leblanc and Anne McIlroy, "Critics Blast Army for Tampering with Files," *The Globe and Mail*, 23 July 1999. Smith was later court-martialled and medically released, ostensibly due to his actions. See Testimony of WO Matthew Stopford, *Croatia Board of Inquiry*, 28 October 1999, vol. XXIII, 9.

68 "Probe to See if Soldiers Ill from Toxins," *The Globe and Mail*, 22 July 1999; Leblanc and McIlroy, 23 July 1999; Graham Fraser and Andrew Mitrovica, "Critics Slam Eggleton over Soldiers' Health," 28 July 1999; Eric Smith, "A Dysfunctional Called Our Military," 29 July 1999. Media reports made it clear that numerous soldiers had drawn a link between their exposure to toxins and their subsequent illnesses as early as April 1997, but an internal investigation into the matter "stalled" in May 1998. The 28 July *Globe* article also contained a picture of a 1994 report that Smith wrote to the DND which mentioned a destroyed bauxite plant. See ibid.

69 See John Ward, "Inquiry Team May Try to Cook Up 'Toxic Soup,'" *The Globe and Mail*, 31 July 1999.

70 Under the National Defence Act, the MND, CDS, or "such other authorities as the Minister" has the authority to call a board of inquiry into "any matter connected with the government, discipline, administration or functions of the Canadian Forces or affecting any officer or non-commissioned member." A board of inquiry has significant legal power in that it can call military *and* civilian persons to give oral or written evidence (on oath) about the matter at hand. A board also has the authority to compel a person to give evidence under oath *even if* that evidence will incriminate them (self-incrimination is usually protected by the Canadian Charter of Rights and Freedoms). See *National Defence Act, Revised Statutes of Canada 1985*, c. N-5, http://laws-lois.justice.gc.ca/eng/acts/n-5/page-18.html#h-32.

71 Sharpe, *Croatia Board of Inquiry*, 1. The board consisted of: Chairman (and Air Force officer) Colonel Joe Sharpe; RCMP Inspector Reg Bonvie; Major J.P. Caron from the Van Doos, also a Croatia veteran; Lieutenant-Colonel Brian Sutherland, reserve adviser to the Chief of the Land Staff; Master Warrant Officer (ret.) Mike Spellen, a Croatia veteran; Major Dave Widdows from the Director General Environment's office; Marc Pilon, CAF ombudsman's representative; Dr Jeff Whitehead, medical adviser to the board; Public Affairs Officer Lieutenant-Colonel Jacques Tremblay; and legal adviser Commander Jane Harrigan.

72 Sharpe, *Croatia Board of Inquiry*, 25.

73 Ibid., 10.

74 Spellen accompanied Sharpe when the latter was called to meet with any-one in the chain of command, from the CDS and MND down to rank-and-file soldiers. This approach led to some "bruised egos" since "Mike [Spellen] was never a diplomat," but in Sharpe's mind, it ensured that the best evidence came out. Sharpe glowingly described Spellen as "honest as the day is long" (e-mail message to author, 17 October 2014). Sharpe's decision proved prescient when one soldier testifying at the Board stated: "The only reason I am here is because Mr Spellen called and asked me because I didn't believe in what was happening. And the only reason why I am here is because of that man there [Spellen]" (Testimony of Sergeant Christopher Byrne, *Croatia Board of Inquiry*, 25 November 1999, vol. XXIX, 8). Another tactic used by Sharpe was to dress in civilian clothes when meeting with the media and rank-and-file soldiers. While perceived as a sign of disloyalty by some "senior members" of the military, it helped to further gain the trust of soldiers, who were more likely to see board members as working on their behalf, instead of representing the military establishment. See Sharpe, *Croatia Board of Inquiry*, 54–8.

75 Sharpe, *Croatia Board of Inquiry*, 10.

76 Spellen interview.

77 Ibid. Sharpe recalled one particularly emotional testimony during which he turned to the back of the room and saw even the board's two translators distraught and in tears. Sharpe, e-mail message to author, 4 November 2014.

78 Sharpe, *Croatia Board of Inquiry*, 27.

79 Ibid., 10. The board was able to use an obscure paragraph in its "terms of reference," which allowed it the freedom of movement to shift its attention toward anything that might be deemed relevant. See English, "From Combat Stress to Operational Stress," 14.

80 Sharpe, *Croatia Board of Inquiry*, 37.

81 English, e-mail message to author, 3 July 2015.

82 Ibid.

83 Sharpe, *Croatia Board of Inquiry*, 37; English, "Historical and Contemporary Interpretations of Combat Stress Reaction."

84 Sharpe, *Croatia Board of Inquiry*, 29.

85 It is important to remember that in 1999 the Internet was not as pervasive as it is in the early twenty-first century, thus making the scanning of documents and availability of all board information online quite a novel feat.

According to Sharpe, the decision to make every aspect of the board's work publicly available helped to create a more cordial relationship with Canadian reporters. This was confirmed by Spellen in an interview with the author. See Sharpe, *Board of Inquiry*, 44–5; Spellen interview.

86 Testimony of Captain Kelly Brett, *Croatia Board of Inquiry*, 22 September 1999, vol. XI, 32.

87 Testimony of Major Dan Drew, *Croatia Board of Inquiry*, 21 October 1999, vol. XXI, 25.

88 English, "From Combat Stress to Operational Stress," 12.

89 See Wood, "Ray Wlasichuk: Colonel," in *The Chance of War*, 174.

90 Testimony of Lieutenant-Commander Gregory Passey, *Croatia Board of Inquiry*, 12 October 1999, vol. XVI, 19.

91 Ibid.

92 Ibid., 18.

93 Wynnyk was specifically responsible for Land Force Area West, which started in Manitoba and ran westward to British Columbia.

94 Testimony of Lieutenant-Colonel Paul Wynnyk, *Croatia Board of Inquiry*, 29 September 1999, vol. XV, 10.

95 As Allan English noted, "Subordinates look to leaders for cues to appropriate behaviour and often emulate leader behaviour." See English, *Understanding Military Culture*, 22.

96 Ibid., 14.

97 Another example is "remf," short for "rear echelon motherfucker," a term used in the US and Canadian militaries to identify those who never leave the forward operating base and/or those who work in ostensibly comfortable circumstances, instead of "in the field."

98 Prodaniuk interview.

99 See aforementioned interview testimony from Westholm, Godin, and Prodaniuk, as well as Dallaire's story.

100 Testimony of Captain Robert Sparks, *Croatia Board of Inquiry*, 21 September 1999, vol. X, 32.

101 Prodaniuk interview.

102 Spellen interview.

103 Ibid. One board member actually recognized a homeless man on the streets of Ottawa as a fellow soldier who had served in Croatia during the early 1990s. The latter was released from the CAF and suffered from severe mental health problems. See Richardson et al., "Operational Stress Injury Social Support," 57.

104 Testimony of Captain Kelly Brett, 31.

105 Prodaniuk interview.

106 The term "weak sister" is an Americanism that dates back to the mid-nine-teenth century, and unsurprisingly, was used to describe a member of a group that was perceived as a weak link. In the 1877 *Dictionary of American-isms* the author defined a weak sister simply as "a person that cannot be relied upon." He used as an example an 1861 quotation from the *New York Tribune* newspaper that discussed the existence of white Unionists in the South: "The rebels assert that the Union has no friends at the South. The assertion is false. There are white Unionists there, but they are *weak sisters*, – overawed, terrorized, silenced." Evidently, at some point the term made its way into Canadian English as well. See John Russell Bartlett, *Dictionary of Americanisms*, 742.

107 Testimony of Dr Mark Tysiaczny, *Croatia Board of Inquiry*, 9 November 1999, vol. XXIV, 15.

108 Ibid.

109 Ibid., 16.

110 Ibid., 9.

111 Ibid; Tysciaczny's statement implied that they usually saw no one above the Army rank of Captain.

112 Spellen interview.

113 Ibid.

114 Ibid.

115 Testimony of Lieutenant-Commander Greg Passey, *Croatia Board of Inquiry*, 12 October 1999, vol. XVI, 17. Doctors in the 2nd Canadian Division made similar claims about preparation, training, and discipline acting as a shield against stress casualties prior to fighting in France in 1944. That argument proved unfounded. History repeated itself in the 1990s. See Shephard, *A War of Nerves*, 254.

116 Spellen interview.

117 Ibid.

118 Testimony of Lieutenant-Commander Greg Passey, 18.

119 Testimony of MWO Ed Larabie, *Croatia Board of Inquiry*, 18 October 1999, vol. XIX, 13.

120 Testimony of Sergeant Christopher Byrne, 8.

121 Testimony of MWO Ed Larabie, 13.

122 Ibid.

123 This point has been made a plethora of times in texts going back to ancient

times. Recently it was stated quite poignantly by journalist/documentarian Sebastian Junger in his book *War*, written during his time "embedded" with US soldiers in the Korengal Valley in Afghanistan from 2007–08. Junger discovered, like many before him, that soldiers' loyalty was primarily to their comrades, and especially those with whom they shared the experience of battle. See Junger, *War*, passim, esp. 232–45.

124 Testimony of Captain Kelly Brett, 34.

125 Testimony of Dr Mark Tysiaczny, 11.

126 Testimony of MWO Randy Northrup, *Croatia Board of Inquiry*, 20 September 1999, vol. IX, 19.

127 Ibid.

128 Dummitt and Holloway, "Canadian Manhood(s)," in *Canadian Men and Masculinities*, 127.

129 Testimony of Karol Wenek, *Croatia Board of Inquiry*, 24 November 1999, vol. XXVIII, 6. As discussed by Wenek in her testimony, this principle was even reflected in an amendment to the Canadian Human Rights Act which makes reference to the principle and interprets it as the liability of CAF members to perform "whatever duties they may be lawfully be called upon to perform." This quite clearly separates the onus placed on serving soldiers from that of civilians. See ibid.

130 Doucette, *Empty Casing*, 207.

131 Sharpe, *Croatia Board of Inquiry*, 6–7.

132 Off, *The Ghosts of Medak Pocket*, 257.

133 Brian Laghi, "Veteran Officer Taking Over Probe Says He's Not Afraid to Buck Superiors," *The Globe and Mail*, 11 August 1999. Sharpe headed a board of inquiry in the mid-1980s into the suicide of a young soldier. The inquiry found fault with a number of the man's superior officers, and demonstrated that Sharpe was unafraid of rocking the boat if necessary.

134 Jeff Sallot, "Sick Soldiers Treatment 'a Disgrace' Probe Finds," *The Globe and Mail*, 17 December 1999.

135 Ibid.

136 Sharpe, e-mail message to author, 10 October 2014.

137 Sharpe, *Croatia Board of Inquiry*, 6.

138 Ibid.

139 Ibid. A peacekeeping operation or multinational operation such as the Gulf War was, since 1949, deemed as a "special duty area"; as opposed to operations within Canada. Those participating were entitled to pensionable benefits in the case of injury or death. Nevertheless, VAC did not even consider

peacekeepers to be veterans after they left the Army. See Granatstein, *Canada's Army*, 397 and 397n.

140 Sharpe, *Croatia Board of Inquiry*, 7.

141 Testimony of Bernard Butler, *Croatia Board of Inquiry*, 9.

142 Ibid.

143 Testimony of Colonel George Oehring (ret.), *Croatia Board of Inquiry*, 10 November 1999, vol. XXV, 23.

144 Testimony of Greg Passey, 14.

145 Testimony of MS Wade Kelloway, *Croatia Board of Inquiry*, 24 September 1999, vol. XIII, 5.

146 Ibid., 16. Kelloway's problems were severed from the testimony document, but PTSD or psychosomatic illnesses were implied several times throughout, particularly in Kelloway's statement that "this is all related to what I've been through in Croatia."

147 Ibid.

148 Testimony of Darrell Menard, *Croatia Board of Inquiry*, 25 November 1999, volume number missing from original document, 14.

149 Testimony of Colonel George Oehring, 22.

150 Sharpe, *Croatia Board of Inquiry*, 74.

151 Off, *The Ghosts of Medak Pocket*, 256.

152 Ibid.

153 Testimony of Master Corporal Phil Tobicoe, *Croatia Board of Inquiry*, 9 November 1999, vol. XXIV, 24.

154 Sharpe, e-mail message to author, 4 November 2014. Sharpe's recollection of Roberts's testimony is supported by the testimony record, which indeed shows that Major Caron, rather than Sharpe himself, thanked Roberts for his appearance. See Testimony of W.D. Roberts, *Croatia Board of Inquiry*, 25 November 1999, vol. XXVII, 25.

155 Ibid.

156 Ibid.

157 Spellen interview. Spellen stated to the author that part of the board's frustration lay in the fact that Roberts seemed to have almost dictatorial power over the outcome of veterans' cases (a point also supported by the testimony transcript), and that he also seemed to revel in it.

158 Ibid.

159 Testimony of Sergeant Gregory Goudie, *Croatia Board of Inquiry*, 25 November 1999, vol. XXIX, 8.

160 Ibid.

161 Sharpe, *Croatia Board of Inquiry*, 3–4.

162 Ibid; Off, *The Ghosts of Medak Pocket*, 231–2.

163 Quoted in Off, *The Ghosts of Medak Pocket*, 274.

164 Wood, "Sergeant Peter Vallée," in *The Chance of War*, 213.

165 Ibid.

166 Ibid.

167 Ibid.

168 Off, *The Ghosts of Medak Pocket*, 207. The use of dark humour during wartime or other harrowing experiences to lighten the mood and deal with overwhelming events is well-documented. See, as just one example, the beginning of Antony Beevor's work on the Battle of Berlin in 1945 in *The Fall of Berlin 1945*, passim, esp. chapter 1. In the Canadian context, veterans at Sunnybrook Hospital in Toronto reported that humour was one of the ways they made it through the Second World War. After the war, humour was also used to suppress the more horrific moments. One veteran at Sunnybrook Hospital stated: "Mostly we joke about the war. That's how we handle it … We look at the jolly side, the women we met, not the cruel side." See *The Toronto Star*, 7 November 2009.

169 Testimony of Lieutenant (Navy) M.J. Brown, *Croatia Board of Inquiry*, 23 September 1999, vol. XII, 49. Another example described by Carol Off was the naming of a reservist's truck as "the Grim Reaper," since the man's surname was Grimmer and his job at one point involved transporting dead bodies. See Off, *The Ghosts of Medak Pocket*, 207.

170 Ibid.

171 Testimony of MWO Randy Northrup, 21.

172 Testimony of Lieutenant (Navy) M.J. Brown, 55.

173 Ibid.

174 Ibid., 58.

175 Testimony of Colonel Jim Calvin, *Croatia Board of Inquiry*, 16 September 1999, vol. VII, 142.

176 Taylor and Nolan, *Tested Mettle*, 231.

177 Ibid.

178 Testimony of Colonel Jim Calvin, 142.

179 Testimony of Sergeant Christopher Byrne, 7.

180 Testimony of Lieutenant-Colonel Craig King, *Croatia Board of Inquiry*, 15 October 1999, vol. XVIII, 23.

181 Ibid.

182 Ibid.

183 Testimony of Sergeant Christopher Byrne, 7.

184 Testimony of Captain John Organ, *Croatia Board of Inquiry*, 24 September 1999, vol. XIII, 7.

185 Spellen interview.

186 Testimony of Colonel Jim Calvin, 122.

187 Testimony of CWO D.F. DesBarres, *Croatia Board of Inquiry*, 19 October 1999, vol. XX, 10.

188 Sharpe, *Croatia Board of Inquiry*, 46.

189 Ibid.

190 Spellen interview.

191 Testimony of MWO Gerald Boyle (ret.), *Croatia Board of Inquiry*, 23 September 1999, vol. XII, 8.

192 Testimony of WO Geoff Crossman, *Croatia Board of Inquiry*, 18 October 1999, vol. XIX, 11–12.

193 Testimony of Corporal Anita Kwasnicki, *Croatia Board of Inquiry*, 18 October 1999, vol. XIX, 11.

194 Ibid., 13.

195 Ibid., 12.

196 Testimony of Captain Kelly Brett, 29.

197 Testimony of CWO D.F. DesBarres, 10.

198 Testimony of Lieutenant-Commander Greg Passey, 8.

199 Ibid.

200 Testimony of MWO Ed Larabie, 17.

201 Off, *The Ghosts of Medak Pocket*, 224.

202 Testimony of Lieutenant Brown, 56.

203 Ibid.

204 Ibid., 60.

205 Testimony of Major Darrell Menard, 16.

206 Testimony of Captain Kelly Brett, 48.

207 Ibid.

208 Ibid.

209 Ibid., 29.

210 Testimony of Captain Alain Guevremont, *Croatia Board of Inquiry*, 23 September 1999, vol. XII, 25.

211 Wood, "Matt Stopford: Warrant Officer," in *The Chance of War*, 143.

212 Testimony of Major Dan Drew, 27.

213 Ibid.

214 Testimony of CWO M.B. McCarthy (ret.), 20.

215 Wood, "Jim Davis: Sergeant," in *The Chance of War*, 50–1.

216 Ibid., 51.

217 Ibid.

218 Ibid.

219 Ibid.

220 Ibid.

221 Godin interview.

222 Wood, "Peter Vallée: Sergeant," in *The Chance of War*, 213.

223 Ibid.

224 Ibid.

225 Testimony of Master Corporal Phil Tobicoe, 15.

226 Ibid.

227 Wood, "Jordie Yeo: Master Corporal," in *The Chance of War*, 226, 230.

228 Ibid., 231.

229 Ibid., 232.

230 Ibid.

231 Sharpe, *Croatia Board of Inquiry*, passim.

232 Ibid., 3.

233 Ibid., 4.

234 Prodaniuk interview.

235 Testimony of Master Warrant Officer Ed Larabie, 15. Unfortunately, the salutary effect of taking the "slow boat" home, while seemingly effective after the First and Second World Wars, did not prevent PTSD among UK troops after the Falklands War.

236 *The Globe and Mail*, 17 December 1999.

237 See Prodaniuk's thoughts at the beginning of this chapter.

238 Brett himself said as much in his testimony. He stated that he conducted a multitude of appointments for Yugoslavia peacekeepers: "in the high thousands, if not into the tens of thousands." See testimony of Captain Kelly Brett, 30.

239 *The Globe and Mail*, 17 December 1999.

240 Ibid.

241 Ibid.

242 Ibid.

243 Graham Fraser, "Inquiry Chief Blasts Veterans Affairs," *The Globe and Mail*, 29 October 1999.

244 Sharpe, *Croatia Board of Inquiry*, 30.

CHAPTER SIX

1 Charlie Gillis, "Armed Forces 'Ignored' Peacekeepers' Illness," *The National Post*, 15 November 2002.
2 Ibid.
3 "Alberta: Soldier With PTSD Charged," *The National Post*, 4 April 2001.
4 *The National Post*, 15 November 2002; 4 April 2001.
5 Ibid., 15 November 2002.
6 Jill Mahoney, "Former Soldier Struggled Alone with Nightmares, Depression," *The Globe and Mail*, 6 February 2002. In this case, McEachern's interference to stop the crimes he witnessed would have compromised the multinational reconnaissance mission Canadian soldiers were a part of.
7 Ibid.
8 *The National Post*, 15 November 2002.
9 Ibid. Passey approached the *National Post* shortly after McEachern's actions in March, hoping to raise awareness of the issue and highlight what he viewed as Ottawa's indifference to the PTSD problem. See James Cudmore, "Peacekeepers Pay High Price, Doctor Says," *The National Post*, 30 March 2001.
10 Marin, *Report to the Minister of National Defence*, 21.
11 Duncan Thorne, "Distraught Corporal Convicted in Garrison Crash," *The National Post*, 4 February 2003.
12 Ibid.
13 James Cudmore, "PM Failed Peacekeepers, Soldier's Mother Says," *The National Post*, 3 April 2001.
14 Ibid.
15 Ombudsman, *Report to the Minister of National Defence*, v; *The National Post*, 11 April 2001. Thanks and acknowledgments to former director of the Special Ombudsman Response Team and lead investigator Gareth Jones, and Mr Sharpe, for clarifications about the McEachern case.
16 Charlie Gillis, "Soldier Not in Robotic State, Psychiatrist Says," *The National Post*, 11 December 2002.
17 Ibid. Boddam also implied in his testimony that McEachern drove into Garrison Headquarters to take $3,000 in accumulated leave pay that he had been denied earlier that day. Boddam stated that "he [McEachern] was driving that evening to the place that would be the source of that money." See *The National Post*, 11 December 2002.

18 Kormos, "The Posttraumatic Stress Defence in Canada," 222.
19 "Prosecutors Question Ex-Soldier's Condition," *The Globe and Mail*, 16 November 2002; *The National Post*, 11 December 2002.
20 *The National Post*, 15 November 2002.
21 Ibid. At the trial, Passey noted, as he had during the Croatia BOI, that the number of psychiatrists in the Canadian Armed Forces had been cut in half from eleven to six, at the same time as he was warning military leaders about an increasing number of peacekeepers returning with psychological problems. See *The National Post*, 30 March 2001.
22 Ibid.
23 "Stressed-Out Soldier Escapes Jail Sentence," *The Globe and Mail*, 8 February 2003.
24 *The National Post*, 4 February 2003.
25 *The Globe and Mail*, 8 February 2003; *The National Post*, 4 February 2003.
26 *The National Post*, 4 February 2003.
27 Ibid.
28 Ombudsman, *Report to the Minister of National Defence*, v. Marin's team interviewed numerous people within and outside the military for its report, including PTSD sufferers' families, members of McEachern's chain of command, senior personnel at NDHQ, staff members at three Operational Trauma and Stress Centres, members of the International Red Cross, and foreign military members. They also consulted Roméo Dallaire and Chief of the Defence Staff Maurice Baril.
29 Ibid., vi.
30 Rosie DiManno, "Bureaucracy Is Soldier's Enemy Number One," *The Toronto Star*, 21 June 2002.
31 Ombudsman, *Report to the Minister of National Defence*, ix.
32 Daniel Leblanc, "Shell Shock to Be Given Priority," *The Globe and Mail*, 6 February 2002.
33 James, *Canada and Conflict*, 85.
34 In a testament to how stretched CAF resources were, Granatstein noted that when soldiers arrived, they had woodland uniforms on instead of a more appropriate desert-style uniform. Canadian soldiers also had to be transported by air and ground vehicles borrowed from the United States. See Granatstein, *Who Killed the Canadian Military?*, 6.
35 Canada, Veterans Affairs Canada, "The Canadian Armed Forces in Afghanistan," http://www.veterans.gc.ca/eng/remembrance/history/canadian-armed-forces/afghanistan. This level of commitment made the Afghanistan

War the largest military operation since the Second World War.

36 Ibid. Operation Medusa was also NATO's first battle since its creation over fifty years earlier. See Horn, *No Lack of Courage*, 13. Medusa cost the Canadians five dead and forty wounded within the first forty-eight hours, a casualty toll unseen in decades. For more on Canadian combat operations see Windsor, Charters, and Wilson, *Kandahar Tour*.

37 Flavelle, *The Patrol*, 51.

38 Ibid.

39 Horn, *No Lack of Courage*, 14.

40 Bélanger and Moore, "Public Opinion and Soldier Identity: Tensions and Resolutions," in Aiken and Bélanger, *Beyond the Line*, 104.

41 Ibid., 103–4.

42 James, *Canada and Conflict*, 35, 53. As James noted, Canadian fatalities, which totalled 157 by the end of combat operations in 2011, were a small fraction of losses endured in single battles in the First and Second World Wars. Nonetheless, after many decades of peacekeeping, during which fatalities were few and far between (and usually caused by accidents), Canadians had become highly sensitized to even a single death.

43 Granatstein, *Who Killed the Canadian Military?*, 171; Michael Petrou, "All of Canada Grieves for Fallen Soldiers," *The Globe and Mail*, 19 April 2002.

44 James, *Canada and Conflict*, 35.

45 In some ways, though, portions of the Canadian participation in the Afghan War did resemble peacekeeping ops. For more see Windsor, Charters, and Wilson, *Kandahar Tour*, passim.

46 James, *Canada and Conflict*, 35.

47 Part of this was the result of the Digital Age, which allowed greater spread of information and a decreased ability to prevent such information from reaching the public.

48 James, *Canada and Conflict*, 2.

49 Brock and Passey, "The Canadian Military and Veteran Experience," 92. Two more OTSSCs were opened at CFBs Petawawa and Gagetown in 2011.

50 Ibid.

51 Canada, Department of National Defence and the Canadian Armed Forces, "Canadian Armed Forces Mental Health Services."

52 Ibid.

53 Brock and Passey, "The Canadian Military and Veteran Experience," 92.

54 Ombudsman, *Follow-Up Report: Review of DND/CF Actions on Operational Stress Injuries*, 21.

55 Ombudsman, *Report to the Minister of National Defence*, 201–2.

56 Ibid., 71.

57 Grenier, e-mail message to author, 22 July 2015.

58 Ibid.

59 Grenier interview. Couture was at that time a two-star general and was at the video unveiling to fill in for Dallaire, who was struggling with his own mental difficulties and unable to attend the event. Couture was later promoted to lieutenant-general. He also in 1999 assisted in the creation of the DND/VAC Centre for the Support of Injured and Retired Members and their Families. See Veterans Affairs Canada, "Christian Couture," accessed 23 January 2015, http://www.veterans.gc.ca/eng/about-us/department-officials /minister/commendation/bio/157. Tragically, Couture died in a snowmobiling accident in January 2006, at the age of fifty-six.

60 Now called Director Casualty Support Management.

61 Grenier, e-mail message to author, 23 July 2015.

62 Ibid.

63 Ibid.

64 Ibid.

65 Grenier interview.

66 See English, "Historical and Contemporary Interpretations of Combat Stress Reaction," cited earlier.

67 Grenier interview.

68 Richardson et al. "Operational Stress Injury Social Support," 62.

69 Ibid.

70 Brock and Passey, "The Canadian Military and Veteran Experience," 93. The definition of OSI was taken from the VAC website. See Veterans Affairs Canada, "Understanding Mental Health," accessed 21 January 2015, http://www.veterans.gc.ca/eng/services/health/mental-health/understanding-mental-health.

71 Brock and Passey, "The Canadian Military and Veteran Experience," 93.

72 Ibid.

73 Grenier interview.

74 Ibid.

75 Ibid.

76 Ibid.

77 Ibid.

78 Brock and Passey, "The Canadian Military and Veteran Experience," 93.

79 Ibid. As the program expanded OSISS later created family peer support coordinators; men or women whose family member served in the CAF and were affected by their family member's OSI.

80 Richardson et al. "Operational Stress Injury Social Support," 59.

81 Ibid.

82 Ibid., 60.

83 Prodaniuk interview.

84 Ibid.

85 Ombudsman, *Follow-Up Report*, 79.

86 Ibid., 81.

87 Ibid.

88 Doucette, *Better Off Dead*, 42.

89 Richardson et al. "Operational Stress Injury Social Support," 61.

90 Grenier interview.

91 Ibid.

92 Sharpe, e-mail message to author, 18 November 2014.

93 Ibid.

94 Barabé interview.

95 Ibid.

96 Ibid.

97 Ibid.

98 Ibid.

99 Ibid. When asked about specifics, Barabé recalled that the resistance in Ottawa stemmed from staff in the research department of the chief of military personnel.

100 Ibid. For more information on the Deployment Support Group see Base Valcartier, "Deployment Support Group," accessed 7 August 2015, http://www.cg.cfpsa.ca/cg-pc/valcartier/en/familyservices/deployment support/Pages/default.aspx.

101 Ibid. Sharpe, e-mail message to author, 18 November 2014.

102 Grenier interview.

103 Richardson et al., "Operational Stress Injury Social Support," 62.

104 Grenier interview.

105 Ibid.

106 Ibid.

107 Ibid.

108 Ibid.

109 Ibid.

110 Department of National Defence and Veterans Affairs Canada, *Interdepartmental Evaluation of the OSISS Peer Support Network*, 1258–138 (CRS), II/V.

111 Grenier interview.

112 Ibid.

113 This topic had been pitched by Navy captain Margaret Kavanagh in the 1990s, and explored by two Canadian military psychologists, Major P.J. Murphy and Captain G. Gingras, in 1997, but it was apparently not taken seriously by CAF and DND officials until the new millennium. See Ombudsman, *Report to the Minister of National Defence*, 131. The most prominent historical comparison usually contrasted the Second World War with Vietnam, with the former being considered a model way of bringing troops home – slowly and amongst comrades. In Vietnam, as with Canadian peacekeeping operations in the 1990s, soldiers were brought home by plane in short order, and often scattered to the winds shortly after their return. See Shephard, *A War of Nerves*, 358; and see also the previous chapter's discussion of reservists' return from peacekeeping ops.

114 Rossignol, "Afghanistan: Military Personnel and Operational Stress Injuries," 1.

115 Ibid.

116 Ibid.

117 Ibid.

118 Ombudsman, *Report to the Minister of National Defence*, 131; Ombudsman, *Follow-Up Report*, i.

119 Bruce Campion-Smith, "R and R Spells Financial Ruin for Canadian Troops," *The Toronto Star*, 7 August 2009.

120 Ibid. Some soldiers also got into trouble, and another report cited in a *Toronto Star* article stated that some had been injured in drinking establishments, while others had damaged hotel furniture, leading to a 3:00 a.m. curfew time. See Allan Woods, "Mental Toll on Soldiers Skyrockets," *The Toronto Star*, 14 April 2009.

121 *The Toronto Star*, 7 August 2009.

122 Hailey interview. According to Lieutenant-Colonel Chris Linford, if soldiers were sick from alcohol during the mandatory morning lectures they were banned from drinking for the remainder of their stay, and in particularly egregious circumstances they faced disciplinary actions. But, as Hailey's testimony demonstrated, some inevitably slipped through the cracks. See Linford, *Warrior Rising*, 301. Hailey's name is a pseudonym because in the long

intervening period between our interview and the book's publication, I was unable to contact him and gain permission for free use of the discussion, and permission to use his real identity.

123 Garber and Zamorski, "Evaluation of a Third-Location Decompression Program for Canadian Forces Members Returning from Afghanistan," 402.

124 Bruce Campion-Smith, "When War Returns with the Soldier," *The Toronto Star*, 17 February 2007.

125 Ibid.

126 Ibid.

127 As noted in chapter 4, the CAF had sent a psychiatric team with the Canadian Naval Task Group during the Gulf War in 1991.

128 Novel and radical, of course, only if one does not include the often forced return to combat of shell-shocked and battle-exhausted soldiers during the First and Second World Wars.

129 Jim Rankin, "Injured Soldiers Reunited with Families, Friends," *The Toronto Star*, 24 April 2002.

130 Ibid. Narratives and opinions expressed during the Croatia Board of Inquiry about the social support provided by the unit were evident.

131 Ibid. This strategy resembled the PIE method utilized in the First and Second World Wars at various points.

132 Jeff Esau, "Stressed-Out Soldiers Sent Back to Kandahar," *The Globe and Mail*, 5 March 2007.

133 Ibid. Boddam's view had support from military leaders and anecdotal evidence. Lieutenant-Colonel Chris Linford wrote that a soldier's heightened worry about failure meant that being pulled early from a mission (or not being sent at all) was even more dreaded than staying in theatre. See Chris Linford, *Warrior Rising*, 156.

134 *The Globe and Mail*, 5 March 2007.

135 Ibid.

136 Ibid.

137 Ibid.

138 Ibid.

139 Joe Friesen, "Standing Guard against a Grim, Invisible Enemy in Afghanistan," *The Globe and Mail*, 19 March 2007.

140 Margaret Kavanagh, "Troops Need to Trust," *The Globe and Mail*, 8 March 2007.

141 Ibid.

142 Once again, it is important to note that in a historical sense this approach

was not new, given that shell-shocked soldiers were sent back to duty as far back as the First World War (and likely even earlier), but since most Canadians were unaware of past practices, it certainly seemed new to many.

143 For more on Rx2000 and an appraisal of its accomplishments and challenges post-2000, see Jung, "Lessons Learned from the War in Afghanistan," S110–S111.

144 Mathieu, director general Health Services, National Defence and the Canadian Armed Forces, "Concept for Canadian Forces Mental Health Care," 14/37. Thanks and acknowledgments to Lieutenant-Colonel Suzanne Bailey, Canadian Forces Health Services Group Headquarters, for providing a copy of this paper.

145 Ibid., ii, viii.

146 Lewis MacKenzie, "Protect Us from 'Touchy Feely' Soldiers," *The National Post*, 10 March 2003. According to Lewis MacKenzie, the name stemmed from the regiment's grey uniforms, adopted during the First World War when the regiment served beside the French Army. On the other hand, according to then 2PPCLI Commanding Officer Lieutenant-Colonel Mike Day, the French Grey Cup went back to the First World War, when Canadian soldiers in France participated in an event involving sports competition and a parade. At that time it was called *Les Folles*. See Ombudsman, *Off the Rails*, 10.

147 The number usually totalled five or six. See ibid.

148 Ibid.

149 For an excellent analysis of such practices during the Second World War, see Jackson, *One of the Boys*, 66–74. For a brief discussion of the same subject during the First World War, see Cook, *At the Sharp End*, 401.

150 Ombudsman, *Off the Rails*, 3.

151 Ibid.

152 Ibid., 12. The float also had, in smaller lettering, a sign saying "CT-01" on it; the CT being short for "Crazy Train." For a picture of the float see ibid., 12.

153 Ibid.

154 Ibid.

155 Ibid., 9. For more on the 2PPCLI leadership's reaction to the float, see ibid., 19–22.

156 Ibid., 10. In an interview with the author, Mike Spellen, who was working with OSISS during the time of the incident, confirmed that the term "crazy train" was well known to 2PPCLI members.

157 Ibid., 9.

158 Spellen interview; Ombudsman, *Off the Rails*, 19.

159 Ombudsman, *Off the Rails*, 19.

160 Spellen interview; Ombudsman, *Off the Rails*, 5.

161 Ombudsman, *Off the Rails*, 3. The incident also, unsurprisingly, made national news. See for example John Ibbitson, "Intolerance Rife for Soldiers on 'Crazy Train,'" *The Globe and Mail*, 6 March 2003.

162 *The National Post*, 10 March 2003.

163 Ibid.

164 Ibid.

165 Ibid. MacKenzie's view also spoke to those who had read about stories of a small number of CAF members fraudulently using PTSD as an excuse for criminal behaviour. One particularly troubling example was the case of Roger Borsch. A Bosnia veteran, Borsch was criminally charged in 2004 for breaking into the home of a co-worker in The Pas, Manitoba, and sexually assaulting the woman's thirteen-year-old daughter at knifepoint. The defence claimed that he suffered from PTSD as a result of his peacekeeping experiences and was unaware of his actions. A Manitoba Court of Queen's Bench in June 2006 initially found Borsch not guilty by reason of mental disorder, marking the first time that a Canadian soldier successfully used PTSD as a defence in a criminal trial. His former commander, retired Colonel Ray Wlasichuk (who also testified at the Croatia BOI several years earlier) became aware of the story and later exposed Borsch's traumatic peacekeeping stories as lies to the *Globe and Mail*. In September 2007 a Manitoba Court of Appeal, citing Justice Nathan Nurgitz's insufficient explanation of his reasoning for ruling Borsch not guilty, overturned the decision. Borsch, sensing his ruse was up, pled guilty at the subsequent trial, stating that it may have been alcohol, not PTSD, which was the precipitating factor in his actions. He was sentenced to two years in prison. Such cases, though rare, did much to fuel the fire of those who believed that malingering and fakery were widespread. See Omar el Akkad, "Ex-Soldier with Stress Disorder Not Culpable in Sex Attack," *The Toronto Star*, 23 June 2006; "Appeal Set for Ex-Soldier in Sex Assault of 13-Year-Old," 6 March 2007; "Court Orders New Trial in War-Trauma Case," 28 September 2007; and Mike McIntyre, "Soldier's War Stories Not on Record, Ex-Officer Says," *The Globe and Mail*, 24 June 2006; Josh Wingrove, "The Courts: Former Soldier Pleads Guilty to Assault," 13 September 2008.

166 *The National Post*, 10 March 2003.

167 Ibid.

168 Hailey interview.

169 Ibid.

170 Those subscribing to that belief could certainly find statistics to back up their argument. For example, in May 2004 the *Toronto Star*, using obtained military documents, reported that depression and PTSD were the highest reasons for sick leave. Depression accounted for one in five sick days, while PTSD accounted for one in ten. This increase was attributed by those preparing the documents for the CAF's chief of Defence Staff to a greater strain being put on a small force. Nonetheless, such documents could also be used to bolster a belief that mental illness was overblown, and that some were abusing the system. See Jeff Esau, "Soldiers Using More Sick Leave," *The Toronto Star*, 3 May 2004.

171 And, one might argue, given the historical evidence, even when made by professionals.

172 Barabé interview.

173 Ibid.

174 Ibid.

175 *War Wounds & Memory*, directed by Brian McKeown (2001; Vancouver: Howe Sound Films Inc., 2001), DVD. Thanks to Mr McKeown for providing a copy of the film, for sharing his recollections of the reasons for its creation, and for kindly sharing his family's military history.

176 McKeown, e-mail message to author, 7 November 2014.

177 Ibid.

178 Ibid.

179 "Broken Heroes," *The Fifth Estate*, CBC, 30 October 2009.

180 Ibid.

181 Ibid.

182 Ibid.

183 Ibid.

184 Ibid.

185 *War in the Mind*, TVOntario (Toronto: TVOntario, 2 August 2011).

186 Ibid.

187 Ibid.

188 Ibid.

189 Ibid.

190 Doucette, *Empty Casing*, 200. Doucette was approached by Grenier to be involved with OSISS in April 2002. See ibid., 210.

191 Ibid., 207.

192 Ibid., 215.

193 Ibid., 214. Doucette further predicted that it would "take a generation of soldiers admitting to OSIs before an OSI is considered an honourable injury and one that you can treat and recover from." See ibid., 218.

194 Ibid., 214.

195 Linford, *Warrior Rising*, passim.

196 Ibid., 189.

197 Ibid., 329.

198 Ibid., 19.

199 Ibid., 171.

200 Ibid., 328.

201 Ibid., 347–9. For more on Outward Bound, see Outward Bound Canada, Veterans' Program, accessed 30 January 2014, http://outwardbound.ca/course _index.asp?Category=110.

202 Linford, *Warrior Rising*, 359.

203 Canada, Veterans Affairs Canada, *Review of Veterans' Care Needs, Phase III, Needs of Canadian Forces Clients,* "Key Findings of Phase III – Review of Veterans' Care Needs."

204 Canada, Veterans Affairs Canada – Canadian Forces Advisory Council, *Honouring Canada's Commitment: "Opportunity with Security" for Canadian Forces Veterans and Their Families in the 21st Century,* 2. For an in-depth treatment of the subject see the above source's companion document, *The Origins and Evolution of Veterans Benefits in Canada 1914–2004.*

205 Canadian Forces Advisory Council, *Honouring Canada's Commitment,* i.

206 Ibid., 6.

207 Canada, Parliament, "The New Veterans Charter."

208 For news coverage see, for example, Bruce Campion-Smith and Allan Woods, "This Is the Face of Our War in Afghanistan That Ottawa Doesn't Want You to See," *The Toronto Star,* 6 November 2010.

209 Ibid.

210 Canada, Veterans Affairs Canada, "New Veterans Charter."

211 Ibid.

212 Ibid.

213 Ibid. For more on the Public Service Health Care Plan, see http://www.pshcp.ca.

214 Ibid.

215 *The Toronto Star,* 6 November 2010.

216 Rosie DiManno, "Shortchanging Wounded Vets," *The Toronto Star,* 20 Sep-

tember 2010. DiManno noted that in the UK total disability carried compensation worth $850,000, while in Australia veterans had the option of choosing either a lump sum or lifetime pension.

217 Spellen interview.

218 *The Toronto Star*, 20 September 2010.

219 Ibid.

220 Ibid., 6 November 2010.

221 Ibid.

222 Ibid., 20 September 2010.

223 Alice Aiken and Amy Buitenhuis, "New Veterans Charter Shortchanges Our Disabled Soldiers," *The Globe and Mail*, 24 August 2010.

224 *The Toronto Star*, 6 November 2010.

225 John Ibbitson, "Veterans Advocate Won't Walk Away Quietly," *The Globe and Mail*, 18 August 2010.

226 Ibid.

227 Bill Curry, "Top General Bolsters Call to Stand Up for Veterans," *The Globe and Mail*, 21 August 2010.

228 Donna Carreiro, "Ex-Veterans' Ombudsman Treated for Post-Traumatic Stress," 5 March 2013, CBC, accessed 15 January 2014, http://www.cbc.ca/news/canada/manitoba/ex-veterans-ombudsman-treated-for-post-traumatic-stress-1.1303470.

229 *The Toronto Star*, 20 September 2010.

230 Ibid. That number included both the physically and mentally wounded.

231 Canada, Veterans Affairs Canada, "Additional Details on the Enhanced New Veterans Charter Act," accessed 23 January 2015, http://www.veterans.gc.ca/eng/news/viewbackgrounder/7.

232 Jane Taber, "Ottawa's New Deal for Injured Veterans," *The Globe and Mail*, 20 September 2010.

233 Ibid.

234 Ibid. For the inspiring story of Franklin's transition after his injuries see Faulder, *The Long Walk Home*.

235 *The Globe and Mail*, 20 September 2010.

236 Ibid.

237 Bruce Campion-Smith, "Clinics to Help Soldiers, Families," *The Toronto Star*, 20 March 2007. The first five clinics were located in Montreal, Quebec City, London, Winnipeg, and Calgary. At the time of writing there are nine clinics.

238 Canada, Veterans Affairs Canada, "Network of OSI Clinics," accessed 28 Jan-

uary 2015, http://www.veterans.gc.ca/eng/services/health/mental-health
/understanding-mental-health/clinics.

239 Ibid.
240 Ibid.
241 Ibid.
242 "Treating Combat Stress," *The Toronto Star*, 20 December 2008.
243 McFadyen, *A Long Road to Recovery*, 13–14.
244 Ibid., 13.
245 Ibid.
246 Ibid., 34.
247 The JPSU replaced the earlier Service Personnel Holding List and even earlier Medical Patient Holding List. For more information on both see Ombudsman, *Systemic Treatment of CF Members with PTSD*, 141–62.
248 Daigle, *On the Homefront*, 27.
249 Canada, National Defence and the Canadian Armed Forces, "The Joint Personnel Support Unit, Backgrounder, May 28, 2009," accessed 22 November 2014, http://www.forces.gc.ca/en/news/article.page?doc=the-joint-personnel-support-unit/hnps1uqv.
250 Ibid.
251 Daigle, *Fortitude under Fatigue*, 20.
252 Ibid.
253 Barabé interview.
254 See earlier discussion of the Universality of Service principle during the Croatia Board of Inquiry.
255 Daigle, *Fortitude under Fatigue*, 22.
256 Ibid., 24.
257 Ibid.
258 Ibid.
259 Westholm interview.
260 Ibid. At that time, those wishing to be employed with the JPSU had to quit the Regular Force and transfer to the Primary Reserves. This was because the JPSU "brass" wanted the stability that the Primary Reserves provided for their frontline positions. Regular Force members were (and are) often posted to different parts of the country, so having the JPSU largely staffed with reservists – who usually stayed in one location – solved that problem. Thanks to Barry Westholm for clarifying this information.
261 Ibid.
262 Ibid.

263 Ibid.
264 Ibid.
265 Ibid.
266 Ibid.
267 Ibid.
268 Ibid.; David Pugliese, "Boards of Inquiry 'Designed to Cover the Military's Butt,'" *The Ottawa Citizen*, 17 October 2014.
269 Westholm interview.
270 Ibid.
271 Ibid.
272 Ibid.
273 Chris Cobb, "DND Buries Report on Care for Ill and Injured Troops," *The Ottawa Citizen*, 29 June, 2015.
274 Chris Cobb, "Advocate Quits Conservative Party as Veterans Groups Prepare to Step Up Pressure," *The Ottawa Citizen*, 3 February 2014.
275 Ombudsman, *Preliminary Assessment – Joint Personnel Support Unit (JPSU)*; Chris Cobb, "Veterans' Support Units Plagued by Understaffing, Despite Promises," *The Ottawa Citizen*, 2 February 2014.
276 Ombudsman, *Preliminary Assessment*.
277 *The Ottawa Citizen*, 2 February 2014.
278 Ibid.
279 Ibid.
280 Chris Cobb, "Veterans Demand Action on Military Suicides after Latest Death," *The Ottawa Citizen*, 19 January 2014.
281 Ibid.
282 David Pugliese, "Injured Ottawa Military Personnel to Wait Longer for Help," *The Ottawa Citizen*, 5 November 2014.
283 Ibid.
284 Ibid.
285 Chris Cobb, "DND Buries Report on Care for Ill and Injured Troops," *The Ottawa Citizen*, 29 June 2015. Defence Minister Jason Kenney later ordered the DND to release data it had gathered during its investigation that began in August 2013.
286 Ibid.
287 Ibid.
288 Ibid. For more on Military Minds, see http://www.militarymindsinc.com.
289 Ibid.

CONCLUSION

1 Alison Auld, "Afghan War Takes Its Toll," *The Toronto Star*, 29 October 2007.

2 Allan Woods, "Mental Toll on Soldiers Skyrockets," *The Toronto Star*, 14 April 2009.

3 Ibid.

4 McFadyen, *A Long Road to Recovery*, 1.

5 Bruce Campion-Smith and Allan Woods, "This Is the Face of Our War in Afghanistan that Ottawa Doesn't Want You to See," *The Toronto Star*, 6 November 2010.

6 Margaret Wente, "Post-Traumatic Stress Is Felling More Troops than the Enemy," *The Globe and Mail*, 6 July 2006. Wente also implied that Second World War or Korean veterans being awarded pensions for PTSD in the early 2000s – "long after the fact" – was further evidence that new CAF/DND initiatives and a national consciousness about PTSD "sometimes increases disability." Such comments flew in the face of overwhelming evidence about PTSD symptoms in many veterans. At Sunnybrook Hospital in Toronto, nursing staff working with Second World War veterans made great efforts to avoid "triggering" flashbacks and traumatic memories for vets still traumatized decades after the war ended. For three such articles on the care of older veterans see *The Toronto Star*, 11 November 2005; 7 November 2009; 12 November 2009.

7 Brock and Passey, 91.

8 "Rash of Suicides among Canadian Soldiers Puts Post-Traumatic Stress in Spotlight," *The Globe and Mail*, 4 December 2013.

9 Ibid.

10 *The Huffington Post*, "Rick Hillier Calls for Public Inquiry in Wake of Soldier Suicides," accessed 25 January 2015, http://www.huffingtonpost.ca/2013/12/14/rick-hillier-soldier-suicides_n_4444402.html.

11 *The Globe and Mail*, 4 December 2013. It is difficult to derive conclusions from these numbers since the DND is, unsurprisingly, very tight-lipped about suicides, and many of the soldiers included in these figures had not deployed to Afghanistan.

12 Bruce Campion-Smith, "Suicide Claims More Soldiers than Those Killed by Afghan Combat," *The Toronto Star*, 16 September 2014; Department of National Defence and the Canadian Armed Forces, "Suicide and Suicide Prevention in the Canadian Armed Forces," accessed 4 April 2015,

http://www.forces.gc.ca/en/news/article.page?doc=suicide-and-suicide-prevention-in-the-canadian-armed-forces/hgq87xvu.

13 *The Toronto Star*, 16 September 2014.

14 Military Police Complaints Commission of Canada, "Backgrounder – Fynes Public Interest Hearing," accessed 3 August 2015, http://www.mpcc-cppm.gc.ca/01/400/fynes/2015-03-10-1-eng.aspx; Chris Cobb, "Inquiry into Veteran's Suicide Cost Taxpayers at Least $3.5M," *The Ottawa Citizen*, 27 March 2015. Thanks to Chris Cobb for discussing details of the case and his investigation by phone and through e-mail.

15 Murray Brewster, "Military Police Withheld Canadian Soldier's Suicide Note in Cover-Up Attempt, Stepfather Alleges," *The National Post*, 6 September 2012; See also Bruce Campion-Smith, "Grieving Mother's Plea Wins Pledge," *The Toronto Star*, 30 October 2010.

16 Murray Brewster, "Canadian Soldier Who Committed Suicide 'Killed by the Military,' Stepfather Says," *The National Post*, 5 September 2013.

17 *The Ottawa Citizen*, 27 March 2015.

18 Ibid.

19 Ibid. Details of the case and the final MPCC report can be viewed online.

20 David Pugliese, "The Canadian Military's War against a Canadian Soldier's Family," *The Ottawa Citizen*, 12 March 2015. Pugliese wrote that he was told that if he did not stop writing about the Langridge case he would no longer be granted interviews with Chief of the Defence Staff Walter Natynczyk. The same article listed other controversial aspects of the case: "Documents clearly naming Sheila and Shaun Fynes as primary and secondary next of kin were ignored. Mistakes were also made on the soldier's death certificate. The Fyneses had to spend $12,000 in legal fees to correct the inaccuracies."

21 Ibid. Arguably, Dallaire's vocal discussions of PTSD and suicide in print and in several documentaries drew a link between the two earlier, but the Langridge case certainly helped to propel it further into the spotlight. Another high-profile suicide case was that of Major Michelle Mendes, who committed suicide in Afghanistan on 23 April 2009. PTSD was not as strongly implied, but it was revealed that she was injured in a friendly fire incident supposedly involving NATO planes in 2006 during her first Afghanistan tour. For three articles on the subject see Christie Blatchford and Jessica Leeder, "'Did We Push Her Too Much?'" *The Globe and Mail*, 20 June 2009; Patrice Bergeron, "NATO Colleagues Bid Final Farewell to Canadian Soldier Maj. Michelle Mendes," *The Toronto Star*, 24 April 2009; Jessica Leeder, "Female Intelligence Specialist Found Dead," *The Toronto Star*, 25 April 2009.

The suicide discussion continued to be a source of controversy, and in 2014 led to another public conflict between Stogran and Mackenzie. For more on the controversy see Lewis MacKenzie, "Canadian Forces: Holding the Line on Mental Health," *The Globe and Mail*, 14 February 2014; David Pugliese, "Pat Stogran to Lewis MacKenzie: Shame on You for Coming Out against the Claims of Veterans," *The Ottawa Citizen*, 17 February 2014.

22 Chris Purdy, "War Veteran Says Justice System Not Equipped to Handle People with PTSD," *The Globe and Mail*, 4 December 2013.

23 Halmrast attempted suicide in his cell, was found, and died in hospital three days later.

24 Ibid.

25 Lee Berthiaume, "PTSD: No Support System for Incarcerated Vets," *Ottawa Citizen*, 5 December 2013.

26 Canada, Correctional Service Canada, "Veterans in Canadian Correctional Systems."

27 Ibid.

28 Ibid.

29 Ibid.

30 United States of America, US Department of Veterans Affairs. PTSD: National Center for PTSD. "Veterans with PTSD in the Justice System." A most kind thanks to the book's (anonymous) reviewer for this suggestion.

31 Ibid.

32 Only those charged with non-violent crimes were eligible.

33 Ibid.

34 Graeme Hamilton, "A Soldier's Spiral from Hero to Accused: How PTSD Led to Criminal Charges and Almost Cost Him His Life," *The National Post*, 27 December 2015.

35 Ibid.

36 Ibid.

37 "Post-Traumatic Stress Disorder and the Mental Health of Military Personnel and Veterans," 1; Canada, Department of National Defence and the Canadian Armed Forces, "The Canadian Armed Forces Legacy in Afghanistan." Figures vary, with the former source by Paré stating 30,000, while both the VAC and CAF/DND websites state 40,000. The latter figures have been used here.

38 Ibid. Four civilians were also killed.

39 Ibid., 2.

40 Brock and Passey, 93. It is important to note that some of these cases were

veterans of earlier conflicts stretching back to the Second World War. Nonetheless, it can be inferred that a high number of them were from Afghanistan and 1990s peacekeeping operations.

41 Thanks to retired chief warrant officer and OSISS national coordinator James Woodley for these figures; James Woodley, e-mail message to author, 6 August 2015.

42 Wounded Warriors Canada, http://woundedwarriors.ca/home/.

43 Barabé interview.

44 English, "From Combat Stress to Operational Stress," 10.

45 This problem is evidently a common one for militaries in the West. For a brief, comparative overview, see Croft, "Emotional Women and Frail Men," in Carden-Coyne, *Gender and Conflict since 1914*, 110–23.

46 Mosse, *The Image of Man*, passim, esp. 180–94.

47 Dummitt and Holloway, "Canadian Manhood(s)," in Greig and Martino, *Canadian Men and Masculinities*, 127.

48 McKay interview.

49 Ibid.

50 Ibid.

51 Prigione interview.

52 Spracklin interview.

53 Ibid.

54 Ibid.

55 Hrechka interview.

56 Ibid.

57 Ibid.

58 Ibid.

59 Testimony of MWO Patrick Lawler, 12.

60 Sharpe, e-mail message to author, 1 June 2015.

61 Ibid.

62 Ibid.

63 Micale, *Hysterical Men*, 284.

64 See Jackson, *One of the Boys*, 3, where he states that earlier in history his book could not have been written.

65 McKay and Swift, *Warrior Nation*, xii.

66 See David Pugliese and Patrick Smith, "Wounded Soldiers Told to Sign Form Agreeing Not to Criticize Military for Their Own Good: Senior Officer," *The National Post*, 2 April 2014; Graham Slaughter, "Canada's Wounded Soldiers Told Not to Criticize Superiors Online," *The Toronto Star*, 20 Sep-

tember 2013; and David Pugliese, "Wounded Vets Asked to Sign Form Saying They Won't Criticize the Military on Social Media," *The Ottawa Citizen*, 25 September 2013.

67 This is demonstrated above all else by the continuing evolution of the *Diagnostic and Statistical Manual of Mental Disorders* and the numerous – too many to list here – criticisms of its expansive growth.

68 Granatstein, *Canada's Army*.

69 Cook, *Warlords*, 4.

70 Grenier interview.

71 Ibid.

72 Sharpe, e-mail message to author, 1 June 2015.

73 Ibid.

74 Ibid.

75 Spellen interview.

76 Godin interview.

77 Ibid.

78 Ibid.

79 Prodaniuk interview.

80 Ibid.

Bibliography

PRIMARY SOURCES – ARCHIVAL

Canada, Department of National Defence. *Board of Inquiry – Potential Exposure of Canadian Forces Personnel to Contaminated Environment – Croatia.*

PRIMARY SOURCES – ORAL INTERVIEWS

Ban, Thomas. Interview by author. Toronto, 1 May 2014.
Barabé, Christian. Interview by author. Telephone. Toronto, 21 November 2014.
Godin, Andrew. Interview by author. Telephone. Toronto, 20 July 2014.
Grenier, Stéphane. Interview by author. Telephone. Toronto, 25 September 2014.
Hailey, Adam [pseud.]. Interview by author. Telephone. Toronto, 21 July 2014.
Hrechka, Daniel. Interview by author. Telephone. Toronto, 24 July 2014.
McKay, Bruce. Interview by author. Telephone. Toronto, 7 August 2014.
Passey, Greg. Interview by author. Telephone. Grimsby, Ontario, 6 August 2015.
Prigione, Toby. Interview by author. Telephone. Toronto, 29 July 2014.
Prodaniuk, Gregory. Interview by author. Telephone. Toronto, 13 August 2014.
Pugliese, David. Interview by author. Telephone. Toronto, 10 November 2014.

Spellen, Mike. Interview by author. Telephone. Toronto, 1 December 2014.
Spracklin, Derek. Interview by author. Telephone. Toronto, 19 August 2014.
Westholm, Barry. Interview by author. Telephone. Toronto, 30 July 2014.

PRIMARY SOURCES – NEWSPAPERS

The Globe
The Globe and Mail
The Huffington Post
The Mail on Sunday
The National Post
The New York Times
The Ottawa Citizen
The Toronto Star

PUBLISHED SOURCES

Aiken, Alice, and Stéphanie Bélanger, eds. *Beyond the Line: Military and Veteran Health Research*. Montreal & Kingston: McGill-Queen's University Press, 2013.

American Psychiatric Association. *Diagnostic and Statistical Manual of Mental Disorders*. Third Edition. Washington, DC: American Psychiatric Association, 1980.

Archibald, Herbert, Dorothy Long, Christine Miller, and Read Tuddenham. "Gross Stress Reaction in Combat – A 15-Year Follow-Up." *American Journal of Psychiatry* 119, no. 4 (1962): 317–22.

Archibald, Herbert, and Read Tuddenham. "Persistent Stress Reaction after Combat: A 20-Year Follow-Up." *Archives of General Psychiatry* 12, no. 5 (1965): 475–81.

Arial, Tracey. *I Volunteered: Canadian Vietnam Vets Remember*. Winnipeg: Watson & Dwyer, 1996.

Artiss, K.L. "Human Behaviour under Stress: From Combat to Social Psychiatry." *Military Medicine* 28, no. 10 (1963): 1011–15.

Barham, Peter. *Forgotten Lunatics of the Great War*. New Haven: Yale University Press, 2004.

Bartlett, John Russell. *Dictionary of Americanisms: A Glossary of Words and Phrases Usually Regarded as Peculiar to the United States*. Boston: Little, Brown and Company, 1877.

Bayer, Ronald. *Homosexuality and American Psychiatry: The Politics of Diagnosis*. New York: Basic Books, 1981.

Beal, A. Lynne. "Post-Traumatic Stress Disorder in Prisoners of War and Combat Veterans of the Dieppe Raid: A 50-Year Follow-Up." *Canadian Journal of Psychiatry* 40, no. 4 (1995): 177–84.

Bercuson, David. *Significant Incident: Canada's Army, the Airborne, and the Murder in Somalia*. Toronto: McClelland & Stewart, 1996.

Biggar, J.L. "The Pensionability of the Disabled Soldier." *Canadian Medical Association Journal* 9, no. 1 (1919): 28–33.

Billings, R.M., F.C.R. Chalke, and L. Shortt. "Battle Exhaustion – A Follow-Up Study." *Canadian Medical Association Journal* 57, no. 2 (1947): 152–5.

Binneveld, Hans. *From Shell Shock to Combat Stress: A Comparative History of Military Psychiatry*. Translated by John O'Kane. Amsterdam: Amsterdam University Press, 1997.

Bird, Will. *And We Go On*. Montreal & Kingston: McGill-Queen's University Press, 2014 [1930].

Birenbaum, Rhonda. "Peacekeeping Stress Prompts New Approaches to Mental-Health Issues in Canadian Military." *Canadian Medical Association Journal* 151, no. 10 (1994): 1484–9.

Bourke, Joanna. "Effeminacy, Ethnicity and the End of Trauma: The Sufferings of 'Shell-Shocked' Men in Great Britain and Ireland, 1914–39." *Journal of Contemporary History* 35, no. 1 (2000): 57–69.

Bourne, Peter. *Men, Stress, and Vietnam*. Boston: Little, Brown, 1970.

Boutros-Ghali, Boutros. *An Agenda for Peace 1995: With the New Supplement and Related UN Documents*. New York: United Nations Publications, 1995 [1992].

Canada, Correctional Service Canada. "Veterans in Canadian Correctional Systems." Accessed 5 May 2015. http://www.csc-scc.gc.ca/research/005008-b46-eng.shtml.

Canada, Department of National Defence. *1994 Defence White Paper*. Ottawa: Department of National Defence, 1994.

– *A Study of the Treatment of Members Released on Medical Grounds*. Ottawa: Department of National Defence, 1997.

Canada, Department of National Defence, Directorate of Medical Policy. *Preparing for Critical Incident Stress*. Ottawa: Department of National Defence, 2000.

Canada, Department of National Defence, Injured Personnel and Family Review Team. *Care of Injured Personnel and their Families Review*. Ottawa: Department of National Defence, 1997.

Canada, Department of National Defence and the Canadian Armed Forces. "The Battle of Medak Pocket." Accessed 22 March 2015. http://www.forces .gc.ca/en/news/article.page?doc=the-battle-of-medak-pocket/hljg3bso.

– "The Canadian Armed Forces Legacy in Afghanistan." Accessed 12 February 2015. http://www.forces.gc.ca/en/operations-abroad-past/cafla.page.

– "Canadian Armed Forces Mental Health Services." Government of Canada. Accessed 14 January 2015. http://www.forces.gc.ca/en/caf-community-health-services-mental/index.page#otssc.

Canada, Department of National Defence and the Canadian Armed Forces, Director General Health Services. "The Canadian Armed Forces in Afghanistan." Accessed 13 January 2015. http://www.veterans.gc.ca/eng /remembrance/history/canadian-armed-forces/afghanistan.

– "Concept for Canadian Forces Mental Health Care." Unpublished Paper. Ottawa: National Defence and the Canadian Armed Forces, 2003.

– "DAOD 5023-0, Universality of Service." Accessed 15 January 2014. http://www.forces.gc.ca/en/about-policies-standards-defence-admin-orders-directives-5000/5023-0.page.

– "DAOD 5023-1, Minimum Operational Standards Related to Universality of Service." Accessed 15 January 2014. http://www.forces.gc.ca/en /about-policies-standards-defence-admin-orders-directives-5000/5023-1 .page.

Canada, Department of National Defence and Veterans Affairs Canada, Chief Review Services. *Interdepartmental Evaluation of the OSISS Peer Support Network*, 1258-138 (CRS). Ottawa: Department of National Defence and Veterans Affairs Canada, 2005.

Canada, Parliament. *Acts of the Parliament of Canada 1919*. 13th Parliament, 2nd Session, vol. 1, chapters 1–76.

– *Moving Forward: A Strategic Plan for Quality of Life Improvements in the Canadian Forces*. Report of the Standing Committee on National Defence and Veterans' Affairs, October 1998.

– "The New Veterans Charter." Library of Parliament Research Publications. Accessed 10 February 2015. http://www.parl.gc.ca/Content/LOP /ResearchPublications/2011-84-e.htm

Canada, Parliament, House of Commons. *Debates*. 19th Parliament, 5th Session, 1944, vol. 239, no. 1, January 27 to February 29, 1944. Accessed 20 April 2016. http://parl.canadiana.ca/view/oop.debates_HOC1905_01 /1?r=0&s=1.

Canada, Veterans Affairs Canada. "Additional Details on the Enhanced New

Veterans Charter Act." Government of Canada. http://www.veterans.gc
.ca/eng/news/viewbackgrounder/7.

Canada, Veterans Affairs Canada. *Review of Veterans' Care Needs, Phase III,
Needs of Canadian Forces Clients, "Key Findings of Phase III – Review of Veterans' Care Needs."* Ottawa: Veterans Affairs Canada, 2000.

Canada, Veterans Affairs Canada – Canadian Forces Advisory Council. *Hon-
ouring Canada's Commitment: "Opportunity with Security" for Canadian
Forces Veterans and Their Families in the 21st Century.* Ottawa: Veterans
Affairs Canada, 2004.

Canada, Veterans Affairs Canada. "The Canadian Armed Forces in
Afghanistan." Accessed 13 January 2015. http://www.veterans.gc.ca/eng
/remembrance/history/canadian-armed-forces/afghanistan.

– "New Veterans Charter." Accessed 2 November 2014. http://www.veterans
.gc.ca/eng/news/vac-responds/just-the-facts/new-veterans-charter.

– *The Origins and Evolution of Veterans Benefits in Canada 1914–2004.*
Ottawa: Veterans Affairs Canada, 2004.

– "2006 Table of Disabilities." Accessed 3 March 2015. http://www.veterans
.gc.ca/eng/services/after-injury/disability-benefits/benefits-determined
/table-of-disabilities.

Carden-Coyne, Ana, ed. *Gender and Conflict since 1914: Historical and Inter-
disciplinary Perspectives.* Basingstoke: Palgrave Macmillan, 2012.

Commission of Inquiry into the Deployment of Canadian Forces to Somalia. *Dishonoured Legacy: The Lessons of the Somalia Affair, Report of the Commission of Inquiry into the Deployment of Canadian Forces to Somalia.*
Ottawa: Canadian Government Publishing, 1997.

Cook, Tim. *At the Sharp End: Canadians Fighting the Great War.* Volume 1.
Toronto: Penguin Canada, 2007.

– *Warlords: Borden, Mackenzie King, and Canada's World Wars.* Toronto:
Penguin Canada, 2013 [2012].

Cooper, Chester. *The Lion's Last Roar: Suez 1956.* New York: Harper & Row,
1978.

Copp, Terry, and Bill McAndrew. *Battle Exhaustion: Soldiers and Psychiatrists
in the Canadian Army, 1939–1945.* Montreal & Kingston: McGill-Queen's
University Press, 1990.

Copp, Terry, and Mark Humphries, eds. *Combat Stress in the 20th Century:
The Commonwealth Perspective.* Kingston: Canadian Defence Academy
Press, 2010.

Coulon, Jocelyn. *Soldiers of Diplomacy: The United Nations, Peacekeeping, and*

the New World Order. Translated by Phyllis Aronoff and Howard Scott.
Toronto: University of Toronto Press, 1998 [1994].

Cowen, Deborah. *Military Workfare: The Soldier and Social Citizenship in Canada*. Toronto: University of Toronto Press, 2008.

Dallaire, Roméo. *Shake Hands with the Devil: The Failure of Humanity in Rwanda*. Toronto: Vintage Canada, 2004 [2003].

Dancey, T.E. "The Interaction of the Welfare State and the Disabled." *Canadian Medical Association Journal* 103, no. 3 (1970): 274–7.

Dancey, T.E., and G.J. Sarwer-Foner. "The Problem of the Secondary Gain Patient in Medical Practice." *Canadian Medical Association Journal* 77, no. 1 (1957): 1108–11.

Davis, James. *The Sharp End: A Canadian Soldier's Story*. Toronto: Douglas & McIntyre, 1997.

Doucette, Fred. *Better Off Dead: Post-Traumatic Stress Disorder and the Canadian Armed Forces*. Halifax: Nimbus Publishing, 2015.

– *Empty Casing: A Soldier's Memoir of Sarajevo Under Siege*. Toronto: Douglas & McIntyre, 2008.

Dummitt, Christopher. *The Manly Modern: Masculinity in Postwar Canada*. Toronto: University of British Columbia Press, 2007.

Dyck, Erika. *Facing Eugenics: Reproduction, Sterilization, and the Politics of Choice*. Toronto: University of Toronto Press, 2013.

Eksteins, Modris. *Rites of Spring: The Great War and the Birth of the Modern Age*. New York: Houghton Mifflin, 2000 [1989].

English, Allan. *The Cream of the Crop: Canadian Aircrew, 1939–1945*. Montreal & Kingston: McGill-Queen's University Press, 1996.

– "From Combat Stress to Operational Stress: The CF's Mental Health Lessons from the 'Decade of Darkness.'" *Canadian Military Journal* 12, no. 4 (2012): 9–17.

– *Understanding Military Culture: A Canadian Perspective*. Montreal & Kingston: McGill-Queen's University Press, 2004.

Erichsen, John Eric. *On Railway and Other Injuries of the Nervous System*. Philadelphia: Henry C. Lea, 1867 [1866].

Faulder, Liane. *The Long Walk Home: Paul Franklin's Journey from Afghanistan – A Soldier's Story*. Victoria: Brindle and Glass Publishing, 2007.

Feighner, John, Eli Robins, Samuel Guze, Robert Woodruff, George Winokur, and Rodrigo Munoz. "Diagnostic Criteria for Use in Psychiatric Research." *Archives of General Psychiatry* 26, no. 1 (1972): 57–63.

Flavelle, Ryan. "Help or Harm: Battle Exhaustion and the RCAMC during the Second World War." *Journal of Military and Strategic Studies* 9, no. 4 (2007): 1–22.

– *The Patrol: Seven Days in the Life of a Canadian Soldier in Afghanistan.* Toronto: HarperCollins, 2011.

Foucault, Michel. *Madness and Civilization: A History of Insanity in the Age of Reason.* Translated by Richard Howard. New York: Vintage Books, 1973 [1964].

Francis, Daniel. *National Dreams: Myth, Memory, and Canadian History.* Vancouver: Arsenal Pulp Press, 1997.

Freud, Sigmund. *The Complete Introductory Lectures on Psychoanalysis.* Translated and edited by James Strachey. New York: W.W. Norton, 1966 [1917].

Fussell, Paul. *The Great War and Modern Memory.* New York: Oxford University Press, 2013 [1975].

Gabriel, Richard. *No More Heroes: Madness and Psychiatry in War.* New York: Hill and Wang, 1987.

Gaffen, Fred. *Unknown Warriors: Canadians in Vietnam.* Toronto: Dundurn Press, 1990.

Garber, Bryan, and Mark Zamorski. "Evaluation of a Third-Location Decompression Program for Canadian Forces Members Returning from Afghanistan." *Military Medicine* 177, no. 4 (2012): 397–403.

Gleason, Mona. *Normalizing the Ideal: Psychology, Schooling, and the Family in Postwar Canada.* Toronto: University of Toronto Press, 1999.

Goffman, Erving. *Asylums: Essays on the Social Situation of Mental Patients and Other Inmates.* Garden City, NY: Anchor Books, 1961.

Governor General of Canada. "Her Excellency the Right Honourable Adrienne Clarkson Speech on the Occasion of a Memorial Ceremony for the Fallen Soldiers of 3 PPCLI." Accessed 6 August 2014. http://archive.gg.ca /media/doc.asp?lang=e&DocID=1056.

Granatstein, J.L. *Canada's Army: Waging War and Keeping the Peace.* Second Edition. Toronto: University of Toronto Press, 2011.

– *Who Killed the Canadian Military?* Toronto: HarperCollins, 2004.

Granatstein, J.L., and Dean Oliver. *The Oxford Companion to Canadian Military History.* Toronto: Oxford University Press, 2011.

Graubard, Stephen, ed. *In Search of Canada.* New Brunswick, NJ: Transaction Publishers, 1989.

Greig, Christopher. *Ontario Boys: Masculinity and the Idea of Boyhood in Postwar Ontario, 1945–1960.* Waterloo: Wilfrid Laurier Press, 2014.

Greig, Christopher, and Wayne Martino, eds. *Canadian Men and Masculini-*

ties: Historical and Contemporary Perspectives. Toronto: Canadian Scholars' Press, 2012.

Griffin, John. *In Search of Sanity: A Chronicle of the Canadian Mental Health Association 1918–1988.* London, ON: Third Eye Canada, 1989.

Grob, Gerald. *Mental Illness and American Society, 1875–1940.* Princeton: Princeton University Press, 1983.

– "Origins of DSM-I: A Study in Appearance and Reality." *American Journal of Psychiatry* 148, no. 4 (1991): 421–31.

– "Psychiatry and Social Activism: The Politics of a Specialty in Postwar America." *Bulletin of the History of Medicine* 60, no. 4 (1986): 477–501.

Gurland, Barry, Joseph Fleiss, John Cooper, Lawrence Sharpe, Robert Kendell, and Pamela Roberts. "Cross-National Study of Diagnosis of Mental Disorders: Hospital Diagnoses and Hospital Patients in New York and London." *Comprehensive Psychiatry* 11, no. 1 (1970): 18–25.

Hale, Nathan. *The Rise and Crisis of Psychoanalysis in the United States: Freud and the Americans, 1917–1985.* New York: Oxford University Press, 1995.

Healy, David. *The Creation of Psychopharmacology.* London: Harvard University Press, 2002.

Hemingway, Ernest. *A Farewell to Arms.* New York: Scribner, 2003 [1929].

Herman, Judith. *Trauma and Recovery: The Aftermath of Violence from Domestic Abuse to Political Terror.* New York: Basic Books, 1992.

Horn, Bernd. *No Lack of Courage: Operation Medusa, Afghanistan.* Toronto: Dundurn Press, 2013.

– ed. *The Canadian Way of War: Serving the National Interest.* Toronto: Dundurn Press, 2006.

– ed. *Forging a Nation: Perspectives on the Canadian Military Experience.* St. Catharines: Vanwell Publishing, 2002.

Horn, Bernd, and Bill Bentley. *Forced to Change: Crisis and Reform in the Canadian Armed Forces.* Toronto: Dundurn Press, 2015.

Horowitz, Mardi. *Stress Response Syndromes.* New York: Jason Aronson, 1976.

Houts, Arthur. "Fifty Years of Psychiatric Nomenclature: Reflections on the 1943 War Department Technical Bulletin, Medical 203." *Journal of Clinical Psychology* 56, no. 7 (2000): 935–67.

Humphries, Mark. "War's Long Shadow: Masculinity, Medicine, and the Gendered Politics of Trauma, 1914–1939." *The Canadian Historical Review* 91, no. 3 (2010): 503–31.

Iacobelli, Teresa. *Death or Deliverance: Canadian Courts Martial in the Great War.* Vancouver: University of British Columbia Press, 2014.

Jackson, Paul. *One of the Boys: Homosexuality in the Military during World War II*. Montreal & Kingston: McGill-Queen's University Press, 2004.

James, Patrick. *Canada and Conflict*. Don Mills, ON: Oxford University Press, 2012.

Jones, Edgar. "Army Psychiatry in the Korean War: The Experience of 1 Commonwealth Division." *Military Medicine* 165, no. 4 (2000): 256–60.

Jones, Edgar, and Simon Wessely. "'Forward Psychiatry' in the Military: Its Origins and Effectiveness." *Journal of Traumatic Stress* 16, no. 4 (2003): 411–19.

– "A Paradigm Shift in the Conceptualization of Psychological Trauma in the 20th Century." *Journal of Anxiety Disorders* 21, no. 2 (2007): 164–75.

– *Shell Shock to PTSD: Military Psychiatry from 1900 to the Gulf War*. New York: Psychology Press, 2005.

Jung, Hans. "Lessons Learned from the War in Afghanistan: A Leader's Perspective." Supplement, *Canadian Journal of Surgery* 54, no. 6 (2011): S110–11.

Junger, Sebastian. *War*. Toronto: HarperCollins, 2010.

Kardiner, Abram. *The Traumatic Neuroses of War*. New York: Paul B. Hoeber, 1941.

Kendler, Kenneth, Rodrigo Munoz, and George Murphy. "The Development of the Feighner Criteria: A Historical Perspective." *American Journal of Psychiatry* 167, no. 2 (2010): 134–42.

Kormos, Benjamin. "The Posttraumatic Stress Defence in Canada: Reconnoitering the Old Lie." *Criminal Law Quarterly* 54, no. 2 (2008): 189–236.

Kuch, Klaus. "Post-Traumatic Stress Disorder after Car Accidents." *Canadian Journal of Psychiatry* 33, no. 1 (1985): 426–7.

Kyle, Keith. *Suez: Britain's End of Empire in the Middle East*. London: I.B. Tauris, 2003 [1991].

Laing, R.D. *The Politics of Experience*. New York: Pantheon Books, 1967.

Lamb, Susan. *Pathologist of the Mind: Adolf Meyer and the Origins of American Psychiatry*. Baltimore: Johns Hopkins University Press, 2014.

Leese, Peter. *Shell Shock: Traumatic Neurosis and the British Soldiers of the First World War*. London: Palgrave Macmillan, 2013 [2002].

Lifton, Robert Jay. *Death in Life: Survivors of Hiroshima*. Chapel Hill: University of North Carolina Press, 1991 [1968].

– *Witness to an Extreme Century: A Memoir*. Toronto: Free Press, 2011.

Linford, Chris. *Warrior Rising: A Soldier's Journey to PTSD and Back*. Victoria: Friesen Press, 2013.

Macphail, Andrew. *Official History of the Canadian Forces in the Great War 1914–19: The Medical Services*. Ottawa: Department of National Defence, 1925.

Manion, R.J. *A Surgeon in Arms*. New York: D. Appleton & Company, 1918.

Marks, John. *The Search for the "Manchurian Candidate": The CIA and Mind Control*. New York: Times Books, 1979.

Mathieu, Lise, Director General Health Services, National Defence and the Canadian Armed Forces. "Concept for Canadian Forces Mental Health Care." Unpublished paper. Ottawa: National Defence and the Canadian Armed Forces, 2003.

Mayes, Rick, and Allan Horwitz. "DSM-III and the Revolution in the Classification of Mental Illness." *Journal of the History of the Behavioural Sciences* 41, no. 3 (2005): 249–67.

McKay, Ian, and Jamie Swift. *Warrior Nation: Rebranding Canada in an Age of Anxiety*. Toronto: Between the Lines, 2012.

McKerracher, D.G. "Psychiatric Problems in the Army." *Canadian Medical Association Journal* 48, no. 5 (1943): 399–404.

McLaren, Angus. *Our Own Master Race: Eugenics in Canada, 1885–1945*. Toronto: McClelland & Stewart, 1990.

Micale, Mark. *Hysterical Men: The Hidden History of Male Nervous Illness*. Cambridge, MA: Harvard University Press, 2008.

– "On the 'Disappearance' of Hysteria: A Study in the Clinical Deconstruction of a Diagnosis." *Isis* 84, no. 3 (1993): 496–526.

Micale, Mark, and Paul Lerner, eds. *Traumatic Pasts: History, Psychiatry, and Trauma in the Modern Age, 1870–1930*. New York: Cambridge University Press, 2001.

Mitchell, J.T. "When Disaster Strikes … The Critical Incident Stress Debriefing Process." *Journal of Emergency Medical Services* 8, no. 1 (1983): 36–9.

Moran, James, and David Wright, eds. *Mental Health and Canadian Society: Historical Perspectives*. Montreal & Kingston: McGill-Queen's University Press, 2006.

Moran, Lord. *The Anatomy of Courage: The Classic WWI Account of the Psychological Effects of War*. New York: Carroll and Graf, 2007 [1945].

Morton, Desmond. *Fight or Pay: Soldiers' Families in the Great War*. Toronto: University of British Columbia Press, 2004.

Morton, Desmond, and Glenn Wright. *Winning the Second Battle: Canadian Veterans and the Return to Civilian Life, 1915–1930*. Toronto: University of Toronto Press, 1987.

Moss, Mark. *Manliness and Militarism: Educating Young Boys in Ontario for War*. Don Mills, ON: Oxford University Press, 2001.

Mosse, George. *The Image of Man: The Creation of Modern Masculinity*. New York: Oxford University Press, 1996.

Mowat, Farley. *And No Birds Sang*. Madeira Park: Douglas & McIntyre, 2013 [1979].

– *The Regiment*. Toronto: McClelland & Stewart, 1955.

Myers, Charles. *Shell Shock in France, 1914–1918*. Cambridge: Cambridge University Press, 1940.

Naylor, C. David., ed. *Canadian Health Care and the State: A Century of Evolution*. Montreal & Kingston: McGill-Queen's University Press, 1992.

Neary, Peter. *On to Civvy Street: Canada's Rehabilitation Program for Veterans of the Second World War*. Montreal & Kingston: McGill-Queen's University Press, 2011.

Neary, Peter, and J.L. Granatstein, eds. *The Veterans Charter and Post-World War II Canada*. Montreal & Kingston: McGill-Queen's University Press, 1998.

Off, Carol. *The Ghosts of Medak Pocket: The Story of Canada's Secret War*. Toronto: Random House of Canada, 2005 [2004].

Office of the Surgeon General, Army Service Forces. "Nomenclature of Psychiatric Disorders and Reactions: War Department Technical Bulletin, Medical 203." *Journal of Clinical Psychology* 2, no. 3 (1946): 289–96.

Ombudsman, National Defence and Canadian Forces. *Follow-Up Report: Review of DND/CF Actions on Operational Stress Injuries*. Ottawa: Department of National Defence, 2002.

– *Fortitude under Fatigue: Assessing the Delivery of Care for Operational Stress Injuries that Canadian Forces Members Need and Deserve*. Ottawa: Department of National Defence, 2012.

– *A Long Road to Recovery: Battling Operational Stress Injuries – Second Review of the Department of National Defence and Canadian Forces' Action on Operational Stress Injuries*. Ottawa: Department of National Defence, 2008.

– *Off the Rails: Crazy Train Mocks Operational Stress Injury Sufferers*. Ottawa: Department of National Defence, 2003.

– *On the Homefront: Assessing the Well-Being of Canada's Military Families in the New Millennium*. Ottawa: Department of National Defence, 2013.

– *Preliminary Assessment – Joint Personnel Support Unit (JPSU)*. Ottawa: Department of National Defence, 2013.

– *Report to the Minister of National Defence, Special Report: Systemic Treatment of CF Members with PTSD, Complainant: Christian McEachern.* Ottawa: Department of National Defence, 2002.

Paré, Jean-Rodrigue, Legal and Social Affairs Division, Parliamentary Information and Research Service. "Post-Traumatic Stress Disorder and the Mental Health of Military Personnel and Veterans." Publication No. 2011-97E. Ottawa: Library of Parliament, 2011 [Revised 2013].

Paris, Joel. "Canadian Psychiatry Across 5 Decades: From Clinical Inference to Evidence-Based Practice." *Canadian Journal of Psychiatry* 45, no. 1 (2000): 34–9.

– *The Fall of an Icon: Psychoanalysis and Academic Psychiatry.* Toronto: University of Toronto Press, 2005.

Parkin, Alan. *A History of Psychoanalysis in Canada.* Toronto: Toronto Psychoanalytic Society, 1987.

Parpart, Jane, and Marysia Zalewski, eds. *Rethinking the Wo/man Question in International Relations.* London: Zed Books, 2008.

Pearson, Lester Bowles. "Nobel Lecture: The Four Faces of Peace." Accessed July 28, 2014. http://www.nobelprize.org/nobel_prizes/peace/laureates/1957/pearson-lecture.html

Rae-Grant, Quentin, ed. *Psychiatry in Canada: 50 Years (1951 to 2001).* Ottawa: Canadian Psychiatric Association, 2001.

Roland, Charles G., ed. *Health, Disease and Medicine: Essays in Canadian History.* Hamilton: McMaster University, Hannah Institute for the History of Medicine, 1984.

Rosenhan, D.L. "On Being Sane in Insane Places." *Science* 19, no. 4070 (1974): 250–8.

Rossignol, Michel, Parliamentary Information and Research Service, PRB 07-20E. "Afghanistan: Military Personnel and Operational Stress Injuries." Ottawa: Library of Parliament, 2007. Accessed 4 August 2014. http://www.parl.gc.ca/HousePublications/Publication.aspx?DocId=1031525&Language=E&Mode=1&Parl=36&Ses=1&File=6.

Russel, Colin. "The Nature of the War Neuroses." *Canadian Medical Association Journal* 41, no. 6 (1939): 549–54.

Rutherdale, Robert. *Hometown Horizons: Local Responses to Canada's Great War.* Toronto: University of British Columbia Press, 2004.

Scheff, Thomas. *Being Mentally Ill: A Sociological Theory.* New York: Aldine de Gruyter, 1999 [1966].

Scott, Wilbur. "PTSD in DSM-III: A Case in the Politics of Diagnosis and Disease." *Social Problems* 37, no. 3 (1990): 294–310.

Scurfield, Raymond, and Katherine Platoni, eds. *War Trauma and Its Wake: Expanding the Circle of Healing.* New York: Routledge, 2013.

Sharpe, G.E. *Croatia Board of Inquiry: Leadership (and Other) Lessons Learned.* Winnipeg: Canadian Forces Leadership Institute, 2002.

Sharpe, G.E., and Allan English. "The Decade of Darkness – The Experience of the Senior Leadership of the Canadian Forces in the 1990s." Unpublished paper written for the Canadian Forces Leadership Institute, 2004.

Shephard, Ben. *A War of Nerves: Soldiers and Psychiatrists in the Twentieth Century.* Cambridge, MA: Harvard University Press, 2001 [2000].

Shorter, Edward. *A History of Psychiatry: From the Era of the Asylum to the Age of Prozac.* Toronto: John Wiley & Sons, 1997.

Showalter, Elaine. *The Female Malady: Women, Madness, and English Culture.* New York: Pantheon Books, 1985.

Spears, Tom. "Psychologic [sic] Scars Remain 50 Years after Dieppe Raid, Study of Canadian Veterans Finds." *Canadian Medical Association Journal* 153, no. 9 (1995): 1324–6.

Spitzer, Robert. "More on Pseudoscience in Science and the Case of Psychiatric Diagnosis." *Archives of General Psychiatry* 33, no. 4 (1976): 459–70.

Spitzer, Robert, Jean Endicott, and Eli Robins. "Research Diagnostic Criteria: Rationale and Reliability." *Archives of General Psychiatry* 35, no. 6 (1978): 773–82.

Spitzer, Robert, Janet Williams, and Andrew Skodol, eds. *International Perspectives on DSM-III.* Washington, DC: American Psychiatric Press, 1983.

Statistics Canada. *The Canadian Persian Gulf Cohort Study: Detailed Report.* Ottawa: Statistics Canada, 2005.

Stretch, Robert. "Effects of Service in Vietnam on Canadian Forces Military Personnel." *Armed Forces and Society* 16, no. 4 (1990): 571–85.

– "Post-Traumatic Stress Disorder and the Canadian Vietnam Veteran." *Journal of Traumatic Stress* 3, no. 2 (1990): 239–54.

– "Psychosocial Readjustment of Canadian Vietnam Veterans." *Journal of Consulting and Clinical Psychology* 59, no. 1 (1991): 188–9.

Sugrue, Thomas. *The Origins of the Urban Crisis: Race and Inequality in Postwar Detroit.* Princeton, NJ: Princeton University Press, 2005 [1996].

Sullivan, Patrick. "War Ended Decades Ago, but PoWs' Problems Continue." *Canadian Medical Association Journal* 137, no. 9 (1987): 837.

Summerfield, Derek. "A Critique of Seven Assumptions behind Psychological Trauma Programmes in War-Affected Areas." *Social Science and Medicine* 48, no. 10 (1999): 1449–62.

Szasz, Thomas. *The Myth of Mental Illness*. New York: Harper Perennial, 2010 [1961].

Taylor, Scott, and Brian Nolan. *Tested Mettle: Canada's Peacekeepers at War*. Ottawa: Esprit de Corps Books, 1998.

Thomas, Gordon. *Journey into Madness*. London: Bantam Press, 1988.

Trimble, Michael. *Post-Traumatic Neurosis: From Railway Spine to the Whiplash*. Toronto: John Wiley & Sons, 1981.

Tyhurst, J.S., F.C.R. Chalke, F.S. Lawson, B.H. McNeel, C.A. Roberts, G.C. Taylor, R.J. Weil, and J.D. Griffin. *More for the Mind: A Study of Psychiatric Services in Canada*. Toronto: Canadian Mental Health Association, 1963.

United Nations. "Resolutions Adopted by the United Nations Security Council in 1964." United Nations Security Council. Accessed 11 May 2015. http://www.un.org/en/sc/documents/resolutions/1964.shtml.

United Nations, Department of Public Information. "Former Yugoslavia – UNPROFOR." United Nations. Accessed March 21, 2015. http://www.un.org/en/peacekeeping/missions/past/unprof_b.htm.

United States of America, US Department of Veterans Affairs. PTSD: National Center for PTSD. "Veterans with PTSD in the Justice System." Accessed 5 May 2016. http://www.ptsd.va.gov/professional/provider-type/community/veterans-PTSD-Justice-System.asp.

Vance, Jonathan. *Death So Noble: Memory, Meaning, and the First World War*. Vancouver: University of British Columbia Press, 1997.

Varadaraj, R. "Management of Post Traumatic Stress Disorder and Ethnicity." *Canadian Journal of Psychiatry* 33, no. 1 (1987): 75.

Watson, Brent Byron. *Far Eastern Tour: The Canadian Infantry in Korea, 1950–1953*. Montreal & Kingston: McGill-Queen's University Press, 2007.

Weaver, John, and David Wright. "Shell Shock and the Politics of Asylum Committal in New Zealand, 1916–22." *Health and History* 7, no. 1 (2005): 17–40.

Whitworth, Sandra. *Men, Militarism and UN Peacekeeping: A Gendered Analysis*. London: Lynne Rienner Publishers, 2004.

Wilson, John. "The Historical Evolution of PTSD Diagnostic Criteria: From Freud to DSM-IV." *Journal of Traumatic Stress* 7, no. 4 (1994): 681–98.

Wilson, Mitchell. "DSM-III and the Transformation of American Psychiatry: A History." *American Journal of Psychiatry* 150, no. 3 (1993): 399–410.

Windsor, Lee, David Charters, and Brent Wilson. *Kandahar Tour: The Turning Point in Canada's Afghan Mission*. Mississauga: Wiley, 2008.

Winslow, Donna. "The Parliamentary Inquiry into the Canadian Peace Mission in Somalia." Paper presented at the fourth Workshop on Strengthening Parliamentary Oversight of International Military Cooperation and Institutions. Brussels, Belgium, July 12–14, 2002.

Winter, Jay. "Shell-Shock and the Cultural History of the Great War." *Journal of Contemporary History* 35, no. 1 (2000): 7–11.

– *Sites of Memory, Sites of Morning: The Great War in European Cultural History*. Cambridge: Cambridge University Press, 1995.

Wood, John, ed. *The Chance of War: Canadian Soldiers in the Balkans, 1992–1995*. Toronto: Breakout Education Network in Association with Dundurn Press, 2003.

Woods, David. "Canadian Physicians in World War II." *Canadian Medical Association Journal* 132, no. 10 (1985): 1103.

Woolf, Virginia. *Mrs Dalloway*. London: Harcourt, 2001 [1925].

Young, Allan. *The Harmony of Illusions: Inventing Post-Traumatic Stress Disorder*. Princeton, NJ: Princeton University Press, 1995.

Index

Index

Page, Herbert (surgeon), 30
Paris, Joel (psychiatrist), 107
Passchendaele, 9–10, 40, 56
Passey, Greg: alcoholism and PTSD, 131, 153–4; Croatia Board of Inquiry testimony, 147, 150; McEachern case, 171–2; on reservists, 162; peacekeeping trauma research, 130–2
Patton, George, 59
peaceable kingdom thesis, 116, 123, 175
peacekeeping: Canadian national identity, 116–17; Pearsonian model, 115, 118, 125; post-Cold War changes, 117–19, 125–7; as traumatic experience, 108, 114–15, 130. See also memory
Pearson, Lester: Nobel Peace Prize, 115–16
Peer Support Coordinator (PSC), 180–1, 183
pensions: British policies, 42; Croatia Board of Inquiry discussion, 152–6; disability scale, 43–4; as emasculating, 42–3, 47, 76; figures, 42, 47; heredity's role in denial, 45–6, 49, 84; as moral crutch, 45, 48, 71; Pension Act, 42; pension-seeking (as transgression), 46. See also masculinity; veterans
physicians: denial of male nervous illness, 11; gender norm protectors, 42, 46, 48, 61, 71–7; as pension gatekeepers, 17–18, 49. See also psychiatry
PIE method, 53, 55
post-traumatic stress disorder (PTSD): as American phenomenon, 19, 107; codification of, 8, 94–100; links to shell shock and battle exhaustion, 12–14; universalization of trauma, 9, 28, 104–5
predisposition, 49, 54, 57, 61, 63, 66–7, 98. See also pensions
Prigione, Toby (master corporal), 211
Princess Patricia's Canadian Light Infantry: 2nd Battalion (2PPCLI), 127–9; casualties in Afghanistan, 175; UN citations, 156, 164. See also Croatia Board of Inquiry; French Grey Cup (Crazy Train) incident; Medak Pocket
Prodaniuk, Greg (corporal), 126–7, 134–6, 148–9, 180, 218–20
psychiatric screening, 58–60, 66, 78, 183–4
psychiatry: anti-psychiatry, 103–4; biological, 19, 84, 87, 94, 100–2; post-Second World War expansion, 79–87; radical psychiatrists, 93–4; rejection by armies, 54–5; social psychiatry, 87
psychoanalysis: decline, 102; Freudian, 84, 87, 100–1. See also Freud, Sigmund
psychodynamics, 52, 70, 72, 83–5, 87–90, 101, 104
psychologists: conflict with psychiatrists, 34, 60; human behaviour research and soldier screening, 57–61
psychotherapy. See psychoanalysis
Pugliese, David (journalist), 141, 159, 207